Download Your Incl
Ebook Today!

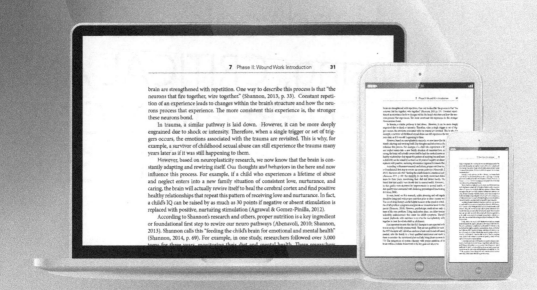

Your print purchase of *Handbook of Clinical Nursing: Critical and Emergency Care Nursing* **includes an ebook download** to the device of your choice—increasing accessibility, portability, and searchability!

Download your ebook today at
http://spubonline.com/emergency
and enter the activation code below:

19THK1R1V

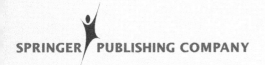

SPRINGER PUBLISHING COMPANY

LS

springerpub.com

Handbook of Clinical Nursing: CRITICAL AND EMERGENCY CARE NURSING

Ronald L. Hickman, Jr., PhD, RN, ACNP-BC, FNAP, FAAN, is an associate professor and a board-certified acute care nurse practitioner at Frances Payne Bolton School of Nursing, Case Western Reserve University (CWRU) in Cleveland, Ohio. He earned a bachelor of arts in biology, a master of science (acute care nurse practitioner), and a doctorate in nursing from CWRU. He has received regional and national distinctions for his commitment and sustained contributions to nursing science and practice. Dr. Hickman is a nationally recognized nurse scientist and advanced practice nurse. In 2015, he was elected a fellow of the American Academy of Nursing and National Academies of Practice. With nearly two decades of clinical experience, he has provided evidence-based nursing care to patients and their families across tertiary care settings. He has authored more than 50 publications and numerous book chapters with a clinical focus, and serves as a contributing editor for the *American Journal of Critical Care*. As an associate editor of *A Guide to Mastery in Clinical Nursing*, Dr. Hickman's clinical expertise in the management of patients requiring life-sustaining care in emergency departments and intensive care units is highlighted in the book's content regarding emergency and critical care, medical–surgical, and nurse anesthesia care.

Celeste M. Alfes, DNP, MSN, RN, CNE, CHSE-A, is associate professor and director of the Center for Nursing Education, Simulation, and Innovation at the Frances Payne Bolton School of Nursing, Case Western Reserve University (CWRU) in Cleveland, Ohio. She earned a bachelor of science in nursing (University of Akron), master of science in nursing (University of Akron), and doctor of nursing practice at CWRU. With a background in critical care nursing, she has 20 years of experience teaching baccalaureate nursing students and has been instrumental in developing high-fidelity simulation programs nationally and internationally. She was instrumental in developing the Dorothy Ebersbach Academic Center for Flight Nursing, which features the nation's first high-fidelity Sikorsky S76® helicopter simulator adapted for interdisciplinary education and crew resource management. She received the National League for Nursing's Simulation Leader in Nursing Education award (2012) and the Joyce Griffin-Sobel Research award (2014). Her research incorporates interprofessional simulations to strengthen clinical reasoning and performance outcomes. Dr. Alfes currently serves as a reviewer for the National Science Foundation, is a coinvestigator on funded research projects with the Laerdal Foundation of Norway and the U.S. Air Force Research Laboratory, is on the editorial board of *Applied Nursing Research*, and is a reviewer for the journals *Nursing Education Perspectives* and *Clinical Simulation in Nursing*.

Joyce J. Fitzpatrick, PhD, MBA, RN, FAAN, FNAP, is Elizabeth Brooks Ford Professor of Nursing, Frances Payne Bolton School of Nursing, Case Western Reserve University (CWRU) in Cleveland, Ohio, where she was the dean from 1982 through 1997. She is also an adjunct professor, Department of Geriatrics, Ichan School of Medicine, Mount Sinai Hospital, New York, New York. She earned a bachelor of science in nursing (Georgetown University), an MS in psychiatric–mental health nursing (The Ohio State University), a PhD in nursing (New York University), and an MBA at CWRU. She was elected a fellow of the American Academy of Nursing (AAN; 1981) and a fellow in the National Academies of Practice (1996). She received the *American Journal of Nursing* Book of the Year award 20 times. Dr. Fitzpatrick received the American Nurses Foundation Distinguished Contribution to Nursing Science award for sustained commitment and contributions to the development of the discipline (2002). She was a Fulbright Scholar at University College Cork, Cork, Ireland (2007–2008), and was inducted into the Sigma Theta Tau International Research Hall of Fame (2014). In 2016, she was named a Living Legend of the AAN. Dr. Fitzpatrick's work is widely disseminated in nursing and health care literature; she has authored or edited more than 300 publications, including more than 80 books. She even served as a coeditor of the *Annual Review of Nursing Research* series, volumes 1 to 26, and she currently edits the journals *Applied Nursing Research, Archives of Psychiatric Nursing,* and *Nursing Education Perspectives,* the official journal of the National League for Nursing.

Handbook of Clinical Nursing: CRITICAL AND EMERGENCY CARE NURSING

Ronald L. Hickman, Jr., PhD, RN, ACNP-BC, FNAP, FAAN

Celeste M. Alfes, DNP, MSN, RN, CNE, CHSE-A

Joyce J. Fitzpatrick, PhD, MBA, RN, FAAN, FNAP

EDITORS

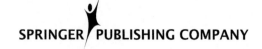
SPRINGER PUBLISHING COMPANY

Springer Publishing Company, LLC
11 West 42nd Street
New York, NY 10036
www.springerpub.com

Acquisitions Editor: Joseph Morita
Compositor: Newgen knowledgeWorks

ISBN: 978-0-8261-3109-6
ebook ISBN: 978-0-8261-3029-7

18 19 20 21 22 / 5 4 3 2 1

Extracted from *A Guide to Mastery in Clinical Nursing: The Comprehensive Reference*

The author and the publisher of this Work have made every effort to use sources believed to be reliable to provide information that is accurate and compatible with the standards generally accepted at the time of publication. Because medical science is continually advancing, our knowledge base continues to expand. Therefore, as new information becomes available, changes in procedures become necessary. We recommend that the reader always consult current research and specific institutional policies before performing any clinical procedure. The author and publisher shall not be liable for any special, consequential, or exemplary damages resulting, in whole or in part, from the readers' use of, or reliance on, the information contained in this book. The publisher has no responsibility for the persistence or accuracy of URLs for external or third-party Internet websites referred to in this publication and does not guarantee that any content on such websites is, or will remain, accurate or appropriate.

Library of Congress Cataloging-in-Publication Data
Names: Hickman, Ronald, editor. | Alfes, Celeste M., editor. | Fitzpatrick, Joyce J., 1944- editor.
Title: Handbook of clinical nursing. Critical and emergency care nursing /
    Ronald L. Hickman, Jr., Celeste M. Alfes, Joyce J. Fitzpatrick, editors.
Other titles: Critical and emergency care nursing | Contained in (work): Guide to mastery in clinical nursing.
Description: New York, NY : Springer Publishing Company, LLC, [2018] |
    Extracted from A guide to mastery in clinical nursing : the comprehensive
    reference / Joyce J. Fitzpatrick, Celeste M. Alfes, Ronald Hickman,
    editors. 2018. | Includes bibliographical references.
Identifiers: LCCN 2017059923 | ISBN 9780826131096 (pbk.) | ISBN 9780826130297 (eISBN)
Subjects: | MESH: Critical Care Nursing | Emergency Nursing
Classification: LCC RT41 | NLM WY 154 | DDC 610.73—dc23
LC record available at https://lccn.loc.gov/2017059923

Contact us to receive discount rates on bulk purchases.
We can also customize our books to meet your needs.
For more information please contact: sales@springerpub.com

Printed in the United States of America.

Contents

Contributors

Kathleen C. Ashton, PhD, RN, ACNS-BC
Clinical Professor of Nursing
College of Nursing and Health Professions
Drexel University
Philadelphia, Pennsylvania
Professor Emeritus
Rutgers, The State University of New Jersey
Camden, New Jersey

Vicki Bacidore, DNP, RN, APRN, ACNP-BC, CEN, TNS
Assistant Professor of Nursing
Loyola University Chicago
Emergency Nurse Practitioner
Loyola University Medical Center
Maywood, Illinois

Laura Stark Bai, MS, RN, FNP-BC
Clinical Nurse Manager
Department of Emergency Medicine
Mount Sinai Hospital
New York, New York

Yolanda Bone, DNP, RN, APRN, FNP-BC
W. Temple Webber Cancer Center
Christus St. Michael
Texarkana, Texas

Kathleen Bradbury-Golas, DNP, RN, FNP-C, ACNS-BC
Associate Clinical Professor
Drexel University
Philadelphia, Pennsylvania
Family Nurse Practitioner
Virtua Medical Group
Hammonton Primary Care
Hammonton, New Jersey
Recovery Centers of America at Lighthouse
Mays Landing, New Jersey

Pamela Harris Bryant, DNP, RN, CRNP, AC-PC
Pediatric Nurse Practitioner
Assistant Professor
School of Nursing
University of Alabama at Birmingham
Birmingham, Alabama

Margaret Jean Carman, DNP, RN, ACNP-BC, ENP-BC, FAEN
Emergency Nurse Practitioner
University of North Carolina Chapel Hill
Department of Emergency Medicine
Chapel Hill, North Carolina
Program Director
Adult-Gerontology Acute Care Nurse Practitioner Program
Georgetown University School of Nursing and Health Studies
Washington, DC

Linda Carson, MSN, RN, APN
Retired Advanced Practice Nurse
Shore Medical Center
Somers Point, New Jersey

Leon Chen, DNP, RN, AGACNP-BC, CCRN, CEN
Clinical Assistant Professor of Nursing
Nurse Practitioner
Critical Care Medicine Service
Rory Meyers College of Nursing
New York University
Department of Anesthesiology and Critical Care Medicine
Memorial Sloan Kettering Cancer Center
New York, New York

Gwendolyn D. Childs, PhD, RN
Associate Professor
School of Nursing
University of Alabama at Birmingham
Birmingham, Alabama

Christopher J. Contino, DNP, RN, ENP-C, FNP-BC, CEN, CRN
Emergency Nurse Practitioner
Atlantic Emergency Associates
Atlantic City, New Jersey

Nancy Jaskowak Cresse, DNP, MSN, RN, ANP-BC
Clinical Assistant Professor
Rutgers School of Nursing–Camden
Camden, New Jersey

Khoa (Joey) Dang, MSN, RN, FNP-C
Assistant Professor/Assistant Director
College of Graduate Nursing
Western University of Health Sciences
Pomona, California

Martha B. Dodd, DNP, RN, FNP-BC, SANE-A, SANE-P
Family Nurse Practitioner
Stephanie V. Blank Center for Safe and Healthy Children
Children's Healthcare of Atlanta
Atlanta, Georgia

Brenda L. Douglass, DNP, RN, APRN, FNP-C, CDE, CTTS
DNP Program Director
Assistant Clinical Professor
Department of Advanced Practice Nursing
Drexel University, College of Nursing & Health Professions
Philadelphia, Pennsylvania
Family Nurse Practitioner
Cape Regional Physician's Associates
Cape May, New Jersey

Andrea Efre, DNP, RN, ARNP, ANP, FNP-C
Owner
Healthcare Education Consultants
Tampa, Florida

Rachell A. Ekroos, PhD, RN, APRN-BC, AFN-BC, DF-IAFN, FAAN
Assistant Professor
School of Nursing
Affiliate Faculty
Center for Biobehavioral Interdisciplinary Science
University of Nevada, Las Vegas
Las Vegas, Nevada

Sherita K. Etheridge, MSN, RN, CPNP-PC
Nursing Instructor
Family, Community, and Health Systems
University of Alabama at Birmingham
Birmingham, Alabama

Diana K. Faugno, MSN, RN, CPN, SANE-A, SANE-P, FAAFS, DF-IAFN
Nurse Examiner
Barbara Sinatra Children's Center
Eisenhower Medical Center
Rancho Mirage, California

Michael D. Gooch, DNP, RN, ACNP-BC, FNP-BC, ENP-BC, ENP-C, CFRN, CTRN, TCRN, CEN, NREMT-P
Assistant Professor of Nursing
Vanderbilt University School of Nursing
Flight Nurse
Vanderbilt University Medical Center's LifeFlight
Emergency Nurse Practitioner
TeamHealth Faculty
Middle Tennessee School of Anesthesia
Nashville, Tennessee

Melanie Gibbons Hallman, DNP, RN, CRNP, CEN, FNP-BC
Instructor/Nurse Practitioner
School of Nursing
University of Alabama at Birmingham
Birmingham, Alabama

Nicole M. Hartman, DNP, MBA, RN, NEA-BC
Magnet Program Director
New York–Presbyterian/Columbia University Irving
Medical Center
New York, New York

Julie E. Herzog, MSN, RN, ACNP-BC, CCRN, CSC
Acute Care Nurse Practitioner
Cardiothoracic Intensive Care Unit
University Hospitals Cleveland Medical Center
Cleveland, Ohio

Breanna Hetland, PhD, RN, CCRN-K
Assistant Professor
University of Nebraska Medical Center
College of Nursing
Omaha, Nebraska

Ronald L. Hickman, Jr., PhD, RN, ACNP-BC, FNAP, FAAN
Associate Professor and Assistant Dean for Research
Frances Payne Bolton School of Nursing
Case Western Reserve University
Cleveland, Ohio

Joyce E. Higgins, MSN, MBA, RN, CCRN
Staff Nurse
Florida Hospital Pepin Heart Institute
Tampa, Florida

Katherine Hornack, MSN, RN, APRN, AGACNP-BC, CCRN
Nurse Practitioner II
University Hospitals Cleveland Medical Center
Cleveland, Ohio

Rita A. Jablonski-Jaudon, PhD, RN, CRNP, FAAN, FGSA
Nurse Practitioner
Memory Disorders Clinic
Professor
School of Nursing
University of Alabama Birmingham
Birmingham, Alabama

Marcia Johansson, DNP, RN, ARNP, ACNP-BC
Assistant Professor
Adult-Gerontology Acute Care Concentration Director
University of South Florida
Tampa, Florida

Qiana A. Johnson, DNP, FNP-C
Family Nurse Practitioner
Children's Healthcare of Atlanta
Stephanie V. Blank Center for Safe and Healthy Children
Atlanta, Georgia

Vicki A. Keough, PhD, RN, FAAN
Dean and Professor
Marcella Niehoff School of Nursing
Loyola University Chicago
Chicago, Illinois

Cindy D. Kumar, MSN, RN, AG-ACNP, FNP, ENP
Emergency Nurse Practitioner
TeamHealth
St. David's South Austin Medical Center Emergency Department
Austin, Texas

Cynthia Ann Leaver, PhD, RN, APRN, FNP-BC
Associate Dean of Faculty and Research
College of Nursing
United States University
San Diego, California

Fidelindo Lim, DNP, RN, CCRN
Clinical Assistant Professor of Nursing
Rory Meyers College of Nursing
New York University
New York, New York

Shannon M. Litten, DNP, RN, ARNP, ACNP-BC, FNP-BC, ENP-C
Lead Regional Director
American Academy of Emergency
Nurse Practitioners
Adjunct Instructor in Nursing
Vanderbilt University School of Nursing
TEAMHealth
Emergency Nurse Practitioner
St. Mary's Medical Center
West Palm Beach, Florida

Lia V. Ludan, DNP, RN, FNP-BC
Family Nurse Practitioner
Department of Emergency
Cape Regional Medical Center
Cape May Courthouse, New Jersey
Penn Presbyterian Medical Center
Philadelphia, Pennsylvania

Virginia Mangolds, MSN, RN, FNP-C, ENP-C, BSED
Instructor
Emergency Medicine
Instructor
Graduate School of Nursing
Assistant Research Director
Department of Emergency Medicine
UMass Memorial Medical Center
Worcester, Massachusetts

Steadman McPeters, DNP, RN, CRNP, CPNP-AC, RNFA
Assistant Professor
Director of Clinical Graduate Program Subspecialty
Tracks and Dual Option & Acute Care Pediatric Nurse
Practitioner Specialty Track Coordinator
Department of Family, Community, and Health Systems
School of Nursing
The University of Alabama at Birmingham
Birmingham, Alabama

Stacey A. Mitchell, DNP, MBA, RN, SANE-A, SANE-P, FAAN
Clinical Associate Professor
Texas A&M University
College of Nursing
Bryan, Texas

Brittany Newberry, PhD, MSN, MPH, APRN, FNP-BC, ENP-BC
Vice President of Education and Clinical Development
Nell Hodgson Woodruff School of Nursing
Emory University
Atlanta, Georgia

Lamon Norton, DNP, RN, FNP, ACNP
Managing Partner
UEE Health Care Consulting Emergency
Nurse Practitioner
Faculty
Samford University
Homewood, Alabama

Marian Nowak, DNP, MPH, RN, CSN, PN, FAAN
Assistant Professor
Rowan University Nursing Program
RN-BSN Program Coordinator
United Nations Nurse Delegate
CICIAMS Pan American President
Glassboro, New Jersey

George Byron Peraza-Smith, DNP, RN, GNP-BC, AGPCNP-C, CNE
Associate Dean of Academic Affairs
United States University
San Diego, California

Grant Pignatiello, BSN, RN
PhD Candidate
Frances Payne Bolton School of Nursing
Case Western Reserve University
Cleveland, Ohio

Sharon R. Rainer, PhD, RN, APRN, FNP-BC
Assistant Professor
Thomas Jefferson University College of Nursing
Nurse Practitioner
Department of Emergency Medicine
Thomas Jefferson University
Philadelphia, Pennsylvania

Janet E. Reilly, DNP, RN, APRN-BC
Nurse Practitioner
Bellin Health Systems
Associate Professor
University of Wisconsin—Green Bay
Green Bay, Wisconsin

Eric Roberts, DNP, RN, FNP-BC, ENP-BC
Assistant Professor
Marcella Niehoff School of Nursing
Loyola University Chicago
Chicago, Illinois

Susanna Rudy, DNP, MFS, RN, AG-ACNP-BC, FNP-BC, ENP, CCRN
Faculty Instructor
Vanderbilt University School of Nursing
Vanderbilt University Medical Center
Emergency Department APRN
Nashville, Tennessee

Al Rundio, PhD, DNP, RN, APRN, CARN-AP, NEA-BC, FNAP, FIAAN, FAAN
Associate Dean for Nursing
Chief Academic Nursing Officer
Clinical Professor of Nursing
Drexel University
College of Nursing & Health Professions
Philadelphia, Pennsylvania

Ian N. Saludares, MPA, BSN, RN, CCRN-K, NEA-BC
ICU/CCU—Nurse Manager
New York Presbyterian—Lawrence Hospital
Bronxville, New York

Megan M. Shifrin, DNP, RN, ACNP-BC
Assistant Professor
School of Nursing
Vanderbilt University
Director of the AGACNP Intensivist Focus
Nashville, Tennessee

Sallie J. Shipman, EdD, MSN, RN, CNL
Assistant Professor
School of Nursing
Family, Community, and Health Systems
University of Alabama at Birmingham
Birmingham, Alabama

Darlie Simerson, DNP, RN, APN, FNP-BC, CEN
Assistant Professor
Marcella Niehoff School of Nursing
Loyola University Chicago
Maywood, Illinois
Family Nurse Practitioner
Northwestern Convenient Care Centers
Northwestern Medicine Central DuPage Hospital
Winfield, Illinois

Tedra S. Smith, DNP, RN, CRNP, CPNP-PC, CNE
Assistant Professor
School of Nursing
University of Alabama at Birmingham
Birmingham, Alabama

Ramona A. Sowers, DNP, RN, FNP-BC, ANP-BC
Family Nurse Practitioner
Neurodiagnostic, Sleep Apnea Clinic
Durham, North Carolina
Adjunct Faculty
Nursing @Simmons Online Programs
School of Nursing and Health Sciences
Simmons College
Boston, Massachusetts

Patricia M. Speck, DNSc, APN, APRN, FNP-BC, DF-IAFN, FAAFS, FAAN
Professor and Coordinator
Advanced Forensic Nursing Department of Family,
Community, & Health Systems
School of Nursing
University of Alabama at Birmingham
Birmingham, Albama

Dustin Spencer, DNP, RN, NRP, NP-C, PMHS, ENP-BC, CNL
Assistant Professor of Nursing
Davenport University
Grand Rapids, Michigan
Lead Advanced Practice Clinician
American Physician Partners
Lancaster, South Carolina

Anita Sundaresh, MS, BSN, RN
Adult Nurse Practitioner
New York Presbyterian Hospital
New York, New York
Adjunct Faculty Member
Adelphi University for Graduate Nursing
Garden City, New York

Diane Fuller Switzer, DNP, ARNP, RN, FNP-BC, ENP-BC, ENP-C, CCRN, CEN, FAEN
Assistant Clinical Professor
Seattle University College of Nursing
Seattle, Washington

Richard Taylor, DNP, RN, CRNP, APN-BC
Associate Scientist
University of Alabama at Birmingham
Center of Palliative and Supportive Care
Assistant Professor
School of Nursing
Department of Acute, Chronic, and
Continuing Care
University of Alabama at Birmingham
Birmingham, Alabama

Rachel Tkaczyk, MSN, RN, CPNP-AC/PC-BC
Pediatric Nurse Practitioner
Assistant Clinical Professor
Drexel University
Philadelphia, Pennsylvania

Kelley Toffoli, DNP, RN, FNP-BC
Drexel University
Philadelphia, Pennsylvania

Rachel K. Vanek, MSN, RN, CNP
Acute Care Nurse Practitioner
Pulmonary Critical Care Medicine
Medical Intensive Care Unit
University Hospitals Cleveland Medical Center
Cleveland, Ohio

Deborah Vinesky, MSN, RN
Assistant Professor
Cuyahoga Community College
Cleveland, Ohio
DNP Student
Frances Payne Bolton School of Nursing
Case Western Reserve University
Cleveland, Ohio

Courtney Vose, DNP, MBA, RN, APRN, NEA-BC
Vice President and Chief Nursing Officer
New York–Presbyterian/Columbia University Irving Medical Center/
    Allen/Ambulatory Care Network
Clinical Instructor
Columbia University School of Nursing
New York, New York

Michael Wichowski, BSN, RN
Hospital Supervisor
St. Nicholas Hospital
Sheboygan, Wisconsin

S. Brian Widmar, PhD, RN, ACNP-BC, CCRN, FAANP
Director
Adult-Gerontology Acute Care Nurse Practitioner Program
Vanderbilt University School of Nursing
Nashville, Tennessee

Jennifer Wilbeck, DNP, RN, ACNP, FNP, ENP, FAANP
Associate Professor
Vanderbilt University School of Nursing
Nashville, Tennessee

Elizabeth Wirth-Tomaszewski, DNP, RN, CRNP, CCRN, ACNP-BC, ACNPC
Assistant Clinical Professor and Track Director
Adult Gerontology Acute Care Nurse Practitioner Program
College of Nursing and Health Professions
Drexel University
Philadelphia, Pennsylvania

Preface

Each year, millions of Americans receive care in emergency departments (EDs) and intensive care units because of acute life-limiting conditions. Nurses working in the ED or intensive care unit are front-line providers who practice in fast-paced health care settings, where a delay in the formulation of a diagnosis or initiation of the plans of care can have damaging consequences for an acutely ill patient. The practice of emergency and critical care nursing requires rapid access to knowledge that spans disciplinary domains, such as the physiological, cognitive, psychosocial, environmental, and behavioral mechanisms, which influence the health and susceptibility to disease among patients requiring life-sustaining care measures in an ED or intensive care unit. The care of these patients and their family systems requires emergency and critical care nurses to maintain an up-to-date knowledge base that guides the formulation of a nursing diagnosis and initiation of evidence-based nursing actions to optimize the health and recovery of acutely ill patients while offering emotional and informational support to their family systems.

The knowledge base of ED and critical care nurses is wide ranging and reflects the diversity of care needs of patients and their family systems. For medical–surgical nurses, the health care environments in which they practice are dynamic, and the complexity of care needs of patients are steadily increasing. Adding to the complexity of providing medical–surgical nursing care, registered nurses are finding it more difficult to acquire and make use of an evolving knowledge base of evidence to guide their nursing practice. Although the challenges of a dynamic health care environment, increasing complexity of patients, and an expanding evidence base for nursing care are not unique, restricted to ED and critical care nurses, these challenges pose a significant threat to the quality of care delivered by novice and even expert nurses in EDs or intensive care units.

The *Handbook of Clinical Nursing: Critical and Emergency Care Nursing* was conceptualized to assist the novice or the expert nurse in accessing up-to-date content on a variety of clinical topics for patients and their families in the ED or the intensive care unit, and is included in *A Guide to Mastery in Clinical Nursing: The Comprehensive Reference*, a comprehensive reference for individuals across the life span. This handbook includes a compendium of clinical topics with a structured format to aid the comprehension and application of the content to nursing practice. The *Handbook of Clinical Nursing:*

Critical and Emergency Care Nursing has selected clinical topics curated by Dr. Theresa Campo and contributions from expert practitioners in specialty areas of emergency and critical care nursing. The objective of the *Handbook of Clinical Nursing: Critical and Emergency Care Nursing* is to provide detailed information on the most important topics in clinical nursing practice for both new registered nurses and those transitioning to a new clinical area.

For each clinical topic, there is an overview of the clinical problem, relevant clinical background, clinical aspects for the nurse (assessment, nursing management and clinical implications, and outcomes), and a summary. Key references are provided for each entry, including both classic references and current citations from clinical and research literature. Although there are a number of comprehensive textbooks, this handbook provides information that is both concise and practical for the students as they enter each clinical area, and for registered nurses searching for up-to-date content, it will guide their nursing practice.

In summary, the *Handbook of Clinical Nursing: Critical and Emergency Care Nursing* has particular relevance to several groups of nurses. Nurse faculty will find it useful because it provides concise synopses of clinical topics relevant to the care of a hospitalized patient. Clinicians transitioning to new clinical areas will have a ready resource for key clinical problems they may face in their new clinical populations. And, importantly, newly licensed registered nurses will find that this guide to clinical mastery will chart their way in addressing the important clinical problems that their patients experience.

Ronald L. Hickman, Jr.
Celeste M. Alfes
Joyce J. Fitzpatrick

Vicki A. Keough

Overview

Aortic aneurysms can become a serious and lethal health crisis. Prior to 2010, aortic aneurysms were the primary cause of death of 15,000 Americans, and were a comorbid condition associated with approximately 17,000 deaths nationwide (Centers for Disease Control and Prevention [CDC], 2016; Go et al., 2014; Hoyert, 2012). Aortic aneurysms disproportionately affect males. Although about one third of aortic aneurysms occur among females, a majority of aortic aneurysms occur among males aged 65 years and older (Kent et al., 2010; Ramanath, Oh, Sundt, & Eagle, 2009). The U.S. Preventive Services Task Force (2005) estimated that aneurysms that occur in the abdominal aorta, abdominal aortic aneurysms (AAAs), annually affect 3.9% to 7.2% of men and 1% to 1.3% of women older than 50 years (LeFevre, 2014). Each year, approximately 55,000 Americans undergo an abdominal aneurysm repair and approximately 1.7 million Americans are screened for abdominal aneurysms (Cowan et al., 2006; LeFevre, 2014). Therefore, nursing care of patients with an AAA is focused on the assessment of disease and symptom progression and implementation of evidence-based care to prevent premature disability or death.

Background

The aorta is the largest artery and blood vessel in the human body, and it extends from the top of the right ventricle to the bifurcation of the iliac arteries in the lower pelvis. The abdominal aorta begins at the diaphragm and extends to the iliac arteries. An aneurysm occurs wherever there is an outpouching and weakness in an arterial vessel. The weakened area of the arterial vessel wall is persistently exposed to shearing forces from blood constantly pumped from the left ventricle through the vascular system. The normal diameters of the abdominal aorta are 1.7 cm in males and 1.5 cm in females (Aggarwal, Qamar, Sharma, & Sharma, 2011; Howell & Rabener, 2016).

When the pressure in the artery exceeds the ability of the weak vessel wall to maintain its integrity, a tear in the vessel wall can occur, causing an outpouching and disruption of the arterial vessel's wall integrity. In the emergent case, the vessel can rupture resulting in sudden, massive blood loss. In a less extreme case, the vessel wall can become weak and bulge, increasing in diameter. Risk of abdominal aortic rupture occurs when the diameter is greater than 3 cm. The Joint Council for the American Association for Vascular Surgery and Society for Vascular Surgery has published an estimation of the risk for rupture of an AAA ranging from 0% risk of rupture when the AAA diameter is less than 4 cm to 30% to 50% risk of rupture when the diameter is greater than or equal to 8 cm (Brewster et al., 2003). The rate at which the AAA expands is also a consideration. If a small AAA expands 0.5 cm or more over 6 months, there is a high rate of rupture. When discovered early enough, very often the vessel can be repaired (Aggarwal et al., 2011; Hirsch et al., 2006; Howell & Rabener, 2016).

Prevention is the best treatment for success. The U.S. Preventive Services Task Force (2005) recommends screening for AAA for males between the ages of 65 and 75 years with a history of smoking and for women of the same age with a history of smoking and hypertension. Having a family history of AAA, as well as a history of either coronary artery disease or atherosclerosis, is indicative of early screening for an AAA. In addition, a family history of repair of AAA in a first-degree relative dramatically increases the risk of AAA. Early detection, surveillance, and appropriate treatment can significantly attenuate the morbidity and mortality associated with AAA.

In cases of hypertension, atherosclerosis, and a positive family or smoking history, there are several less common contributing factors that predispose adults to an AAA. In adults, infants, and children, AAA has been associated with "seatbelt syndrome," whereby the seatbelt can cause injury to the abdominal aorta during a high-speed crash. Other possible causes of AAA include cystic medial necrosis, trauma, and syphilis. Finally, a *Chlamydia pneumoniae* infection has been implicated as a causative factor in weakening of the abdominal aortic wall (Guirguis-Blake & Wolff, 2005; Keisler & Carter, 2015; Kokje, Hamming, & Lindeman, 2016; Kurosawa, Matsumura, & Yamanouchi, 2013; LeFevre, 2014; Motte, 2015; Salo, Soisalon-Soininen, Bondestam, & Matilla, 1999).

Clinical Aspects

ASSESSMENT

As the mainstay of therapy is focused on screening and rapid intervention, early detection is essential. AAAs can occasionally be found on a physical examination; however, this occurs in only about 50% of confirmed cases. It is more difficult to palpate AAAs if the patient is obese. When a palpable AAA mass is found, it is most likely in the epigastric and left hypochondriac area of the abdomen (Howell & Rabner, 2016). Auscultation is another physical assessment technique that is helpful in the diagnosis of AAA. The presence of a bruit over the abdominal aorta should alert the clinician to do further tests for AAA (Aggarwal et al., 2011). Palpating distal pulses, such as popliteal and pedal, gives the nurse an indication of distal perfusion. In addition, the nurse should examine the skin for signs of adequate perfusion such as warmth, pink color, and good capillary refill. Ominous signs that the skin is not being perfused adequately are cool, pale skin, diaphoresis, and mottling (Aggarwal et al., 2011; Hirsch et al., 2006).

The majority of AAAs are found serendipitously. Often, adults with an AAA present without signs or symptoms until the vessel wall has ruptured and their circumstances are life-threatening. AAAs are often detected during abdominal imaging studies, such as CT, ultrasound, or MRI, as part of a workup for an unrelated complaint. The most common symptom of an AAA is pain and tenderness around the abdomen, flank, or back. Some patients also report epigastric discomfort and altered bowel elimination. Pain on palpation is predictive of a serious risk for rupture. If AAA is suspected, the clinician should be careful not to palpate too vigorously in order to prevent a rupture. A ruptured AAA represents a medical emergency. Once the AAA ruptures, patients often report severe, sharp abdominal or back pain, and a pulsatile abdominal mass may appear. AAA rupture is associated with severe hypotension resulting from hypovolemic shock and consequently results in manifestations such as mottled skin, decreased level of consciousness, diaphoresis, and oliguria. The abdomen may become distended with ecchymosis or a palpable hematoma. For patients who present with clinical findings consistent with a ruptured AAA, half of these patients will survive (Aggarwal et al., 2011; Creager & Loscalzo, 2008; Harris, Faggioli, Fiedler, Curl, & Ricotta, 1991; Keisler & Carter, 2015).

NURSING INTERVENTIONS, MANAGEMENT, AND IMPLICATIONS

Interventions for AAA are focused on serial observation, medical management, and surgical repair or endovascular stenting. Observation can be tricky. The American College of Cardiology/American Heart Association (ACC/AHA) guidelines recommend monitoring aneurysms that are 3 to 4 cm in diameter every 2 to 3 years and those with a diameter of 4.0 to 5.4 cm should be monitored every 6 to 12 months (Hirsch et al., 2006).

Medical management is focused on smoking cessation; management of hypertension, atherosclerosis and coronary artery diseases; treatment of infection; and surveillance. As infection has been implicated as a possible cause of AAA, the administration of pathogen-specific antibiotics has demonstrated some success in treating aneurysms (Kurosawa et al., 2013). Pharmacologic interventions that have been used in the treatment of AAAs that are not within standards for surgical or endovascular repair include managing hypertension, atherosclerosis, and antibiotics (Baxter, Terrin, & Dalman, 2008; Hirsch et al., 2006; Kurosawa et al., 2013).

Surgical or endovascular repair is recommended for patients with an AAA measuring 5.5 cm or greater that is asymptomatic, patients who are symptomatic, and for those patients with an aneurysm that increased in size at a rate greater than 0.5 cm over 6 months (Hirsch et al., 2006). Poor long-term survival for surgical AAA repair has been associated with end-stage renal disease, chronic lung disease, and cardiovascular disease (Khashram, Williman, Hider, Jones, & Roake, 2016). In general, patients do well after an AAA repair.

A ruptured AAA presents a life-threatening emergency. Once the nurse has completed a thorough assessment and AAA is suspected, the provider must be alerted to the emergency. As it is often an emergent life-threatening situation, keeping the patient calm and informing the family of the emergent nature of the repair is of high priority. Nursing interventions include providing adequate oxygenation, cardiovascular support in the form of fluid (blood and/or blood products), vasopressors, and emergent transport to repair the ruptured artery. Managing of extreme anxiety and pain is crucial at this time. Keeping the family informed and providing family-centered care are critical as the patient is facing a life-threatening emergency.

However, if the AAA has been identified as stable, then educating the patient and family about the risk factors, signs, and symptoms of an expanding or ruptured AAA is important. The patients and their families must be given clear and specific follow-up instructions that include follow-up appointments and instructions for ameliorating the risk factors for AAA such as smoking cessation, healthy eating, and close adherence to medication. The patient and family should be informed of the seriousness of the disease. Patients and their families should also understand that they can lead a normal and healthy life as long as they reduce or eliminate risk factors and follow-up as instructed.

OUTCOMES

The goals of nursing care with a patient with an AAA are focused on positive patient outcomes and prevention of complications. Early identification and intervention of an AAA are foundational to emergency nursing. Performing a rapid but thorough health history, including past medical history and risk factors, and physical examination will assist the nurse in not only identification of an AAA but also other life-threatening disorders. Nurses must closely monitor these patients for abrupt changes in mental status, vital signs, and symptoms in order to prevent complications.

Summary

Emergency and critical care nurses play a vital role in the early detection of AAAs as they can often be discovered during the initial nursing assessment. If the AAA is discovered before rupture, quick diagnosis and immediate intervention can be a lifesaving measure. Once the AAA has progressed to the point of rupture, a life-threatening emergency exists. Even in the best of circumstances, once a rupture has occurred, survival is only about 50%. It is important for the emergency or critical care nurse to have knowledge of the pathophysiology, signs, symptoms, and quick interventions for AAA so that they can intervene appropriately. In addition, knowledge of the best practice recommendations for AAA screening, prevention, and treatment is essential for emergency nurses.

Aggarwal, S., Qamar, A., Sharma, V., & Sharma, A. (2011). Abdominal aortic aneurysm: A comprehensive review. *Experimental Clinical Cardiology*, *16*(1), 11–15.

Baxter, B. T., Terrin, M. C., & Dalman, R. L. (2008). Medical management of small abdominal aortic aneurysms. *Circulation*, *117*, 1883–1889.

Brewster, D. C., Cronenwett, J. L., Hallett, J. W., Johnston, K. W., Kupski, W.C., & Matsumura, J. S. (2003). Guidelines for the treatment of abdominal aortic aneurysms. Report of a subcommittee of the Joint Council of the American Association for Vascular Surgery and Society for Vascular Surgery. *Journal of Vascular Surgery*, *37*, 1106–1117.

Centers for Disease Control and Prevention. (2016). Deaths, percent of total deaths, and death rates for the 15 leading causes of death in 5-year age groups, by race, and sex: United States, 2013. Retrieved from https://www.cdc.gov/nchs/data/dvs/lcwk1_2013.pdf

Cowan, J. A., Dimick, J. B., Henke, P. K., Rectenwald, J., Stanley, J. C., & Upchurch, G. R., Jr. (2006). Epidemiology of aortic aneurysm repair in the United States from 1993–2003. *Annals of the New York Academy of Sciences, 1082,* 1–10.

Creager, M. A., & Loscalzo, J. (2008). Diseases of the aorta. In A. S. Fauci, E. Braumwald, D. L. Kasper, S. L. Hauser, D. L. Longo, J. L. Jameson, & J. Loscalzo (Eds.), *Harrison's principles of internal medicine* (17th ed., pp. 736–738). Columbus, OH: McGraw-Hill.

Go, A. S., Mozaffarian, D., Roger V. L., Benjamin E. J., Berry J. D., Blaha, M. J., . . . Turner, M. B. (2014). Heart disease and stroke statistics—2013 update: A report from the American Heart Association. *Circulation, 127,* e6–e245.

Guirguis-Blake, J., & Wolff, T. A. (2005). Screening for abdominal aortic aneurism. *American Family Physician, 71,* 2154–2155.

Harris, L. M., Faggioli, G. L., Fiedler, R., Curl, G. R., & Ricotta, J. J. (1991). Ruptured abdominal aortic aneurysms: Factors affecting mortality rates. *Journal of Vascular Surgery, 14,* 812–818.

Hirsch, A. T., Haskal, Z. J., Hertzer, N. R., Bakal, C. W., Creager, M. A., Halpern, J. L., . . . Riegel, B. (2006). ACC/AHA 2005 Practice Guidelines for the management of patients with peripheral arterial disease (lower extremity, renal, mesenteric, and abdominal aortic): A collaborative report from the American Association for Vascular Surgery/Society for Vascular Surgery, Society for Cardiovascular Angiography and Interventions, Society for Vascular Medicine and Biology, Society of Interventional Radiology, and the ACC/AHA Task Force on Practice Guidelines (Writing Committee to Develop Guidelines for the Management of Patients With Peripheral Arterial Disease): Endorsed by the American Association of Cardiovascular and Pulmonary Rehabilitation; National Heart, Lung, and Blood Institute; Society for Vascular Nursing; Trans-Atlantic Inter-Society Consensus; and Vascular Disease Foundation. *Circulation, 113,* e463–e654.

Howell, C. M., & Rabener, M. J. (2016). Abdominal aortic aneurysm: A ticking time bomb. *Journal of the American Association of Physician Assistants, 26,* 3.

Hoyert, D. L. (2012). National vital statistics reports. NCHS. *National Vital Statistics Reports, 61,* 1–52.

Keisler, B., & Carter, C. (2015). Abdominal aortic aneurysm. *American Family Physician, 91*(8), 538–543.

Kent, K. C., Zwolak, R. M., Egorova, N. N., Riles, T. S., Manganaro, A., Moskowitz, A. J., & Greco, G. (2010). Analysis of risk factors for abdominal aortic aneurysm in a cohort of more than 3 million individuals. *Journal of Vascular Surgery, 52,* 539–548.

Khashram, M., Williman, J. A., Hider, P. N., Jones, G. T., & Roake, J. A. (2016). Systematic review and meta-analysis of factors influencing survival following abdominal aortic aneurysm repair. *European Journal of Vascular and Endovascular Surgery, 51,* 203–215.

Kokje, V. B., Hamming, J. F., & Lindeman, J. H. (2016). Pharmaceutical management of small abdominal aortic aneurysms: A systematic review of the clinical evidence. *European Journal of Vascular and Endovascular Surgery, 51*(1), 64–75. doi:10.1016/j.ejvs.2015.09.006

Kurosawa, K., Matsurmura, J. S., & Yamanouchi, D. (2013). Current status of medical treatment for abdominal aortic aneurysm. *Circulation, 77,* 2860–2866.

LeFevre, M. I. (2014). Screening for abdominal aortic aneurysm: U.S. Preventive Services Task Force recommendation statement. *Annals of Internal Medicine, 161,* 281–290.

Motte, S. (2015). What is the evidence to support screening for abdominal aortic aneurysm and what is the role of the primary care physician? *Radiology Clinics of North America, 53*(6), 1209–1224. doi:10.1016/j.rcl.2015.06.007

Ramanath, V. S., Oh, J. K., Sundt, T. M., & Eagle, K. A. (2009). Acute aortic syndromes and thoracic aortic aneurysm. *Mayo Clinic Proceedings, 84*(5), 465–481.

Salo, J. A., Soisalon-Soininen, S., Bondestam, S., & Matilla, P. S. (1999). Familial occurrence of abdominal aortic aneurysm. *Annals of Internal Medicine, 130,* 637–642.

U.S. Preventive Services Task Force. (2005). Screening for abdominal aortic aneurysm: Recommendation statement. *Annals of Internal Medicine, 142,* 198–202.

■ ABDOMINAL PAIN

Christopher J. Contino

Overview

Abdominal pain is a complicated complaint in the emergency care setting. The chief complaint of abdominal pain comprises approximately 5% to 10% of emergency department visits annually (Kendall & Moreira, 2016). The most recent data from the Centers for Disease Control and Prevention (CDC) indicates that 8.1% of patients who seek care in an emergency department have a chief complaint of stomach or abdominal pain, which translates into more than 11 million visits related to the complaints of abdominal pain (CDC, 2011). Although many cases of abdominal pain are not life-threatening and are self-limited, there are a multitude of cases that may require emergent intervention from emergency room nurses.

Background

Abdominal pain comprises a significant portion of emergency department visits annually (Kendall & Moreira, 2016). Although abdominal pain affects all patient populations, there are key demographics that may have a more significant course, and include the *elderly*, defined as those older than 65 years, and immunocompromised patients, such as individuals living with HIV. Individuals from these at-risk populations have disproportionately higher rates of mortality and morbidity compared to younger adults with a functioning immune system. In the emergency department, nurses are usually the first point of contact for the patients, and it is important that they are able to recognize life-threatening emergencies and care for the patients appropriately (Cole, Lynch, & Cugnoni, 2006).

The abdomen can be broadly divided into four quadrants: right upper, left upper, right lower, and left lower. In addition, the epigastric area, just under the xiphoid process, is a key area for assessment. Understanding the location of pain may help in determining the cause of the origin of the pain. Right upper quadrant pain may be due to cholecystitis, hepatitis, or ulcers. Left upper quadrant pain may involve the spleen or stomach. Right lower quadrant pain may be appendicitis or diverticulitis, and left lower quadrant pain may be from colitis or diverticulitis. Depending on the gender of the patient, lower abdominal pain can stem from genitourinary processes such as ectopic pregnancy and pelvic inflammatory disease in the female, or testicular disease in the male patient. Diffuse abdominal pain can occur from a multitude of causes (Penner, Mary, & Majumdar, 2016).

The differential diagnoses of abdominal pain can vary widely and include causes arising from the abdominal or extra-abdominal etiologies (O'Brien, 2015). The complete discussion of all causes of abdominal pain is vast and exceeds the scope of this entry; therefore, this discussion will focus on the most common causes of life-threatening abdominal pain. These include bowel obstruction, abdominal aortic aneurism, bowel perforation, ectopic pregnancy, placental abruption, splenic rupture, mesenteric ischemia, and myocardial infarction.

Pediatric patients with abdominal pain pose a challenge with diagnosis and may vary widely with age. In the infant through toddler years, patients may not be able to adequately describe their pain. Many of the differential diagnoses remain salient; however, in the very young infant, consider pyloric stenosis, intussusception, Hirschsprung's disease, and Meckel's diverticulitis. Pediatric patients may become dehydrated faster than adults, so fluid balance is key. Also, pediatric patients can cardiovascular compensate longer than adults; however, when the decompensation occurs, it happens rapidly. Assess a pediatric patient frequently and thoroughly, and keep a high index of suspicion for serious disease.

Clinical Aspects

ASSESSMENT

The key to managing patients with a chief complaint of abdominal pain is performing a thorough history and physical examination that can narrow the list of suspicious etiologies. As with all patient encounters, an initial assessment should focus on airway, breathing, and circulation (ABC), and generate a rapid sense of whether the patient is critically ill or unstable before proceeding to further assessment. Any abnormalities during the initial evaluation should be addressed immediately, and only after this should further assessment be performed. Findings that may indicate that a patient is critical include tachycardia, hypertension, fever, extreme tenderness, abdominal rigidity, or pain elicited by minor touch. In these cases, it is important to ensure that the provider is aware and is at the bedside to evaluate the patient concurrently.

Once it has been established that the patient is otherwise stable, a thorough history and physical examination may commence. All patients should receive a thorough SAMPLE history, which includes signs and symptoms, allergies, medications, past illnesses, last oral intake, and events leading up to the present illness. The patient's pain should be characterized utilizing the OPQRST mnemonic, which evaluates onset, provocative and palliative factors, quality, radiation, site or location, associated signs and symptoms, and time. In case of abdominal pain, the location of pain may help to narrow the differential diagnosis, although it should not be relied on as many etiologies of abdominal pain can vary from patient to patient. The character and nature of the pain can also help to narrow the diagnosis. There are three main types of pain described as visceral, somatic, and referred. Visceral pain is typically described as dull and hard to localize, and it usually originates from solid organs and the walls of hollow organs. Somatic pain is usually described as sharp and can be localized, and is usually caused by inflammation, ischemia, or peritoneal irritation. Referred pain is pain that is felt at a location distant from its originating source. This is a key concept to remember as several potentially life-threatening disease processes may be felt as abdominal pain but do not originate in the abdominal area; a key example of this would be myocardial ischemia presenting as epigastric pain.

NURSING INTERVENTIONS, MANAGEMENT, AND IMPLICATIONS

Initial nursing interventions should ensure that the ABC status is adequate and secure. All undifferentiated abdominal pain patients should have nothing by mouth (NPO) in case surgery may be necessary. Patients should have intravenous (IV) access secured, preferably with a large-bore IV catheter in the antecubital region. This is important should fluid resuscitation be necessary and many diagnostic imaging modalities require this for IV contrast administration. The nurse should prepare to obtain diagnostic samples of blood and urine. Local protocol should dictate when and how to obtain the samples. Laboratory evaluation should be tailored to the individual patient to avoid unnecessary testing; however, in some clinical settings, there are established nursing protocols that should dictate the nurse's plan of care. It is important to note that in the case of abdominal pain, all females of childbearing age should receive a rapid test for pregnancy, as a potentially life-threatening diagnosis of ectopic pregnancy may be the cause of pain or pregnancy may prohibit certain diagnostic medical imaging tests from being performed. An emergency department adage is to always consider a female of childbearing age with abdominal pain to have an ectopic pregnancy until proven otherwise.

OUTCOMES

When discussing any clinical disease process, it is important to discuss outcomes. With regard to abdominal pain, the main outcome in the emergency department setting is rapid exclusion of life-threatening causes of pain that require emergent intervention. This includes timely diagnosis; early consultation with specialists, including surgery; and collaboration with ancillary departments. Pain control is also a significant outcome measure (Kendall & Moreira, 2016). Once an appropriate physical exam has been conducted, pain control should be a priority. Pain should be assessed and reassessed frequently by utilizing a standard pain scale. The ultimate outcome is to reduce mortality and morbidity.

Summary

Abdominal pain is a common complaint in the emergency department, with a wide variety of potential causes. Although a large portion of patients with abdominal pain do not have a specific cause of their pain, there are a few disease processes that are immediately life-threatening. It is crucial that emergency department nurses are able to recognize the spectrum of possible causes of pain, recognize unstable or ill patients, and institute appropriate interventions. The key to most abdominal pain complaints is a thorough history and physical examination, with assistance from appropriate labs and imaging as necessary. Be aware of special populations such as the elderly, immunocompromised, and women of childbearing age.

Centers for Disease Control and Prevention. (2011). National Hospital Ambulatory Medical Care Survey: 2010 emergency department summary tables (pp. 1–39). Retrieved from https://www.cdc.gov/nchs/data/ahcd/nhamcs_emergency/2011_ed_web_tables.pdf

Cole, E., Lynch, A., & Cugnoni, H. (2006). Assessment of the patient with acute abdominal pain. *Nursing Standard*, 20(39), 67–75.

Kendall, J. L., & Moreira, M. E. (2016). Evaluation of the adult with abdominal pain in the emergency department. In R. Hockberger & J. Grayzel (Eds.), *UptoDate* (pp. 1–51). Retrieved from https://www.uptodate.com/contents/evaluation-of-the-adult-with-abdominal-pain-in-the-emergency-department

O'Brien, M. C. (2015). Gastrointestinal emergencies. In J. Tintinalli, J. S. Stapczynski, O. J. Ma, D. Cline, R. K. Cydulka, & G. Meckler (Eds.), *Tintinalli's emergency medicine: A comprehensive study guide* (8th ed.). New York, NY: McGraw-Hill.

Penner, R., Mary, F., & Majumdar, S. (2016). Evaluation of the adult with abdominal pain. In A. Auerbach, M. Aronson, & H. N. Sokol (Eds.), *UptoDate* (pp. 1–31). Retrieved from https://www.uptodate.com/contents/evaluation-of-the-adult-with-abdominal-pain

■ ACID–BASE IMBALANCES

Michael D. Gooch

Overview

Acid–base balance is key for all physiological processes and functions. An imbalance occurs when the pH falls outside the normal range and leads to organ dysfunction, for example, coagulopathy, electrolyte disturbances, and organ failure. The potential of hydrogen (pH) is a measure of the concentration of hydrogen ions (H⁺) in the body and is based on a 0-to-14 scale. There is an inverse relationship between the pH and H⁺ concentration: The lower the number, the higher the H⁺ concentration of the body fluid. An acid–base imbalance, acidosis, results from an accumulation of acids or a loss of base and is often defined as a pH less than 7.35. Whereas, alkalosis is often specified as a pH greater than 7.45 and occurs due to an excess amount of base/alkali or deficiency of the body's acids. A prolonged pH of less than 6.8 or greater than 7.8 is not compatible with life (Berend, de Vries, & Gans, 2014; Hall, 2016; Kamel & Halperin, 2017).

Acid–base imbalances may occur in patients of any age and result from numerous processes, including pulmonary and renal disease, toxicological and endocrine emergencies, and shock (Berend et al., 2014; Gooch, 2015). Identification and management of these imbalances are important to reduce complications and improve patient outcomes. Nurses should be able to recognize the diagnostics needed to properly identify an imbalance, the associated clinical manifestations, and initial management of these derangements.

Background

For equilibrium to be maintained, there must be a balance between the intake or production and the excretion of both acids and bases. Acid is used to describe any compound capable of donating an H⁺. A base is a substance capable of accepting an H⁺ (Hall, 2016; Kamel & Halperin, 2017). Without acid–base balance, the pH will not be maintained at a level that supports homeostasis. Acids can be classified as carbonic or respiratory and noncarbonic or metabolic acids. Metabolic acids include ketones and lactate, which often results from the oxidation or metabolism of carbohydrates, proteins, and fats. Foods containing phosphates and sulfates also contribute to the metabolic acid load. Carbonic acid (H_2CO_3) is a weak acid that plays a major role in this balance. Bicarbonate (HCO_3^-) is the body's primary base. Bicarbonate is formed during the metabolism of some fruits and vegetables, and by the kidneys (Gooch, 2015; Hall, 2016; Kamel & Halperin, 2017).

There are three processes that regulate acid–base balance. First is the chemical buffer system. This process can quickly alter the pH by reversibly changing the concentration and state of H⁺. In the setting of acidosis, H⁺ is combined with a buffer. As the concentration decreases or, in the case of alkalosis, it is released from the buffer. Bicarbonate is the most abundant extracellular buffer. This reaction is summarized by the formula: $H_2CO_3 \leftrightarrow H^+ + HCO_3^-$. Phosphate and proteins, including hemoglobin, are key intracellular buffers (Cho, 2017; Gooch, 2015; Hall, 2016; Kamel & Halperin, 2017).

In addition to the chemical buffering system, there is physiological buffering or compensation. Carbon dioxide (CO_2) is a by-product of the body's metabolic processes. There is a direct relationship between the H^+ concentration and the CO_2 level, and an inverse relationship between the CO_2 level and the pH. The medulla and chemoreceptors regulate the respiratory rate in response to changes in the H^+ concentration. As CO_2 levels increase, the respiratory rate increases to blow off more CO_2, lowering the level and increasing the pH. As the respiratory rate slows, the CO_2 concentration increases and the pH decreases. This buffer can quickly adjust the CO_2 level to compensate for an imbalance over minutes to hours, though it is not as potent as chemical buffering (Gooch, 2015; Hall, 2016; Kamel & Halperin, 2017).

Lastly, the kidneys regulate the excretion of noncarbonic acids and H^+, as well as the reabsorption of almost 100% of the excreted HCO_3^-. The kidneys produce HCO_3^- during the excretion of ammonium, if needed, to maintain a normal pH. Unlike the lungs, the renal or metabolic pathway is much slower and may take hours to days to complete the process. The lungs expel 150 times more acid each day than the kidneys (Rice, Ismail, & Pillow, 2014). If there is an increase in the H^+ concentration, the kidneys can increase the excretion of acids and increase the reabsorption and production of HCO_3^- to help stabilize the pH. Just the opposite can occur if there is an accumulation of HCO_3^-. This entire balance process is demonstrated by the formula: $CO_2 + H_2O \leftrightarrow H_2CO_3 \leftrightarrow H^+ + HCO_3^-$. Carbonic anhydrase, an enzyme found primarily in red blood cells, the lungs, and renal tubules, increases the rate of these reactions. In the case of lung or renal disease, these physiological buffer systems are altered (Gooch, 2015; Hall, 2016; Kamel & Halperin, 2017).

Clinical Aspects

Imbalances are categorized as metabolic or respiratory in nature. Evaluation of the patient's blood gas is needed to properly identify the imbalance. An arterial blood gas is not always needed and in most patients a venous gas is acceptable. Primary respiratory imbalances affect the pH because of an altered CO_2 level (normal range: 35–45 mmHg), in which primary metabolic imbalances are due to an altered HCO3- level (normal range: 22–26 mEq/L). A patient may present with one of four acid–base imbalances, referred to as a *simple imbalance*, or a combination of metabolic and respiratory imbalances, referred to as a *mixed imbalance*. A primary imbalance is most often accompanied by secondary compensation of the physiological buffer systems; however, this compensation may not be enough to return the pH to a normal range (Berend et al., 2014; Cho, 2017; Hall, 2016; Kamel & Halperin, 2017).

Respiratory acidosis often develops due to impaired gas exchange or hypoventilation from pulmonary disease or injury, or altered central nervous system control, for example, an opioid or sedation agent. If there is impaired exhalation of CO_2, there will be an increase in the H^+ concentration and a drop in the pH leading to acidosis. Respiratory alkalosis develops from hyperventilation. As the CO_2 level decreases due to the increased respiratory rate, the pH increases due to a drop in the H^+ concentration. Hyperventilation can be related to hypoxia, the stress response, or could be iatrogenic, for example, incorrect mechanical ventilation (Al-Jaghbeer & Kellum, 2014; Cho, 2017; Gooch, 2015; Hall, 2016; Kamel & Halperin, 2017).

Respiratory imbalances are best managed by managing the airway. As with any patient, the history and physical exam are essential to identifying the cause, managing the patient, and preventing complications. In the setting of a respiratory acidosis, measures may be needed to improve ventilations, gas exchange, and expiration of CO_2. This may include beta agonists, assisting ventilations, or administration of a reversal agent, for example, naloxone (Narcan), to improve the respiratory rate and effort. For the patients with hyperventilation, which has led to a respiratory alkalosis, the respiratory rate should be slowed. The nurse should consider reasons why the patient is hyperventilating and address the cause, not just the rate, for example, hypoxia, anxiety, and pain. Hyperventilation may be compensatory for an impending metabolic acidosis, for example, Kussmaul's respirations (Cho, 2017; Gooch, 2015; Kamel & Halperin, 2017). Once the cause of the respiratory imbalance is identified, the disarrangement can usually be quickly reversed.

A metabolic acidosis results from the buildup of acids or the loss of base, leading to an increase in the H^+ concentration that shifts the pH downward. This may result from renal impairment, that is, renal failure, in which the kidneys are unable to excrete acids or reabsorb and produce adequate amounts of bicarbonate. Metabolic acidosis is often defined based on the anion gap, which represents the difference between the measured serum cations and anions. It may be calculated using this formula: sodium − (chloride + bicarbonate). A normal gap is considered by some to be 8 ± 4 mEq/L; this as well as the formula varies from lab to lab. A nongap acidosis results from bicarbonate loss due to gastrointestinal, renal, or iatrogenic causes. Bicarbonate is lost as a result of excessive vomiting or diarrhea. Hyperchloremia, which leads to increased renal excretion of bicarbonate, may result from excessive administration of intravenous (IV) normal saline solution (iatrogenic) or renal tubular acidosis (Al-Jaghbeer & Kellum, 2014; Berend et al., 2014; Cho, 2017; Gooch, 2015; Hall, 2016; Kamel & Halperin, 2017; Rice et al, 2014).

An anion gap metabolic acidosis results from the increased production or accumulation of noncarbonic acids, which cannot be buffered by the respiratory system. A gap indicates there are anions present that are not evaluated during routine laboratory analysis. A mnemonic sometimes used to recall common causes of a gap acidosis is CAT MUDPILES: carbon monoxide, cyanide, alcoholic ketoacidosis, toluene, methanol, metformin, uremia, diabetic ketoacidosis, propylene glycol, ingestion of iron or isoniazid, lactic acidosis, ethylene glycol, and salicylates (Al-Jaghbeer & Kellum, 2014; Cho, 2017; Gooch, 2015; Rice et al., 2014). As these anions accumulate, they shift the pH downward, impair the body's buffering systems, and disrupt cellular activities.

The initial management of a patient with a metabolic acidosis should focus on restoring perfusion with IV fluids and identifying the cause. Improving cellular and especially renal perfusion will improve energy production and elimination of acids. The specific treatment will depend on the cause of the acidosis. The administration of IV sodium bicarbonate is rarely indicated and should only be used in the setting of severe acidosis, that is, a pH less than 7.0 with organ dysfunction (Al-Jaghbeer & Kellum, 2014; Berend et al., 2014; Cho, 2017, 2014; Gooch, 2015; Kamel & Halperin, 2017; Rice et al., 2014).

The last imbalance is metabolic alkalosis, which develops as the result of excessive acid loss or accumulation of base, shifting the pH upward. The causes of this imbalance are separated based on the urine chloride level: low—referred to as saline or chloride responsive or elevated—referred to as saline or chloride unresponsive. Saline-responsive conditions are often due to an increase in bicarbonate due to a loss of hydrochloric acid, chloride, and potassium caused by excessive vomiting, diarrhea, or suctioning, or from diuresis. Saline-unresponsive alkalosis is less common and is often related to the excess production or intake of mineralocorticoids (Al-Jaghbeer & Kellum, 2014; Berend et al., 2014; Cho, 2017; Gooch, 2015; Hall, 2016; Kamel & Halperin, 2017; Soifer & Kim, 2014).

The management of a metabolic alkalosis also varies with the cause. If the patient has a chloride-responsive condition, the administration of IV normal saline may be indicated to restore renal perfusion and replace chloride. In the setting of a chloride-unresponsive alkalosis, acetazolamide (Diamox), a carbonic anhydrase inhibitor, is sometimes administered to increase urinary bicarbonate excretion (Al-Jaghbeer & Kellum, 2014; Berend et al., 2014; Cho, 2017; Gooch, 2015; Kamel & Halperin, 2017; Soifer & Kim, 2014).

Summary

Acid–base balance is essential to maintaining normal cellular function. Given the narrow range of a normal pH, a small change may lead to organ dysfunction. A patient may have a simple or a mixed imbalance. Analysis of the pH, CO_2, and HCO_3^- from the blood gas and assessment findings help identify the problem and guide treatment to correct the imbalance. Most respiratory imbalances are corrected by managing the airway and improving gas exchange. Metabolic problems are corrected based on the cause, but often involve restoring vascular volume and restoring perfusion. Acid–base imbalances are associated with various diseases and may be encountered in any patient. Prompt recognition and management are essential to limiting complications and improving patient outcomes.

Al-Jaghbeer, M., & Kellum, J. A. (2015). Acid–base disturbances in intensive care patients: Etiology, pathophysiology and treatment. *Nephrology, Dialysis, Transplantation, 30*(7), 1104–1111. doi:10.1093/ndt/gfu289

Berend, K., de Vries, A. P. J., & Gans, R. O. B. (2014). Physiological approach to assessment of acid-base disturbances. *New England Journal of Medicine, 371*(15), 1434–1445. doi:10.1056/NEJMra1003327

Cho, K. C. (2017). Electrolyte and acid–base disorders. In M. A. Papadakis, S. J., McPhee, & M. W. Rabow (Eds.), *Current medical diagnosis and treatment 2017* (56th ed., pp. 884–912). New York, NY: McGraw-Hill.

Gooch, M. D. (2015). Identifying acid-base and electrolyte imbalances. *Nurse Practitioner, 40*(8), 37–42. doi:10.1097/01.NPR.0000469255.98119.82

Hall, J. E. (2016). *Guyton and hall textbook of medical physiology* (13th ed.). Philadelphia, PA: Elsevier.

Kamel, K. S., & Halperin, M. L. (2017). *Fluid, electrolytes, and acid-base physiology: A problem-based approach* (5th ed.). Philadelphia, PA: Elsevier.

Rice, M., Ismail, B., & Pillow, M. T. (2014). Approach to metabolic acidosis in the emergency department. *Emergency Medicine Clinics of North America, 32*(2), 403–420. doi:10.1016/j.emc.2014.01.002

Soifer, J. T., & Kim, H. T. (2014). Approach to metabolic alkalosis. *Emergency Medicine Clinics of North America, 32*(2), 453–463. doi:10.1016/j.emc.2014.01.005

■ ACUTE ABDOMEN

Susanna Rudy

Overview

An acute abdomen can be defined as a sudden or spontaneous onset of severe non-traumatic abdominal pain lasting longer than 6 hours and typically less than 24 hours, which can be associated with potentially life-threatening intra-abdominal pathology in a relatively healthy person. The acute abdomen can be caused by the progression of nontraumatic disorders that are benign or self-limited to conditions that require emergent surgical intervention. A thorough history and focused physical exam will be the cornerstone of diagnoses and treatment of a presenting acute abdominal complaint.

Background

Acute abdominal pain (AAP) has been generally defined as nontraumatic abdominal pain of limited duration. It is the most common diagnosis for emergency department (ED) visits, accounting for approximately 7.7% of 130 million ED visits in 2013. It is also the number one listed diagnosis for ED visits in women aged 15 to 65 years and the third leading diagnosis in men and women older than 65 years who present to the ED (Centers for Disease Control and Prevention, 2013; Cervellin et al., 2016; Jiang, Weiss, & Barrett, 2017; Macaluso & McNamara, 2012).

The incidence of adults presenting with AAP symptoms to the ED has steadily increased across the past two decades and is expected to maintain an upward trajectory with the influx of the newly insured into the health care system (Skinner, Blanchard, & Elixhauser, 2014). Nonsurgical cases of abdominal pain account for nearly 30% of inpatient hospital admissions (Cervellin et al., 2012). The primary symptom in an acute abdomen is most often how the pain is expressed or presents. Although many cases are benign, a rapid onset of severe pain can indicate a serious medical problem. The differential diagnoses of abdominal pain can be a challenge and therefore, the type and location of the pain are indicators of the direction to take when narrowing down a diagnosis (Papadakis & McPhee, 2017). Not all pain is the same; the different types are rooted within our embryologic development and are expressed differently, dependent on the organ or structure innervated. Pain can be caused by infection, inflammation, obstruction, muscle contraction, or decreased blood flow to the organs.

The type and location of pain is a helpful diagnostic tool. Visceral pain originates from innervations of nociceptors within the abdominal organs that respond to stretch and contraction, distention or ischemia such as gas, bloating, and microvascular occlusion. This pain is often difficult to pinpoint, characterized as dull, aching, colicky, gnawing, vague, and creating a nauseating sensation. Visceral pain in the upper epigastric area of the abdomen may reflect disorders of the stomach, duodenum, pancreas, and liver (Macaluso & McNamara, 2012). Umbilical pain may indicate disorders of the small intestine, upper colon, or appendix. Lower abdominal suprapubic visceral pain may be related to the lower colon or issues with the aorta, bladder, or kidneys. Somatic pain is described as sharp, stabbing, and localized and is triggered by noxious stimulation of the nerves lining the peritoneal cavity. Blood or chemical irritants from a perforated bowel or ruptured ectopic pregnancy can lead to peritonitis, a painful acute abdomen and a life-threatening condition if treatment is delayed. Referred pain is a perception of pain distant from the source. Some abdominal pain can be referred, or felt in another area due to irritation to the same nerve distribution. Examples of referred pain are kidney stones that are felt in the groin, and free air or blood causing irritation to the diaphragm that may be felt in the shoulder. A perforated stomach, bowel, or ruptured appendix, ectopic pregnancy, and abdominal aortic aneurysm (AAA) are life-threatening surgical emergencies requiring urgent diagnosis and management. Intestinal obstruction and pancreatitis can also present as an acute abdomen requiring prompt diagnosis and medical management to prevent deterioration in status.

The time of onset of pain and severity can determine progression. A severe and sudden onset of pain could indicate an intra-abdominal catastrophe such as a dissecting or ruptured AAA, perforated ulcer, or torsion. Gradual, insidious onset of pain can be seen with inflammatory disease and infections as well as mechanical obstructions such as volvulus and mesenteric ischemia from occlusions. Referred pain, and patterns of pain, may be diagnostic but any persistent pain should raise concern for a potentially life-threatening process. Noting exertional or alleviating factors can also help lead to a diagnosis. Abdominal pain relieved or exacerbated by eating fatty or spicy foods could indicate gallbladder or peptic ulcer disease. Pain exacerbated by jarring, jumping up and down, ambulation, or with coughing can be indicative of peritoneal irritation from free fluid in the abdomen (Macaluso & McNamara, 2012).

Abdominal pain accompanied by the time of onset of associated symptoms, such as nausea, vomiting, diarrhea, or urinary retention, can also indicate a primary intra-abdominal pathology and help narrow the differential list. In an acute abdomen, pain will typically precede vomiting but not in all cases. Vomiting should be evaluated for the presence of blood or bile. Vomiting is rarely seen in large-bowel obstructions but is almost always present in small-bowel obstructions, which can progress to feculent emesis as the obstruction progresses (Macaluso & McNamara, 2012). Diarrhea is common with abdominal complaints but is serious in conditions that can cause an acute abdomen such as mesenteric ischemia, appendicitis, and colon and bowel obstructions. Absence of bowel sounds (BS), inability to pass flatus, and blood in stool can indicate serious underlying conditions that can lead to an acute abdomen.

Clinical Aspects

ASSESSMENT

A structured approach must be used with any patient with abdominal pain. A thorough history and physical examination are a priority and will guide the overall management and determine the necessary lab and diagnostic tests to rule out any life-threating causes for presentation.

Previous medical, surgical, and social history should be queried from the non-sedated patients. A previous history of abdominal surgery in patients presenting with acute abdomen raises concerns of obstruction from adhesions. Underlying medical conditions, such as metabolic derangements, toxic ingestions, autoimmune diseases, diabetic ketoacidosis, and illicit drug use, can affect the heart as well as the integrity of the gastrointestinal (GI) tract and obstruction of the mesenteric arterial circulation, which may result in GI bleeding, decreased motility, and bowel ischemia (Macaluso & McNamara, 2012). An atypical presentation of abdominal pain is of greater concern in patients who abuse narcotics, have a history of gastric bypass, and those who are immunocompromised due to medication or underlying immune system pathology (Makrauer & Greenberger, 2016).

Comprehensive nursing care involves an overall assessment of the patient with AAP. A toxic-appearing patient may present with altered mental status, be anxious, diaphoretic, in severe pain, have a distended and rigid abdomen with severe pain indicating the possibility of a surgical abdomen, and signs of shock. This presentation warrants immediate stabilization, surgical consultation, and further diagnostic and lab workup (Jacobs & Silen, 2016).

Evaluation begins with a history of presenting illness and an assessment of pain in terms of location, quality or character, onset, intensity, presence of radiation, duration, progression, exacerbating and alleviating factors, as well as determining the presence of associated symptoms, reviewing the medical and surgical history, and conducting a thorough focused physical examination. Physical assessment involves evaluating the patients overall general appearance, vital signs, and assessment of the abdomen through inspection, auscultation, percussion, and palpation (Macaluso & McNamara, 2012; Makrauer & Greenberger, 2016).

A focused visual inspection of the exposed abdomen is done to evaluate for the presence of masses, pulsations, symmetry, scarring from previous injury or surgery, ecchymosis, distention, or ascites. Auscultation of an acute abdomen may reveal high, low-pitched, or absent BS. Often of low utility and reliability, absent BS can be a late sign indicating ileus, bowel obstruction, or an ominous finding in abdominal catastrophe (Macaluso & McNamara, 2012). Percussion of the abdomen can illicit pain in peritonitis as well as differentiate tympany between small- and large-bowel obstructions. Palpation of the abdomen should be conducted with the patient supine and the knees in a flexed position to help relax the abdominal muscles. Palpation will help identify the location of pain; determine the presence of a rigid abdomen, guarding, and rebound tenderness, all of which are indications of an acute abdomen. In addition, nurses should be familiar with the specialty abdominal examination techniques used by providers to identify the etiology of abdominal pain, which include but are not limited to Carnett's sign, cough test, closed eyes sign, Murphy's sign, psoas sign, obturator sign, and Roving's sign (Jacobs & Silen, 2016; Macaluso & McNamara, 2012; Papadakis & McPhee, 2017).

Appropriate lab techniques and diagnostics are dictated by the physical exam and presenting symptoms; however, many are of limited value in evaluating a patient with AAP due to the high rate of false-negative results. The baseline lab tests to consider are urinalysis, urine pregnancy test in women of childbearing age, a complete metabolic panel (CMP), complete blood count (CBC) with differential, liver function tests (LFTs), lipase, prothrombin time (PT)/partial thromboplastin time (PTT), and international normalized ratio (INR), lactate, blood cultures if sepsis is suspected, arterial blood gas (ABG), and a type and screen if the patient has an acute abdomen and surgery is anticipated (Jacobs & Silen, 2016; Makrauer & Greenberger, 2016; Papadakis & McPhee, 2017).

Initial diagnostic imaging exams are dictated by the location of pain. Plain abdominal films are of limited value in the acute abdomen. Abdominal ultrasonography (US) can be used as a focused assessment with sonography for trauma (FAST) and has the advantages of rapid point-of-care testing, is less expensive than a contrast scan, and has no risk of exposure to radiation or contrast dye that can adversely affect the kidneys (Jacobs & Silen, 2016; Makrauer & Greenberger, 2016; O'Brien, 2016). A CT scan with contrast is recommended over US in certain cases of AAP. Reliance on this advanced medical imaging is commonplace in part due to a high degree of sensitivity (89%) and a specificity of approximately 77%, increasing the chances of identifying the underlying condition when compared with ultrasound (Brownson & Mandell, 2014; Cartwright & Knudson, 2015; Gans, Pols, & Boermeester, 2015).

NURSING INTERVENTIONS, MANAGEMENT, AND IMPLICATIONS

Nursing care of patients with an acute abdomen centers on reliance on prompt identification of an acute intra-abdominal emergency and identification of signs and symptoms of early sepsis. Competence in IV insertion and nursing-related procedural skills will facilitate treatment for stabilizing hemodynamics, facilitating labs, diagnostics, and antibiotic administration, as well as placement of a nasogastric tube for gastric decompression and management of nausea with an antiemetic. Attention to guidelines for GI and deep vein thrombosis (DVT) prophylaxis in preparation for emergent surgical intervention or admission is standard of care.

The management of abdominal pain management is a priority and an achievable goal for optimizing patient care. Addressing pain management is one of the most important contributing factors to removing barriers to care. Research indicates that pain medication should not be withheld from patients experiencing AAP as pain relief can help remove the physical and emotional barriers associated with pain that can limit obtaining an accurate history and physical exam (Thomas, 2013). Family-centered care should be encouraged for overall compassionate support of the patient and family.

OUTCOMES

Early recognition of the acute abdomen with surgical consultation is helpful for both patient and surgeon in establishing a definitive diagnosis for prompt treatment and management for improving patient outcomes and decreasing mortality. Evidence-based identification of an acute abdomen with intra-abdominal sepsis has a 50% mortality rate; if sepsis progresses and results in multiple organ failure (three organs), the mortality rate approaches 100% (Arumugam et al., 2015). Ongoing assessment and serial repeat examination of the patient can trend toward improvement with current management or identify failed therapy. When a diagnosis remains in question, the patient should be continually observed in a monitored ED setting or admitted under observation. Patients who are found to be stable enough to discharge should be given strict instructions to return immediately for any worsening of symptoms, persistent pain beyond 8 hours, the development of a fever, or new-onset vomiting that could indicate the progression of an early appendicitis or bowel obstruction (Brownson & Mandell, 2014; Macaluso & McNamara, 2012).

Summary

AAP is the most common presenting symptom in the ED. An acute abdomen is associated with severe and sudden onset of abdominal pain with associated symptoms with an onset of less than 24 hours, likely requiring surgical intervention. Rapid assessment and diagnosis are priority. Despite advances in medical technology and diagnostics, a delay in the diagnosis and treatment of an acute abdomen can adversely affect outcomes, leading to misdiagnosis, increased morbidity and mortality, and subsequent medicolegal litigation (Macaluso & McNamara, 2012).

Arumugam, S., Al-Hassani, A., El-Menyar, A., Abdelrahman, H., Parchani, A., Peralta, R., . . . Al-Thani, H. (2015). Frequency, causes and pattern of abdominal trauma: A 4-year descriptive analysis. *Journal of Emergencies, Trauma, and Shock, 8*(4), 193–198. doi:10.4103/0974-2700.166590

Brownson E. G., & Mandell, K. (2014) The acute abdomen. In G. M. Doherty (Ed.), *Current diagnosis & treatment: Surgery* (14th ed., Chapter 21). New York, NY: McGraw-Hill. Retrieved from http://accessmedicine.mhmedical.com/content .aspx?bookid=1202&section id=71519979

Cartwright, S., & Knudson, M. (2015, April 1). Diagnostic imaging of acute abdominal pain in adults. *American Family Physician, 91*(7), 452–459. Retrieved from http:// www.aafp.org/afp/2015/0401/p452.html

Centers for Disease Control and Prevention. (2013). Emergency department visits. Retrieved from https://www.cdc.gov/nchs/data/ahcd/nhamcs_emergency/2013_ed_ web_tables.pdf

Cervellin, G., Mora, R., Ticinesi, A., Meschi, T., Comelli, I., Catena, F., & Lippi, G. (2016). Epidemiology and outcomes of acute abdominal pain in a large urban emergency department: Retrospective analysis of 5,340 cases. *Annals of Translational Medicine, 4*(19), 362. doi:10.21037/atm.2016.09.10

Gans, S. L., Pols, M. A., & Boermeester, M. A. (2015). Guideline for the diagnostic pathway in patients with acute abdominal pain [Review Article]. *Digestive Surgery, 32*(1), 23–31. doi:10.1159/000871583

Jacobs, D. O., & Silen, W. (2016). Abdominal pain. In D. L. Kasper, A. S. Fauci, S. L. Hauser, D. Longo, J. Jameson, & J. Loscalzo (Eds.), *Harrison's manual of medicine* (19th ed., pp. 154–157). New York: NY: McGraw-Hill.

Jiang, H. J., Weiss, A. J., & Barrett, M. L. (2017). Characteristics of emergency department visits for super-utilizers by payer, 2014. [Statistical Brief #221]. Retrieved from https://www.hcup-us.ahrq.gov/reports/statbriefs/sb221-Super-Utilizer-ED-Visits-Payer-2014.pdf

Macaluso, C. R., & McNamara, R. M. (2012). Evaluation and management of acute abdominal pain in the emergency department. *International Journal of General Medicine, 5*, 789–797. doi:10.2147/IJGM.S25936

Makrauer, F. L., & Greenberger, N. J. (2016). Acute abdominal pain: Basic principles & current challenges. In N. J. Greenberger, R. S. Blumberg, & R. Burakoff (Eds.), *Current diagnosis & treatment: Gastroenterology, hepatology, & endoscopy* (3rd ed., Chapter 1). New York, NY: McGraw-Hill. Retrieved from http://accessmedicine.mhmedical.com/content.aspx?bookid=1621&Section id=105181134

O'Brien, M. C. (2016). Acute abdominal pain. In J. E. Tintinalli (Ed.), *Tintinalli's emergency medicine: A comprehensive study guide* (8th ed.). New York, NY: McGraw-Hill. Retrieved from http://accessmedicine.mhmedical.com.proxy.library.vanderbilt.edu/book.aspx?bookid=1658

Papadakis, M. A., & McPhee, S. J. (2017). *Current medical diagnosis and treatment.* New York, NY: McGraw-Hill.

Skinner, H. G, Blanchard, J, & Elixhauser, A. (2014). Trends in emergency department visits, 2006–2011 [Statistical Brief #179]. Retrieved from https://www.hcup-us.ahrq.gov/reports/statbriefs/sb179-Emergency-Department-Trends.pdf

Thomas, S. H. (2013). Management of pain in the emergency department [Review Article]. *International Scholarly Research Notices [ISRN] Emergency Medicine, 2013.* doi:10.1155/2013/583132

■ ACUTE CORONARY SYNDROME

Andrea Efre

Overview

Acute coronary syndrome (ACS) is an umbrella term used to describe a range of coronary artery emergencies, including myocardial infarction (MI) and unstable angina (UA). It is caused by a sudden reduction or blockage of blood flow to the cardiac muscle, frequently caused by atherosclerosis, and most prevalent in older adults. The blockage limits blood flow to the myocardium (heart muscle) that usually causes chest pain. The treatment goal is to improve blood flow (revascularization) as quickly as possible and may be achieved with pharmacology or interventional cardiac catheterization depending on the available facilities. Rapid identification of diagnostic criteria and initiation of emergency treatment by the nurse is essential to save the coronary muscle, prevent further cardiac damage, and improve outcomes.

Background

ACS refers to a spectrum of conditions that are divided into three categories:

1. ST-elevation MI (STEMI), also known as *acute myocardial infarction (AMI)*
2. Non-ST elevation MI (NSTEMI)
3. UA

The latter two categories of NSTEMI and UA were combined into a new title of non-ST elevation ACS (NSTE) in the American Heart Association and American College of Cardiologists 2014 practice guidelines to emphasizes the continuum between UA and NSTEMI (Amsterdam et al., 2014). Therefore, you may see the terms and treatment plans used interchangeably. Almost three quarters of all ACS patients present as NSTE-ACS (greater than 625,000 patients annually) in the United States (Amsterdam et al., 2014). As a common presentation of coronary heart disease, NSTE-ACS is the leading cause of global cardiovascular morbidity and mortality (Rodriguez & Mahaffey, 2016).

Risk factors associated with ACS are the same as those involved in coronary heart disease and include age, gender, family history, smoking, hypertension, dyslipidemia, physical inactivity, obesity, diabetes mellitus, and recreational drugs such as cocaine. An estimated 15.5 million Americans older than 20 years of age have CHD, and from that number 550,000 have MIs annually, and 200,000 have recurrent attacks (Mozaffarinini et al., 2016). The older adult is most at risk from ACS. In the United States, the average age at the first MI is 65 years for men and 72 years for women (Mozaffarinini et al., 2016).

The cause of ACS is typically related to the formation of a thrombus that occludes the coronary vessel and prevents blood flow to the myocardium. The STEMI suggests that the coronary artery is fully occluded and is the most life-threatening and time-sensitive presentation of ACS. In NSTEMI or

UA, the thrombus may partially or intermittently occlude the coronary artery, which is why the symptoms may be less severe or difficult to determine. The limited coronary blood flow is most often characterized by sternal or central chest pain.

Diagnosis of ACS is determined by the 12-lead EKG findings and serum cardiac enzymes. A 12-lead EKG should be performed and interpreted in 10 minutes of symptom onset or arrival to the emergency facility (Amsterdam et al., 2014). The EKG determine whether there is an acute injury to the myocardium identified by ST-elevation, T wave changes, or a new onset of left bundle branch block. The STEMI has elevations of ST segment in grouped leads on the 12-lead EKG, which identify the location of the affected myocardium and the coronary artery most likely involved. No ST elevations are noted in NSTEMI or UA, but it should be noted that ST depression or T wave inversions may be present in either.

Cardiac biomarkers are released into the blood when myocardial tissue damage (necrosis) occurs, and are found in both STEMI and NSTEMI. The biomarkers of troponin, myoglobin, and creatine kinase may remain elevated in the circulation following the infarction, but troponin has a longer period of detection (up to 10 days) and is thought to be the more sensitive and specific of the other biomarkers (Roffi et al., 2015). No increase in serum biomarkers is found in UA.

Immediate identification and differentiation of STEMI or NSTE-ACS are needed to define the treatment plan. Rapid intervention is necessary to restore coronary blood flow with percutaneous coronary intervention (PCI) in a cardiac catheterization laboratory. Delays in treatment enhance the progression of the coronary blockage, which leads to the loss of myocardial muscle and a potential cardiac arrest or death.

Clinical Aspects

ASSESSMENT

Acute, central (substernal) chest pain is the typical primary symptom of ACS. The pain may radiate to the left arm, shoulders, back, neck, jaw, or abdomen. It is important to ask open-ended questions and ask the patient to describe the chest pain and any other symptoms. Establish the location, onset, duration, and characteristics of the pain. Both STEMI and NSTE-ACS are most commonly present as a pressure-type chest pain that typically occurs at rest or with minimal exertion, and lasting for more than 10 minutes, whereas angina is typically relieved in 5 minutes of stopping the offending activity or with short-acting nitroglycerin (Amsterdam et al., 2014).

Determine whether there are associated symptoms such as shortness of breath, diaphoresis, lightheadedness, nausea, vomiting, or apprehension. Also, ask the patient whether anything aggravates or relieves the symptoms, what they were doing at the time of symptom onset, and whether they have attempted any treatments before telling you about the pain. When a patient arrives in the emergency room it is common that he or she has attempted treatments at home (e.g., taking other people's prescriptions, or using illicit drugs to self-medicate), they may not openly offer this information initially without probing questions being asked.

Women, older adults, patients with diabetes, or patients with a history of heart failure may present with more subtle symptoms often without severe chest pain, which makes the diagnosis much more challenging and may lead to delay in treatment. Symptoms include shortness of breath, fatigue, lethargy, indigestion, anxiety, or sleep disturbances. If chest pain is present, it may be atypical and be reported as numbness, burning, or stabbing pain.

The physical examination should remain relatively unchanged from before the onset of the symptom. It is advisable to reassess the heart and lungs to identify deterioration, for example, rales on lung examination and development of S3 heart sound (found in fluid overload) suggest pulmonary edema or heart failure. Finding new murmurs or S4 heart sound (related to a noncompliant ventricle) could be caused by cardiac ischemia and should be further evaluated.

A change in vital signs may be noted in ACS, such as tachycardia, hypotension, hypertension, tachypnea, and possibly decreased oxygen saturation. Continuous cardiac monitoring for dysrhythmias and ST or T wave changes identify lethal rhythms or evolution of the ischemia. EKG changes are related to the location of myocardial impairment and lack of blood flow. If the right coronary artery is occluded, then ST changes may be noted in the inferior leads (II, III, and AVF), plus atrial dysrhythmias may be seen because of the lack of blood supply to the right atria, the sinoatrial node, or atrioventricular node. These rhythms may include new-onset atrial fibrillation, tachycardia, bradycardia, or a heart block. If the circumflex artery is involved the ST changes are usually noted in the lateral leads (I, AVL, V5, and V6). If the left coronary artery is affected by occlusion, anterior changes are seen in the 12-lead EKG throughout the chest leads (V1–V4), plus the left ventricle may be affected causing ventricular arrhythmias, including the life-threatening ventricular tachycardia or ventricular fibrillation.

NURSING INTERVENTIONS, MANAGEMENT, AND IMPLICATIONS

The goal for the management of STEMI is PCI, which should be performed within 90 minutes of arrival to the emergency facility (or from the symptom onset if inpatient). If PCI is not available, arrangements should be made to transfer the patient to a facility that can perform PCI in 120 minutes. If the transfer takes longer than 2 hours, then a fibrinolytic agent (such as tenecteplase, reteplase, or alteplase) should be administered and arrangements made to transfer for PCI in 3 to 24 hours (O'Gara et al., 2013). Primary PCI is also considered reasonable in patients with STEMI if there is clinical or EKG evidence of ongoing ischemia between 12 and 24 hours after symptom onset (O'Gara et al., 2013).

Dual antiplatelet therapy with aspirin and platelet inhibitors (known as *P2Y12 inhibitors*) is used in the initial treatment of STEMI and remains the cornerstone for the treatment of NSTE-ACS (Rodriguez & Mahaffey, 2016).

An aspirin loading dose of 325 mg is given, followed by 81 mg daily, and loading doses of clopidogrel 300 mg to 600 mg followed by daily doses of 75 mg. If desired, prasugrel or ticagrelor may be used instead of clopidogrel.

Adjunct pharmacological treatments for ischemia to decrease myocardial oxygen demand and increase myocardial oxygen supply are considered. These include nitrates (sublingual or intravenous), antiplatelet therapy, morphine, and beta-blockers. Beta-blockers should be avoided if cocaine use is suspected, or in patients with vasospastic angina (Roffi et al., 2015).

Following a successful PCI, the expected outcome of the ACS patient is to be discharged home with education on lifestyle modifications, medication compliance, and committing to cardiac rehabilitation and continued care. Underlying disorders, such as hypertension, diabetes mellitus, or dyslipidemia, need to be controlled. Beta- blockers, ACE inhibitors, angiotensin receptor blockers (ARB), and statins are often prescribed. Lifestyle modifications to reduce overall cardiovascular risk include smoking cessation, regular physical activity, weight reduction in patients with high body mass index, and dietary changes to include reduced intake of salt and saturated fat, and increase in fruit, vegetables, wholegrain cereals, and fish (Amsterdam et al., 2014; O'Gara et al., 2013).

OUTCOMES

A rapid assessment by the nurse ensures early intervention and improved outcomes. Delays in assessment, diagnosis, or intervention can be prevented with the use of standing orders and algorithms to initiate care. Cardiogenic shock may occur in up to 3% of NSTE-ACS patients, for whom immediate PCI is most often used for revascularization (Roffi et al., 2015). Primary PCI is also indicated for cardiogenic shock or acute severe heart failure in STEMI patients, irrespective of time delay from onset (O'Gara et al., 2013). Revascularization with PCI is not always possible, such as in multiple vessel diseases, or difficult positioning of the coronary occlusion. For those who are not candidates for PCI or fibrinolytic therapy, emergency coronary artery bypass graft (CABG) in 6 hours of symptom onset may be considered in STEMI (O'Gara et al., 2013).

Summary

In summary, the priority of the nurse is to rapidly gather accurate information, including symptoms, vital signs, physical assessment, and a 12-lead EKG. Initial treatments should be started during the assessment period, including continuous cardiac monitoring, supplemental oxygen, dual antiplatelet therapy, and consideration of nitroglycerine administration if available and the patient is normotensive. Early intervention improves outcomes and therefore contacting the provider and transmitting a copy of the 12-lead EKG if the provider is not physically available speeds up the diagnostic process. Every effort should be made to reach the revascularization goal to undergo PCI within 90 minutes of symptom onset.

Amsterdam, E. A., Wenger, N. K., Brindis, R. G., Casey, D. E., Ganiats, T. G., Holmes, D. R., . . . Zieman, S. J.; American College of Cardiology; American Heart Association Task Force on Practice Guidelines; Society for Cardiovascular Angiography and Interventions; Society of Thoracic Surgeons; American Association for Clinical Chemistry. (2014). 2014 AHA/ACC guideline for the management of patients with non-ST-elevation acute coronary syndromes: A report of the American College of Cardiology/American Heart Association Task Force on Practice Guidelines. *Journal of the American College of Cardiology, 64*(24), e139–e228.

Jacobs, A. K., Kushner, F. G., Ettinger, S. M., Guyton, R. A., Anderson, J. L., Ohman, E. M., . . . Somerfield, M. R. (2013). ACCF/AHA clinical practice guideline methodology summit report: A report of the American College of Cardiology Foundation/American Heart Association Task Force on Practice Guidelines. *Journal of the American College of Cardiology, 61*(2), 213–265.

Mozaffarian, D., Benjamin, E. J., Arnett, D. K., Blaha, M. J., Cushman, M., Das, S. R., . . . Turner, M. B.; American Heart Association Statistics Committee and Stroke Statistics Subcommittee. (2016). Heart disease and stroke statistic—2016 update: A report from the American Heart Association. *Circulation, 133*(4), e38–e360. doi:10.1161/cir.0000000000000350

O'Gara, P. T., Kushner, F. G., Ascheim, D. D., Casey, D. E., Chung, M. K., DeLemos, J. A., . . . Yancy, C. W.; American College of Cardiology Foundation/American Heart Association Task Force on Practice Guidelines. (2013). 2013 ACCF/AHA guidelines for the management of ST-elevation myocardial infarction: A report of the American college of cardiology foundation/American Heart Association Task Force on Practice Guidelines. *Circulation, 127*(4), e362–e425. doi:10.1161/CIR.0b013e3182742cf6

Rodriguez, F., & Mahaffey, K. W. (2016). Management of patients with NSTE-ACS: A comparison of the recent AHA/ACC and ESC guidelines. *Journal of the American College of Cardiology, 68*(3), 313–321.

Roffi, M., Patrono, C., Collet, J. P., Mueller, C., Valgimigli, M., Andreotti, F., . . . Windecker, S. (2015). 2015 ESC guidelines for the management of acute coronary syndromes in patients presenting without persistent ST-segment elevation. *Revista Espanola de Cardiologia, 68*(12), 1125.

■ ACUTE EXACERBATION OF A CHRONIC CONDITION

Brenda L. Douglass

Overview

Across the United States, chronic health conditions have escalated over the past decade. In 2016, about one in four Americans had more than one chronic health condition and for individuals aged 65 years and older, prevalence rises to three in four Americans (Centers for Disease Control and Prevention [CDC], 2016, November 14). According to the National Health Council (2016), a chronic condition is defined as a disease lasting 3 months or more. Chronic health conditions have a profound impact on quality of life, often leading to premature disability. Chronic conditions cause heightened rates of mortality and considerable economic burdens to the patient, family, and society (CDC, 2016a). An acute exacerbation of a chronic condition occurs when there is an increase in severity of the chronic condition over baseline symptoms and physiologic decline.

Chronic conditions and acute exacerbations are often preventable, thus presenting an opportunity for nursing professionals to intervene to restore an individual's health status and provide education on the prevention of future exacerbations. One of the most common chronic conditions with episodes of acute exacerbations in the setting of emergency or critical care is chronic obstructive pulmonary disease (COPD). The recognition and management of patients with an acute exacerbation of COPD is the principal focus of this discussion.

Background

The clinical trajectory of adults with COPD is often marked with acute exacerbations requiring hospitalization. An acute exacerbation of COPD is an event characterized by worsening respiratory symptoms beyond the normal daily variations and lending to a change in the medication regimen (World Health Organization [WHO], 2017). Acute exacerbations of COPD are critical events that denote physiologic instability and worsening in the obstructive ventilation, which contributes to an increase in an individual's risk of death (Global Initiative for Chronic Obstructive Lung Disease [GOLD], 2017; Wedzicha, 2015). Risk factors for COPD exacerbation include advanced age, duration of COPD, productive cough, chronic mucous hypersecretion, history of exacerbations and antibiotic use, COPD-related hospitalization in the prior year, and one or more comorbid conditions (Stoller, 2017). Comorbidities, such as cardiovascular disease, diabetes mellitus, and hypertension, are common in patients with COPD, further raising the risk of the need for hospitalization and mortality (GOLD, 2017; Stoller, 2017).

Acute exacerbations of COPD are typically classified by the range of the severity of dyspnea, from mild (e.g., increased dyspnea or cough), moderate (e.g., chest tightness, wheezing), to severe worsening in dyspnea (e.g., hypoxemia, acute respiratory failure; GOLD, 2017; Stoller, 2017). In 70% of cases, COPD exacerbations are associated with acute respiratory infections (Stoller, 2017). COPD exacerbations are disabling, necessitate urgent medical care and hospitalizations, as well as heighten an individual's risk of death (CDC, 2016b; GOLD, 2017). In addition to devastating personal costs, there is a significant societal burden associated with COPD exacerbations with direct costs estimated at $32 billion and indirect costs at $20.4 billion (CDC, 2016b).

According to the Global Initiative for Chronic Obstructive Lung Disease (GOLD) guidelines (2017), goals of therapy in the management of COPD exacerbations are directed at minimizing the negative impact of the current exacerbation and to prevent recurrent episodes. The severity of the exacerbation and underlying disease determines whether the patient can be managed in an inpatient or outpatient setting (GOLD, 2017). About 80% of patients experiencing COPD exacerbations can be managed in the outpatient setting with pharmacologic therapies (GOLD, 2017). Classification of the level of severity for the COPD exacerbation is crucial to optimal intervention. COPD exacerbations are classified into three categories: (a) mild (administration of short-acting beta agonist [SABA]), (b) moderate (administration of a SABA, antibiotic, and/or oral corticosteroid), and (c) severe (pharmacologic management and/or positive ventilation; GOLD, 2017). Acute respiratory failure associated with severe COPD exacerbations mandates aggressive intervention, such as those often delivered in the emergency and critical care settings.

Clinical Aspects

ASSESSMENT

To guide nursing care, a comprehensive assessment of signs and symptoms is recommended to determine the level of airflow limitation and presence of comorbid health issues during an acute exacerbation of COPD. Emphasis on assessing the severity of symptoms as changes from the individual's baseline symptom profile is recommended. Specifically, nurses should assess for worsening dyspnea, wheeze, increased cough, sputum characteristics, work of breathing, mental status, and indications of an upper respiratory infection. This information should be used to classify the severity of the COPD exacerbation (e.g., mild, moderate, or severe), as well as the frequency of and time since last acute exacerbation: a thorough review of preexisting comorbid conditions (e.g., pneumonia, cardiovascular disease, obstructive sleep apnea, respiratory failure requiring mechanical ventilation) and assessment for symptoms of comorbid conditions (e.g. chest pain/ pressure, peripheral edema), environmental factors (e.g., smoking history, exposure to smoke and other pollutants), and current medication regimen with attention to medications for the management of COPD, including medication dosages, devices, adherence, and responsiveness to these therapies. On physical examination, attention to vital signs (e.g., blood pressure, heart rate, respiratory rate, level of consciousness) may help to inform a nurse's ability to specify the severity of the COPD exacerbation. To further specify the severity of an acute exacerbation, pulse oximetry, arterial blood gas analysis, and a chest radiograph are useful objective and diagnostic measures that guide nursing care for individuals with a COPD exacerbation.

NURSING INTERVENTIONS, MANAGEMENT, AND IMPLICATIONS

Nursing interventions provide opportunities to set goals in the clinical management of chronic conditions manifested by an acute exacerbation. An emphasis is placed on prevention, early recognition, and engaging the patient through patient-centered care (CDC, 2016a; GOLD, 2017). Providing education to patients on self-management goals to include in early recognition of worsening symptoms and when to seek medical care is integral to prevent or minimize impairment. Key points to effective nursing management include assessment of severity and providing the level of intervention necessary according to evidence-based guidelines for the most optimal treatment strategy (GOLD, 2017).

OUTCOMES

Acute exacerbations of chronic conditions, such as COPD, are often intertwined with comorbid conditions, precipitated by triggers, and present complexities in care of the patient with chronic conditions (GOLD, 2017). The delivery of nursing care from a holistic perspective, blending in physical, emotional, and spiritual care with integration of evidence-based practices, presents an opportunity to improve the health outcomes of individuals experiencing an acute exacerbation of COPD.

Summary

An acute exacerbation of COPD is a leading cause of death in the United States (CDC, 2016a). COPD exacerbations have negative impact on an individual's health and quality of life—leading to premature disability and shortened life spans (CDC, 2016a; GOLD, 2017). The cost of chronic conditions and acute exacerbations of chronic disease pose an economic burden to the nation. Acute exacerbation of COPD provides an illustration of a chronic health condition in which prevention and early intervention are key to improving health outcomes.

Centers for Disease Control and Prevention. (2016a). Chronic disease prevention and health promotion. Retrieved from https://www.cdc.gov/chronicdisease

Centers for Disease Control and Prevention. (2016b). Chronic obstructive pulmonary disease (COPD). Retrieved from https://www.cdc.gov/copd/index.html

Global Initiative for Chronic Obstructive Lung Disease. (2017). Global strategy for the diagnosis, management and prevention of COPD, GOLD 2017 report. Retrieved from http://goldcopd.org

Han, M. K., Dransfield, M., & Martinez, F. (2016). Chronic obstructive pulmonary disease: Definition, clinical manifestations, diagnosis, and staging. In J. Stoller & H. Hollingsworth (Eds.), *UpToDate*. Retrieved from http://www.uptodate.com/contents/chronic-obstructive-pulmonary-disease-definition-clinical-manifestations-diagnosis-and-staging

National Health Council. (2016). About chronic health conditions. Retrieved from http://www.nationalhealthcouncil.org/newsroom/about-chronic-conditions

Stoller, J. (2017). Management of exacerbations of chronic obstructive pulmonary disease. In P. Barnes & H. Holingsworth (Eds.), *UpToDate*. Retrieved from http://www.uptodate.com/contents/management-of-exacerbations-of-chronic-obstructive-pulmonary-disease

Wedzicha, J. (2015). Mechanisms of chronic obstructive pulmonary disease exacerbations. *Annals of the American Thoracic Society*, 12(2), 157–159. doi:10.1513/AnnulsATS.201507-427AW

World Health Organization. (2017). Chronic respiratory diseases. Retrieved from http://www.who.int/respiratory/copd/en

■ ACUTE PANCREATITIS IN ADULTS

Virginia Mangolds

Overview

Acute pancreatitis (AP) is an inflammatory process of the pancreas involving the activation of intrapancreatic enzymes that further exacerbate pancreatic tissue injury and altered organ function. The diagnosis of AP is made using elevations in pancreatic enzymes, clinical symptoms, and a variety of diagnostic imaging. Nursing care for adults with AP is focused on hemodynamic monitoring, prevention of pancreatic stimulation, electrolyte monitoring, pain control, identifying and treating local complications in the pancreas, identifying and treating multisystem failure, emotional support, patient education and discharge preparation with outpatient support if necessary (Burns, 2014; Krenzer, 2016).

Background

AP is the most common gastrointestinal diagnosis for acute hospitalizations in the United States. In fact, more than 270,000 annual admissions were attributed to AP in 2012 and the estimated cost of these hospitalizations totaled $2.6 billion (Peery et al., 2012). Despite the need for inpatient care, the mortality rate of patients with AP is 2% to 10%, which is related to shock, anoxia, hypotension, or fluid or electrolyte imbalance. This high mortality rate may be attributed to the 10% to 30% of patients exhibiting severe AP associated with pancreatic and peripancreatic necrosis (Talukdar, Clemens, & Vege, 2012).

The diagnosis of AP is made by fulfilling two of the three following criteria: (a) abdominal pain; (b) elevated serum lipase or amylase (more than three times the upper limit of normal); and (c) characteristic findings of AP on imaging, usually contrast-enhanced CT (Banks et al., 2013). Gallstones and chronic alcohol abuse account for 90% of AP. Drug-induced causes have been linked to metronidazole, tetracycline, azathioprine, and estrogens. Other less common etiologies are vascular, genetic, infectious, autoimmune, traumatic, and idiopathic, and may include hyperlipidemia, hypercalcemia, and pancreatic neoplasms (Burns, 2014). Laboratory evaluation and treatment consist of obtaining and analyzing multiple laboratory values, including amylase, lipase, complete blood cell count with differential, electrolytes, blood urea nitrogen (BUN), creatinine, glucose, coagulation studies, lactate, calcium, magnesium, albumin, and liver enzymes (Van Leeuwen & Bladh, 2015).

Common diagnostic imaging consists of ultrasound, CT and CT angiography (CTA; Catanzano, 2009) and/or MRI (Tenner, Baillie, DeWitt, Vege, & American College of Gastroenterology, 2013). Imaging recommendations indicate that ultrasound should be the initial diagnostic study (Catanzano, 2009; Krenzer, 2016; Sarr, 2013), which is particularly sensitive to AP as a result of cholelithiasis. CT imaging is recommended for later in the course of the disease, for patients whose symptoms do not improve or worsen (Catanzano, 2009; Sarr, 2013). Early in the course of the disease, CT findings may be minimal or absent. CT is used with contrast to confirm an unclear diagnosis and to evaluate the extent of damage to the pancreas and surrounding area. It can be used to separate the pancreatic parenchyma from the surrounding duodenum and to evaluate for pancreatic necrosis. It is also useful for identifying and evaluating a suspected or known pancreatic mass. CTA may be performed in cases of known pancreatic neoplasm; complicated pancreatitis, such as pancreatic necrosis, abscess, or hemorrhage; or evaluation of pseudocyst formation (Catanzano, 2009).

The classification of severity has been broken down to mild, moderately severe, and severe (Sarr, 2013). Mild AP is associated with nonorgan failure and lack of local or systemic complication. Moderately severe AP is associated with organ failure that resolves in 48 hours (transient) and local or systemic complications without persistent organ failure. Severe AP is associated with persistent single or multiple organ failure for more than 48 hours (Banks et al., 2013; Krenzer, 2016).

Clinical Aspects

According to Ackley, Ladwig, and Makic (2017), based on the North American Nursing Diagnosis Association International (NANDA International), patients being cared for in the inpatient setting may benefit from the following nursing diagnosis and treatment, based on the assess, diagnose, plan, implement care, evaluate the outcomes (ADPIE) plan and from making necessary improvements in (a) ineffective breathing pattern, (b) deficient fluid volume, (c) acute pain, (d) diarrhea, (e) nausea, and (f) ineffective denial.

ASSESSMENT

Ineffective breathing pattern occurs when inspiration and/or expiration does not provide adequate ventilation. Monitor respiratory rate, depth, and ease of respiration; note the amount of anxiety associated with dyspnea; attempt to determine whether the client's dyspnea is physiological or psychological; note the rapidity of the development of dyspnea, which may be an indicator of the severity of the condition. Treatment of dyspnea includes positioning the patient in an upright or semi-Fowler's position, and administering oxygen as ordered.

Deficient fluid volume occurs when there is decreased intravascular, interstitial, and/or intracellular fluid. Monitor for thirst, restlessness, headaches, and difficulty concentrating. Notify the provider of any indication of deficient fluid volume, and assist in adjusting the fluid replacement as indicated.

NURSING INTERVENTIONS, MANAGEMENT, AND IMPLICATIONS

To identify acute pain, perform a comprehensive assessment of pain, which includes location, characteristics, onset/duration, frequency, quality, intensity, and severity of pain. Work with the medical provider to ensure adequate pain control.

Diarrhea is the passage of loose, unformed stools. Document frequency and amount of stool. Follow dietary orders as written by the patient's providers and notify them if the diarrhea continues, despite of their diet.

Nausea is a subjective, phenomenon of an unpleasant feeling in the back of the throat and stomach, which does not result in vomiting. Implement appropriate dietary measures, such as NPO (nothing by mouth) status as appropriate, small frequent meals, and low-fat meals.

Ineffective denial is the conscious or unconscious attempt to disavow knowledge or meaning of an event to reduce anxiety and/or fear, leading to the detriment of health. Assess the patient's and family's understanding of the illness, treatments, and expected outcomes. Aid the patient in making choices regarding treatment and actively invite him or her into the decision-making process.

OUTCOMES

Outcomes to aim for, using nursing diagnoses, are related to breathing patterns, urine output, pain control, diarrhea control, nausea and vomiting control, and active participation in outpatient treatment programs if the AP is related to substance abuse (Ackley et al., 2017). Specifically, the suggested outcomes include that (a) the patient demonstrates a breathing pattern that supports blood gas results within his or her normal parameters; (b) maintains urine output of 0.5 mL/kg/hour; (c) maintains normal blood pressure, heart rate, and body temperature; (d) maintains elastic skin turgor and moist mucous membranes and orientation to person, place, and time; (e) expresses satisfaction with pain control; (f) has solid, formed stool with defecation; (g) has the ability to tolerate normal oral intake without vomiting; (h) seeks out appropriate health care attention when needed; and (i) actively engages in a treatment program related to identified "substance abuse" if applicable (Ackley et al., 2017).

Summary

AP is the most common gastrointestinal cause for acute hospitalization with more than 270,000 annual admissions and an estimated cost of $2.6 billion. The classification of severity has been broken down to mild, moderately severe, and severe. The diagnosis includes clinical, laboratory, and diagnostic findings. Nursing outcome goals can be used to evaluate the patient's progression toward reaching a normal functioning and a good health status.

Ackley, B. J., Ladwig, G. B., & Makic, M. F. (2017). *Nursing diagnosis handbook—An evidence-based guide to planning care* (11th ed.). St. Louis, MO: Elsevier.

Banks, P. A., Bollen, T. L., Dervenis, C., Gooszen, H. G., Johnson, C. D., Sarr, M. G., . . . Acute Pancreatitis Classification Working Group. (2013). Classification of acute pancreatitis—2012: Revision of the Atlanta classification and definitions by international consensus. *Gut, 62*(1), 102–111. doi:10.1136/gutjnl-2012-302779

Burns, S. M. (2014). *AACN essentials of critical care nursing* (3rd ed.). New York NY: McGraw-Hill.

Catanzano, T. M. (2009). *How to think like a radiologist—Ordering imaging studies.* New York, NY: Cambridge University Press.

Krenzer, M. E. (2016). Understanding acute pancreatitis. *Nursing, 46*(8), 34–40. doi:10.1097/01.NURSE.0000484959.78110.98

Peery, A. F., Dellon, E. S., Lund, J., Crockett, S. D., McGowan, C. E., Bulsiewicz, W. J., . . . Shaheen, N. J. (2012). Burden of gastrointestinal disease in the United States: 2012 update. *Gastroenterology, 143*(5), 1179–1187; e1171–e1173. doi:10.1053/j.gastro.2012.08.002

Sarr, M. G. (2013). 2012 revision of the Atlanta classification of acute pancreatitis. *Polish Archives of Internal Medicine, 123*(3), 118–124.

Talukdar, R., Clemens, M., & Vege, S. S. (2012). Moderately severe acute pancreatitis: prospective validation of this new subgroup of acute pancreatitis. *Pancreas, 41*(2), 306–309. doi:10.1097/MPA.0b013e318229794e

Tenner, S., Baillie, J., DeWitt, J., Vege, S. S.; American College of, G. (2013). American College of Gastroenterology guideline: Management of acute pancreatitis. *American Journal of Gastroenterology, 108*(9), 1400–1415; 1416. doi:10.1038/ajg.2013.218

Van Leeuwen, A. M., & Bladh, M. L. (2015). *Davis's comprehensive handbook of laboratory and diagnostic tests with nursing implications* (6th ed.). Philadelphia, PA: F. A. Davis.

■ ACUTE RESPIRATORY DISTRESS SYNDROME

Kathleen C. Ashton

Overview

In the spectrum of illnesses associated with the respiratory system, acute respiratory distress syndrome (ARDS) is one of the most life-threatening and potentially fatal acute respiratory conditions. Formerly known as adult respiratory distress syndrome, ARDS results from either direct or indirect trauma to the lungs and affects both children and adults who are hospitalized with other conditions. It can also occur following an acute medical problem or procedure. The nursing care for patients with ARDS is primarily supportive and includes monitoring positive pressure ventilation, avoiding fluid overload, as well as a careful assessment and evaluation of the patient's treatment response. Based on the current literature, the mortality rate for ARDS is approximately 30%, and survivors of ARDS suffer high rates of morbidity (Mehta & Povoa, 2017; Sweeney & McAuley, 2016).

Background

Several conditions are implicated in the development of ARDS, including sepsis, smoke inhalation, near-drowning, severe pneumonia, major trauma, and any conditions resulting in a profound systemic inflammatory response. Sepsis is a leading cause of ARDS that tends to stimulate a systemic inflammatory response (Vidyasagar, 2016). In general, there are a variety of pathophysiologic conditions that activate the innate immune response, which in turn activates a physiologic reaction to that and, as a result, releases proinflammatory substances into the bloodstream to combat the infection or aid the recovery from a traumatic injury. An otherwise protective process, a systemic inflammatory response can have broad effects on the blood vessels, in particular the pulmonary vessels, which experience increased permeability. As the changes in the permeability of pulmonary vessels lead to the diffusion of fluid into alveoli, it reduces the affected alveoli's ability to promote blood oxygenation effectively. As more alveoli are affected, hypoxemia can be captured on chest imaging as bilateral pulmonary infiltrates that are not fully associated with heart failure (Mehta & Povoa, 2017).

First described by Ashbaugh, Bigelow, Petty, and Levine (1967), ARDS is classified as noncardiogenic pulmonary edema that leads to decreased lung compliance and hypoxia (Vidyasagar, 2016). The American–European Consensus Conference (AECC) defined the syndrome in 1994, and the Berlin Definition was established in 2011 by a panel convened by the European Society of Intensive Care Medicine, the American Thoracic Society, and the Society of Critical Care Medicine (Raneri et al., 2012). The Berlin Definition was validated in more than 4,000 patients' data (Sweeney & McAuley, 2016) and delineates the three stages of ARDS, mild, moderate, and severe, based on the degree of hypoxemia with the associated mortality for each stage. The corresponding mortality rates are 27% for mild, 32% for moderate, and 47% for the severe stage (Fanelli et al., 2013).

Risk factors for the development of ARDS include numerous illnesses and injuries, both pulmonary and systemic with pneumonia being the most common risk factor (Sweeney & McAuley, 2016). Pneumonia and aspiration have the highest associated mortality in ARDS. There are currently about 200,000 cases of ARDS reported annually in the United States.

Over the past 50 years, there have been numerous studies addressing the pathogenesis and clinical aspects of the syndrome, including underlying mechanisms, biomarkers, genetic predisposition, risk factors, epidemiology, and treatment. Genetics is now recognized to play a role in the predisposition to the development of ARDS (Fanelli et al., 2013). Despite the plethora of research studies, there are currently very few effective therapies for ARDS, other than the use of protective lung strategies (Fanelli et al., 2013).

Clinical Aspects

ASSESSMENT

Critical care nurses are the frontline nurses regarding the surveillance of the progression of ARDS. The assessment of patients for changes in the respiratory status is an ongoing responsibility of the nurses to alert physicians and others to changes in the patient's ability to effectively deliver oxygenated blood to the tissues. Breath sounds must be assessed at frequent intervals to ascertain any changes that could signal an increase in fluid and the effects of inflammation. Oxygen saturation, as measured by pulse oximetry, is a crucial measurement to assist in recognition of changes. Invasive lines to measure pressure changes and fluid status are a mainstay of critically ill patients in intensive care units. Individuals may begin to show signs of respiratory compromise even before they land in an intensive care unit, so it is imperative that nurses assess patients to look for signs showing that they could be developing ARDS.

NURSING INTERVENTIONS, MANAGEMENT, AND IMPLICATIONS

The treatment for ARDS is supportive and centered on mechanical ventilation. In the setting of lung injury associated with ARDS, this modality can treat both the condition and contribute to lung injury, too. However, the positive pressure mechanical ventilation is the cornerstone of management; it can also incite lung injury and contribute to both the morbidity and mortality seen in ARDS (Fanelli et al., 2013). Thus, a judicious management of positive pressure ventilation is recommended among patients with ARDS.

Results of recent studies point to the use of lower tidal volumes and maintenance of plateau pressures in a specified range to reduce mortality and provide a survival benefit (Fanelli et al., 2013, p. 327). Tidal volumes of 6 mL/kg are now recommended as opposed to 10 mL/kg used previously (Vidyasagar, 2016). Lower tidal volumes help prevent ventilator-induced lung injury (VILI) caused by volutrauma (Vidyasagar, 2016). One recent and very significant change in ventilator strategy is the acceptance of lesser arterial oxygen tension (PaO$_2$) in the range of 85% to 90% for patient survival and hemodynamic stability (Vidyasagar, 2016). Lower tidal volumes and acceptance of lesser oxygen tension reduce lung overdistension and help prevent additional injury.

Another problem of management is the cyclic opening and closing of small airways and alveolar units, known as *atelectatic trauma*. Clinical trials have measured the effects of using higher levels of positive-end expiratory pressure (PEEP). The results are inconclusive, but there is limited evidence that higher (between 5 and 9 cm H$_2$O) levels of PEEP may reduce mortality (Fanelli et al., 2013).

Many other unconventional therapies are also used to manage ARDS, with varying success. Prone positioning exploits gravity and repositioning of the heart in the thorax to promote lung reexpansion and improve ventilation, thus improving oxygenation. Its impact on mortality remains controversial (Fanelli et al., 2013). The recent PROSEVA (Proning Severe ARDS Patients) trial demonstrated a significant benefit in mortality with the use of ventilation in the prone position (Scholten, Beitler, Prisk, & Malhotra, 2017).

High-frequency oscillatory ventilation (HFOV) is a technique that delivers extremely small tidal volumes using a relatively high mean airway pressure at high respiratory frequencies to avoid tidal overstretch (Fanelli et al., 2013). In two large multicenter clinical trials, HFOV failed to demonstrate improvement in survival, and its use is currently quite controversial (Fanelli et al., 2013).

In the case of severe hypoxemia and respiratory failure, extracorporeal membrane oxygenation (ECMO) is used as a rescue therapy. The objective is to overcome severe hypoxemia and respiratory acidosis while maintaining the lungs in a state of complete rest (Fanelli et al., 2013). However, ECMO is a scarce and expensive resource available only in major specialty centers. Regarding pharmacologic interventions, neuromuscular blockade and sedatives are often administered to decrease the patient's work of breathing, thereby improving respiratory mechanics and lowering oxygen consumption (Sweeney & McAuley, 2016).

As ARDS is a form of pulmonary edema, fluid therapy is an essential component of management. Fluids are provided for resuscitation and organ rescue during the early stages of the illness, followed by fluid unloading (deresuscitation)—either spontaneous or induced—after hemodynamic stability has been achieved (Sweeney & McAuley, 2016). The nursing role in intake and output measurement is paramount is this aspect of management.

OUTCOMES

Individuals who survive ARDS have significant morbidity and look on the clinicians to provide interventions to reduce the sequelae. Survivors experience exercise limitation, physical and psychological sequelae, decreased physical quality of life, and increased costs and use of health care services that may persist for

5 years or more (Mehta & Povoa, 2017). Interventions are aimed at identifying modifiable risk factors and addressing specific needs such as rehabilitation, nutrition, and support for caregivers.

Summary

ARDS is an acute process that can occur rapidly. Nursing vigilance can contribute to early identification and excellence in management to reduce morbidity and mortality. Prevention includes vaccination and other methods to reduce predisposing factors.

Ashbaugh, D. G., Bigelow, D. B., Petty, T. L., & Levine, B. E. (1967). Acute respiratory distress in adults. *Lancet, 12*(2), 319–323.

Fanelli, V., Vlachou, A., Ghannadian, S., Simonetti, U., Slutsky, A. S., & Zhang, H. (2013). Acute respiratory distress syndrome: New definition, current and future therapeutic options. *Journal of Thoracic Disease, 5*(3), 326–334.

Mehta, S., & Povoa, P. (2017). Long-term physical morbidity in ARDS survivors. *Intensive Care Medicine, 43*(1), 101–103.

Raneri, V. M., Rubenfeld, G. D., Thompson, B. T., Ferguson, N. D., Caldwell, E., Fan, E., . . . Slutsky, A. S.; ARDS Definition Task Force. (2012). ARDS definition task force: Acute respiratory syndrome: The Berlin definition. *Journal of the American Medical Association, 307,* 2526–2533.

Scholten, E. L., Beitler, J. R., Prisk, G. K., & Malhotra, A. (2017). Treatment of ARDS with prone positioning. *Chest, 151*(1), 215–224.

Sweeney, R. M., & McAuley, D. F. (2016). Acute respiratory distress syndrome. *Lancet, 388*(10058), 2416–2430.

Vidyasagar, S. (2016). Emerging concepts in acute respiratory distress syndrome: Implications for clinicians. *Journal of Clinical Science and Research, 5,* 202–204. doi:10.15380/22775706.JCSR.16.09.001

■ ACUTE RESPIRATORY FAILURE

Breanna Hetland

Overview

Acute respiratory failure (ARF) is characterized by a sudden onset of respiratory distress. It occurs when the lungs fail to maintain adequate exchange of oxygen and carbon dioxide to meet the body's metabolic needs. ARF is classified as either hypoxemic (insufficient oxygen) or hypercapnic (excessive carbon dioxide). It may result from inadequate air movement, insufficient gas diffusions in the alveoli, and/or poor pulmonary blood flow. Conditions, such as pneumonia, chronic obstructive pulmonary disease (COPD), acute respiratory distress syndrome (ARDS), and congestive heart failure (CHF), commonly lead to ARF (Fourneir, 2014; Peter, 2016; Rehder, Turi, & Cheifetz, 2014).

In the United States, the number of hospitalizations for ARF has increased to approximately 2 million each year. Although a reduction in inpatient mortality has been noted, ARF still carries an annual cost of more than $50 billion (Stefan et al., 2013). Due to the two different types of ARF, knowledge of the physiologic cause of ARF is crucial to selecting appropriate treatments. Targeted management of ARF is dependent on the extent and duration of symptoms, but nursing management should focus on providing symptom support until the underlying cause of ARF can be identified and treated (Fourneir, 2014; Peter, 2016; Rehder et al., 2014).

Background

Respiration, the act of inhaling and exhaling air to transport oxygen to the lung alveoli, includes (a) ventilation, (b) oxygenation, (c) perfusion, (d) ventilation/perfusion relationship. Ventilation, the movement of air in and out of the lungs through inspiration and expiration, is affected by airway compliance and airway resistance. Oxygenation involves the exchange of carbon dioxide and oxygen at the alveoli. Perfusion is the movement of blood through the pulmonary capillaries. The ventilation/perfusion relationship encompasses the balance between the amount of air reaching the alveoli (ventilation) and the amount of blood reaching the alveoli (perfusion). These processes involve the conducting airways (nose, pharynx, larynx, trachea, bronchi, bronchioles, and terminal bronchioles), alveoli (tiny sacs within the lungs where gas exchange occurs), pulmonary circulation (portion of the cardiovascular system that oxygenates the blood), and respiratory pump (thorax, respiratory musculature, and nervous system). They are regulated by neurological, chemical, and mechanical control systems within the body, and dysfunction in any of these control systems can lead to ARF (Fourneir, 2014; Peter, 2016; Rehder et al., 2014).

ARF is classified as hypoxemic, a lack of circulating oxygen in the blood characterized by an arterial oxygen concentration of PaO_2 less than 60 mmHg, or hypercapnic, an excess of circulating carbon dioxide in the blood, characterized by an atrial carbon dioxide concentration of $PaCO_2$ greater than 40mmHg. Hypoxemic ARF occurs in conditions that cause lung atelectasis and those that lead to fluid in the lungs such as pulmonary edema, pneumonia, alveolar hemorrhage, ARDS. Hypercapnic ARF happens when there is hypoperfusion of the respiratory muscles during shock states as well as when processes in the central nervous system (CNS), peripheral nerves, muscles, neuromuscular junction, or alveoli malfunction. These conditions include: CNS depression (drug overdose, stroke), spinal cord infections or transection, peripheral nerve weakness (Guillain–Barré Syndrome), chest wall deformities, muscle weakness (myasthenia gravis, hypokalemia, hypophosphatemia), and alveolar hypoventilation (COPD, cystic fibrosis, airway obstruction, pulmonary fibrosis) (Fourneir, 2014; Peter, 2016; Rehder et al., 2014).

ARF is the most frequent reason for admission of hospitalized patients to the intensive care unit with 2.5% of cases requiring ventilatory support. ARF requires an average hospital length of stay of 7.1 days and results in more than 350,000 in-hospital deaths each year. The most common etiologies noted in hospitalized patients with ARF include: pneumonia, CHF, COPD, ARDS, asthma, drug ingestion, trauma, and sepsis. Mortality rates were highest in patients 85 years of age and older (Stefan et al., 2013). Patients with severe ARF requiring mechanical ventilation report a multitude of distressing symptoms, including anxiety, pain, delirium, and lack of sleep (Puntillo et al., 2010). In addition, after hospital discharge, patients report symptoms of posttraumatic stress disorder (PTSD) and rate their quality of life significantly lower than comparative controls (Bienvenu et al., 2013).

Clinical Aspects

ASSESSMENT

Clinical signs of acute respiratory distress are often nonspecific, but early detection through comprehensive nursing assessment can help prevent progression to ARF. Tachypnea and shortness of breath are often the first signs of respiratory distress. Clinical indications of worsening condition include nasal flaring, use of accessory muscles, paradoxical abdominal movements, prolonged expiratory phase, expiratory grunting, cyanosis, decrease in pulse oximetry despite increasing the administration of supplemental oxygen, anxiety, diminished lung sounds, inability to speak in full sentences, tripod positioning to further expand the chest, feelings of impending doom, and altered mental status. In addition to clinical presentation, pulse oximetry, arterial blood gasses, and capnography are important physiologic measurements to consider (Fourneir, 2014; Peter, 2016; Rehder et al., 2014).

The goals of treatment for ARF depend on its pathophysiologic cause, but should aim to treat the underlying cause of the respiratory failure, improve oxygen delivery to the tissues, decrease oxygen demand in the tissues, reduce the production of carbon dioxide, promote the elimination of carbon dioxide, and limit damaging therapies. Treatment of the underlying cause may include antibiotics (infection), steroids and bronchodilators (acute asthma, COPD), medications to reverse CNS or peripheral nerve problems that caused the respiratory failure (i.e., Narcan for a drug overdose). Oxygen delivery to the tissues can be enhanced by applying supplemental oxygen through low-flow devices, high-flow devices, or noninvasive or invasive mechanical ventilation. Ventilator support may be required for patients with severe or hypoxic respiratory failure with progressing respiratory fatigue. Extracorporeal life support may also be necessary to treat ARF when conventional ventilatory strategies are not sufficient. In addition to supplemental oxygen delivery, it is important to maintain hemoglobin and optimize cardiac output as well as reduce fever and control sepsis in order to decrease oxygen demand of the tissues (Fourneir, 2014; Peter, 2016; Rehder et al., 2014).

Carbon dioxide production can be reduced, controlling excess motor activity (anticonvulsants for seizures). The elimination of carbon dioxide can be promoted by increasing respiratory drive (reduce sedatives; give CNS stimulants) and improving lung mechanics. Upright positioning, analgesics for chest pain, bronchodilators and bronchial hygiene for airway resistance, and interventions to reduce abdominal distention can all improve lung mechanics. In addition, respiratory muscle performance can be enhanced by ensuring adequate oxygenation and tissue perfusion, correcting electrolyte abnormalities, and administering medications to improve diaphragmatic contractility. Special care should be given to limit therapies that may potentially damage lung tissue such as using high oxygen concentrations for protracted periods and failing to implement lung-protective ventilator strategies (Fourneir, 2014; Peter, 2016; Rehder et al., 2014).

NURSING INTERVENTIONS, MANAGEMENT, AND IMPLICATIONS

When caring for a patient with ARF, it is imperative to perform continuous assessments and provide appropriate symptom support measures to promote relaxation and facilitate oxygenation. Supplemental oxygen should be applied immediately and the airway must be evaluated for patency. The airway should be clear of secretions or mechanical obstructions and the head of bed upright. If a patient continues to decompensate, an oral or nasal airway may be placed and mechanical ventilation applied. The need for mechanical ventilation should be assessed with attention to the clinical scenario, rate of clinical deterioration, and the patient's response to previously attempted therapies (Fourneir, 2014; Peter, 2016; Rehder et al., 2014).

OUTCOMES

Nurses must be aware of physiologic symptoms of inadequate tissue oxygenation, such as angina and mental status changes, as well as conditions that may impair oxygen delivery. It is important to turn the patient regularly to maintain the ventilation/perfusion relationship. Efforts to minimize and remove secretions in addition to liberal use of an incentive spirometer will maximize tissue oxygenation and help prevent atelectasis. Malnutrition can impair respiratory muscle function and reduce ventilator drive. Patients with ARF can easily become malnourished due to increased metabolic demands and inadequate nutrition intake, therefore nutritional expertise should be sought. Lastly, nurses should offer the patient and family pertinent education related to medications, the purpose of nursing measures, signs of clinical decompensation, patient risk factors, and appropriate follow-up (Fourneir, 2014; Peter, 2016; Rehder et al., 2014).

Summary

Treating ARF requires knowledge of the specific mechanisms that cause respiratory failure and a systematic approach to supportive symptom management. As the number of ARF cases continues to rise, nurses must be acutely aware of the signs, symptoms, and appropriate nursing interventions for ARF in order to reduce the morbidity and mortality related to ARF (Fourneir, 2014; Peter, 2016; Rehder et al., 2014).

Bienvenu, O. J., Gellar, J., Althouse, B. M., Colantuoni, E., Sricharoenchai, T., Mendez-Tellez, P. A., . . . Needham, D. M. (2013). Post-traumatic stress disorder symptoms after acute lung injury: A 2-year prospective longitudinal study. *Psychological Medicine, 43*(12), 2657–2671. doi:10.1017/S0033291713000214

Fourneir, M. (2014). Caring for patients in respiratory failure. *American Nurse Today, 9*(11), 18–23.

Peter, J. V. (2016). Acute respiratory failure. *Clinical Pathways in Emergency Medicine,* 167–178. Retrieved from https://link.springer.com/chapter/10.1007/978-81 -322-2710-6_13/fulltext.html

Puntillo, K. A., Arai, S., Cohen, N. H., Gropper, M. A., Neuhaus, J., Paul, S. M., & Miaskowski, C. (2010). Symptoms experienced by intensive care unit patients at high risk of dying. *Critical Care Medicine, 38*(11), 2155–2160. doi:10.1097/ CCM.0b013e3181f267ee

Rehder, K. J., Turi, J. L., & Cheifetz, I. M. (2014). Acute respiratory failure. *Pediatric Critical Care Medicine,* 401–411. Retrieved from https://link.springer.com/chapter/ 10.1007/978-1-4471-6362-6_31

Stefan, M. S., Shieh, M. S., Pekow, P. S., Rothberg, M. B., Steingrub, J. S., Lagu, T., & Lindenauer, P. K. (2013). Epidemiology and outcomes of acute respiratory failure in the United States, 2001 to 2009: A national survey. *Journal of Hospital Medicine, 8*(2), 76–82. doi:10.1002/jhm.2004

■ ADRENAL INSUFFICIENCY

Rachel K. Vanek

Overview

Adrenal insufficiency (AI) can be an acute or chronic illness affecting patients in the acute care, office, long-term care, or home care settings. It can either be a primary disorder due to destruction of the adrenal cortex or a secondary disorder due to disruption of hypothalamic–pituitary functions. Its signs and symptoms are a consequence of the failure of the hypothalamic–pituitary–adrenal axis (HPA) to secrete adequate amounts of essential hormones and of the adrenal gland to respond properly. It is a rare disease, often undiagnosed, thought to occur in one person in 100,000; it occurs equally in men and women in the United States. It is often an overlooked disorder that has myriad symptoms that mimic other acute and chronic illnesses (National Organization for Rare Disorders, 2017).

Background

The Endocrine Society's clinical practice guidelines define primary adrenal insufficiency as "the inability of the adrenal cortex to produce sufficient amounts of glucocorticoids and/or mineralocorticoids. It is a severe and potentially life-threatening condition due to the central role of these hormones in energy, salt, and fluid homeostasis" (Bornstein et al., 2016, p. 367).

This hypothalamic–pituitary–adrenal axis is essential for the regulation of homeostasis and an individual's stress response. Any alteration affecting a component of the HPA axis can lead to insufficient adrenal hormone secretion. Under physiologic conditions, the HPA axis is regulated by negative feedback control mechanisms. When there is insufficient circulating cortisol, the hypothalamus secretes corticotropin-releasing hormone, which stimulates the release of adrenocorticotropic hormone (ACTH) from the anterior pituitary. ACTH affects the cortex of the adrenal gland to stimulate the secretion of cortisol until there is an adequate concentration of circulating cortisol to maintain homeostasis (Charmandari, Nicolaides, & Chrousos, 2014.)

In primary AI, the adrenal cortex is either destroyed or does not function properly. This can be caused by infiltrative disease destroying the adrenal cortex. Bleeding into the adrenal gland, systemic fungal or bacterial infection, HIV infection, tuberculosis, autoimmune disease, metastatic disease, and amyloidosis can result in adrenal destruction. Secondary AI occurs when damage to the hypothalamus or pituitary gland occurs. Surgery to remove the pituitary, radiation to the pituitary, tumors of the hypothalamus, metastatic disease involving the pituitary or hypothalamus, chronic systemic steroid use, and pituitary necrosis are some examples of pathological states that can lead to the development of secondary deficiency of adrenal hormones. These disorders can be seen in pediatric and adult populations (Oelkers, 1996).

AI can have vague and insidious symptoms and signs. They often overlap with symptoms of other disorders and can be difficult to characterize as caused by AI alone. In general, AI symptoms impact quality of life by rendering the patient at baseline tired, weak, dizzy from orthostasis, anorexic, and depressed. The patient can have skin changes, constipation, diarrhea, loss of libido, arthralgia, myalgia, and electrolyte disturbances. Acutely, the patient can have fever, abdominal pain, mental status changes, encephalopathy, delirium, and shock. Refractory hypotension can lead to multisystem organ dysfunction and failure (Bornstein et al., 2016).

Clinical Aspects

ASSESSMENT

History of the patient or family may reflect fatigue, loss of energy, perhaps recent infection, or pregnancy. Heat or cold intolerance can also be a common complaint. Recent changes in appetite, bowel habits, or abdominal pain are common. Dizziness is often a trigger prompting patients to seek medical care. Physical exam may reveal patients with evidence of recent weight loss. Their skin may be very dry or have changes in pigmentation, such as hyperpigmentation in areas of skin exposed to the sun or constant friction (think "waistband, socks"). Blood pressure and heart rate should be checked with the patient sitting and standing to evaluate orthostasis. Mucous membranes may be dry and appear dusky in color. Patients may have loss of axillary or pubic hair (Bornstein et al., 2016).

Laboratory findings may reveal hyponatremia, hypoglycemia, and hyperkalemia. Chloride may also be elevated. Elevated blood urea nitrogen and creatinine due to dehydration may also be noticed. Hemoglobin usually is normal but in up to 15% of the patients with AI normocytic anemia may occur. An early-morning cortisol level may be collected and, if it is less than 10, AI should be considered (Oelkers, 1996).

An ACTH stimulation test may also be done. In this test, the patient's baseline cortisol is measured. The patient is then given a dose of intravenous ACTH and cortisol is checked at 30 and 60 minutes. If the levels increase above 20 mcg/mL, then adrenal function is normal. Plasma ACTH, renin, or aldosterone levels may be measured as well in patients who are not in extremis. Laboratory studies to rule out autoimmune disease may also be ordered. Abdominal CT can be performed to evaluate for disruptions in adrenal anatomy. The test can identify enlarged, calcified, or acute hemorrhage in the adrenal glands (Oelkers, 1996).

NURSING INTERVENTIONS, MANAGEMENT, AND IMPLICATIONS

Risk for falls and risk for injury may be related to volume depletion. Oftentimes, changing position slowly and allowing time for equilibration lessens this risk while the disorder is being evaluated. Once treatment has commenced, orthostatic changes should improve.

Ongoing monitoring of orthostatic blood pressure and pulse helps assess response. Assessing adequate oral hydration and administering any ordered intravenous fluids while monitoring for signs of fluid overload are within the nursing realm. Proper administration of glucocorticoid and mineralocorticoid is key to treatment. The patient must be taught signs of symptoms of treatment failure, how and when to take medications, and what symptoms to report to the health care provider (National Organization for rare disorders, 2017).

Weight loss and poor appetite are key signs of nutritional imbalance and should begin to improve with treatment. Weighing patients, assessing for weight loss, and appetite changes are part of the ongoing nursing assessment. The patient may have a knowledge deficiency of AI as a new diagnosis or even as a previously existing problem (The Complete List of NANDA Nursing Diagnosis for 2012–2014, with 16 New Diagnoses, 2014. The nurse should assess the patient's knowledge and provide education for a positive outcome. Key education requirements for patients are proper medication management, when to call the provider, side effects, and warning signs of infection. Patients must be taught to keep an up-to-date medication list for all providers who participate in their care. Informing other providers of the diagnosis of AI will allow proper treatment during surgery or other interventions that can precipitate an adrenal crisis. Patients and their caregivers need to recognize signs of adrenal crisis and know what to do to intervene (Charmandari et al., 2014).

OUTCOMES

Nurses should be astute to the subtle signs of renal insufficiency (RI) on laboratory analysis to help identify the patient with RI and help to prevent progression to kidney injury and chronic failure. These signs may not be apparent but the nurse can use measures that encourage RI from occurring or progressing through hydration, avoidance of renal damaging medication administration, and diet. These measures can promote positive outcomes.

Summary

AI is a rare disorder that can lead to life-threatening symptoms related to the actions of the HPA axis, the most severe being refractory hypotension leading to organ damage. Nursing actions and management are key to establishing proper diagnosis and supporting recovery. Proper administration and timing of diagnostic tests are essential. Restoration of volume and correction of electrolyte disturbances facilitate resumption of life activities and improved satisfaction with the improved quality of life. Teaching the patients and their caregivers about the diagnosis, treatment aims, medications actions, and warning signs of failing treatment are all essential to positive outcomes.

Bornstein S. R., Allolio B., Arlt W., Barthel A., Don-Wauchope A., Hammer G. D., . . . Tory D. J. (2016). Diagnosis and treatment of primary adrenal insufficiency: An Endocrine Society clinical practice guideline. *Journal of Clinical Endocrinology and Metabolism*, *101*(2), 364–389.

Charmandari E., Nicolaides N. C., & Chrousos G. P. (2014). Adrenal insufficiency. *Lancet*, *383*(9935), 2152–2167.

The Complete list of NANDA nursing diagnoses for 2012–2014, with 16 new diagnoses. (2014). Retrieved from http://www.kc-courses.com/fundamentals/week2process/nanda2012.pdf

National Organization for Rare Disorders. (2015). Addison's disease. Retrieved from https://rarediseases.org/rare-diseases/addisons-disease

Oelkers, W. (1996). Adrenal insufficiency. *New England Journal of Medicine*, *335*(16), 1206–1212.

■ BACK PAIN

Sharon R. Rainer

Overview

Back pain is one of the most common conditions for which patients seek medical treatment from a health care professional. Most people older than 18 years experience at least one episode of acute low-back pain (ALBP) during a lifetime. According to data from the National Electronic Injury Surveillance System, the incidence of back pain is 139 per 100,000 person-years in the United States. According to the Centers for Disease Control and Prevention's (CDC) National Center for Health Statistics (NCHS), 28.4% of adults older than 18 years had experienced lower back pain in the previous 3 months (Ma, Chan, & Carruthers, 2014). In addition, approximately 6 million people annually are evaluated in emergency departments (EDs) for back pain (Perina, 2017).

Back pain is costly to treat and manage. Along with high incidence and prevalence, back pain is the third most costly medical condition followed by cancer and heart disease (Perina, 2017). The cost of treatment increases considerably with chronicity. The economic impact of chronic low-back pain (CLBP) includes decreased function and mobility that results in lost productivity, high treatment costs, and disability payments. Chronic back pain (CBP) is the most common cause of disability in Americans younger than 45 years (Allen & Hulbert, 2009). Each year, 3% to 4% of the U.S. population is temporarily disabled, and 1% of the working-age population is totally and permanently disabled due to back pain (Ma et al., 2014). Low-back pain (LBP) is the second most frequent reason to visit an outpatient office, the fifth most common cause for hospitalization, and the third most frequent reason for a surgical procedure (Wheeler & Berman, 2016). Estimates of the cost of back pain treatment and management have reached $100 to $200 billion annually (Allen & Hulbert, 2009, p. 1067; Ma et al., 2014, p. 4).

Background

ALBP is defined as pain with duration of less than 6 weeks in the posterior area between the costal angles and gluteal folds (Kinkade, 2007). Typically, in adults, the first episode of LBP will occur between the ages of 20 and 40 and resolve within 6 to 12 weeks (Kinkade, 2007). Episodes of LBP may be nonspecific in nature or may be the result of an underlying illness or injury. Most acute episodes of musculoskeletal LBP are self-limited and resolve quickly requiring minimal interventions. Typically, strains and sprains of the back are described as nonspecific. However, pain associated with the condition can be moderate to severe and in some cases debilitating, causing the patient limited activity and mobility and lost time from work. Moreover, within 1 to 2 years, recurrent back pain occurs in approximately 25% to 62% of patients (Casazza, 2012).

Pain that persists longer than 3 months is defined as CLBP (Allen & Hulbert, 2009, p. 1067). As with ALBP, CLBP can be related to an underlying chronic condition. Sometimes, the underlying chronic condition may be serious in nature and therefore patients warrant a careful clinical evaluation. In many cases, CLBP impacts a patient's quality of life. It is common for psychosocial issues to play a role in treatment of patients with CLBP. Patients with chronic, persistent pain that is not well controlled may experience clinical, psychological, and social problems associated with chronic pain. The consequences of unrelieved pain include limitations in daily activities, lost work productivity, reduced quality of life, and stigma (Dowell, Haegerich, & Chou, 2016). Patients with CLBP may also experience a reduced sense of control, disturbed mood, negative self-efficacy, anxiety, and other mental health disorders (Last & Hulbert, 2009), including opioid use disorder (Dowell et al., 2016). Opioids are commonly prescribed to patients with CLBP in spite of a lack of evidence to support the efficacy of these medications. In fact, opioids are commonly prescribed for adults with both acute and chronic pain. An estimated 20% of patients seen by a primary care provider with noncancer pain will obtain an opioid prescription (Dowell et al., 2016).

Clinical Aspects

ASSESSMENT

A careful and accurate focused health history and physical examination are essential for all patients experiencing back pain. A thorough evaluation of a patient's symptoms by a clinician is essential to identify potentially serious underlying causes of back pain. Generally, back pain can be placed into four broad categories. They are nonspecific LBP, including sprains/strains; pain associated with radiculopathy or spinal stenosis (spine related); referred pain from a nonspinal source such as aortic aneurysm, gynecologic, or renal conditions; and pain associated with another cause such as cancer, arthritis, or infection (Last & Hulbert, 2009).

Although back pain associated with a serious underlying pathology is rare, health care providers (HCPs) are obligated to assess patients for "red flags," which are symptoms that raise clinical suspicion of a serious underlying etiology (Casazza, 2012). Red flags will prompt a clinician to investigate further, initiate aggressive treatment, and/or make a referral to the ED or spine specialist. Examples of chief complaints involving LBP that raise clinical suspicion about serious red flags include significant trauma such as motor vehicle crash, falls in the elderly, falls from significant heights in younger patients, and heavy lifting in patients with osteoporosis (Casazza, 2012).

Likewise, patients with back pain need to be assessed for the presence or absence of sciatica indicating a mechanical spinal condition, which in some cases may be serious, and indicates a need for a specialist referral. Sciatica or sciatic neuralgia is defined as pain in the distribution of the sciatic nerve often associated with a lumbar herniated disc (Stafford, Peng, & Hill, 2007). It is important to differentiate between leg pain and sciatica that involves pain traveling below the knee. Neurological symptoms, including progressive motor or sensory deficits in the extremities, raise serious concerns and may indicate the need for urgent surgical intervention. Patients need to be assessed quickly for signs of cauda equina syndrome (CES). CES is a rare but serious condition that results from pressure and swelling of the nerves at the end of the spinal cord. CES is a medical emergency requiring urgent surgical intervention to relieve pressure of the spinal nerves (Spector, Madigan, Rhyne, Darden, & Kim, 2008). Without emergency intervention, patients with CES may experience adverse results, including paralysis, impaired bladder and/or bowel control, difficulty walking, and/or other neurological and physical problems. Although CES is an uncommon condition, it is important that patients are screened quickly for signs of the disorder. Signs and symptoms include bowel and bladder dysfunction or urinary retention, loss of anal sphincter tone, saddle anesthesia, progressive leg weakness, bilateral sciatica, or numbness in the legs. Decreased rectal tone may be a relatively late finding. Early signs and symptoms of a developing postoperative CES are often attributed to common postoperative findings. Therefore, HCPs in the perioperative setting are urged to have a high level of suspicion of potential CES in postoperative spine patients with back and/or leg pain refractory to analgesia, especially with urinary retention (Spector et al., 2008).

Additional assessment of the patient with back pain includes a thorough history of any cancer that may have metastasized to bone and risk factors for suspected spinal infections. Spinal infections are of high clinical suspicion in patients injecting intravenous (IV) drugs such as heroin and crack cocaine. A complete health history must also specifically include questions about bone health (osteoporosis, arthritis, prior fractures, or injuries), fever, weight loss, and any prior imaging to help determine whether any underlying cause can be identified (Wheeler & Berman, 2016).

The goal of a focused history and physical examination is to help clinicians stratify patients into back pain categories—nonspecific, spine related, referred from nonspine source, or other causes as described previously. Clinicians are obligated to identify and treat the cause of back pain. One important test to help identify a possible herniated disc is the straight leg raise (SLR). The SLR is a screening test used by clinicians to detect a herniated lumbar disk and it has high sensitivity and moderate specificity (Perina, 2017). The test is performed with the patient sitting or lying; however, the supine position is preferred. The knee is kept extended while the clinician raises one leg at a time to assess for pain in the posterior leg radiating below the knee caused by irritation or inflammation of the sciatic nerve. The SLR test is positive only when the maneuver elicits pain that radiates to below the knee. It is not considered a positive test, indicating a possible herniated disc, if the pain remains localized in the back or there is pain in the hamstrings when the leg is raised. In addition to the SLR, the patient should have strength and reflexes in the lower extremities assessed as part of a thorough physical examination. The basic examination of a patient with back pain includes observation of movement and palpation of the spine for tenderness, range of motion of the back and extremities; SLR; and neurological examination, including deep tendon reflexes, muscle strength, and sensation in the lower extremities.

NURSING INTERVENTIONS, MANAGEMENT, AND IMPLICATIONS

Providing nursing care to patients with back pain can be challenging across all settings. The aim of treatment for LBP is to provide adequate pain care and improve function, reduce time away from work or activities, and develop coping strategies in the event of chronic, persistent pain or surgical intervention (Casazza, 2012). Most often, clinicians will not order imaging, such as radiographs, for patients presenting with back pain in the absence of trauma and red-flag symptoms. If the clinician suspects a serious underlying condition, he or she will order an MRI, which is the study of choice. CT is an alternative diagnostic test when MRI is contraindicated or unavailable. Radiography may be helpful to screen for serious conditions but usually has little diagnostic value. If spinal infection is suspected, the clinician may order laboratory tests. These tests would likely include a complete blood count with differential, erythrocyte sedimentation rate (ESR), and C-reactive protein (CRP) level. In the case of nonspecific LBP, clinicians will not typically order any laboratory testing or imaging; however, in some cases of LBP that are not clearly musculoskeletal, a urinalysis may be useful. Other laboratory studies are rarely needed unless the clinician strongly suspects a disorder other than back pain (Kinkade, 2007).

Treatment of back pain depends on the suspected underlying cause. Generally, patients with back pain are treated conservatively and surgical referral is a last resort. Treatment for CBP encompasses conservative management with both pharmacological and nonpharmacological pain care. Remaining active with exercise and physical therapy may be beneficial for patients with CLBP (Perina, 2017). Recommended first-line treatment for nonspecific back pain includes nonsteroidal anti-inflammatory drugs (NSAIDs) and acetaminophen. There is conflicting evidence about NSAIDs being more effective than acetaminophen in the treatment of ALBP. Used by patients in recommended dosages, acetaminophen can be a helpful adjunct that avoids the renal and gastrointestinal toxicities of NSAIDs (Perina, 2017). This is a particularly important consideration for the treatment of back pain in older adults who are at higher risk for adverse drug reactions. For patients experiencing sciatica, opioids may be required to control pain when first-line medications fail. Tramadol (Ultram) is an analgesic that has weak opioid and serotonin–norepinephrine-reuptake inhibitor (SNRI) activity. Studies show some short-term improvements in pain and function with Tramadol but there is a lack of evidence to support long-term use in chronic pain sufferers. Opioids should be considered a second- or third-line analgesic for a short period of time. It is important to note that studies have shown no significant advantage of opioid use in symptom relief or return to work when compared with NSAIDs or acetaminophen (Kinkade, 2007).

Muscle relaxants are another class of drugs that may be prescribed in the treatment of back pain. Patients may be prescribed cyclobenzaprine (Flexeril) in the first 1 to 2 weeks of treatment. There is some evidence that suggest skeletal muscle relaxants lead to better relief of symptoms when used with NSAIDs. However, studies do not show benefit of long-term use of muscle relaxants to treat CBP. The use of benzodiazepines and carisoprodol (Soma) carries risk of dependency. Clinicians will often refer people with CLBP to pain management and/or a spine specialist.

Nurses are an important and integral part of the interprofessional team involved in the care of patients with LBP. Often, nurses have a significant impact on a patient's ability to self-manage their pain. Education around self-management is important to help prevent back pain relapses and in managing pain that lasts longer than 3 months. Patient education that has shown to have some benefit in preventing CLBP includes exercise and activity, promoting weight loss where indicated, increasing overall physical conditioning, recognizing and avoiding aggravating factors, the natural history of the disease, and expected time frame for improvement in pain and function (Kinkade, 2007; Perina, 2017).

OUTCOMES

Back pain relapses are common and the socioeconomic burden of CBP is sizable. Therefore, efforts to prevent relapse and reduce the incidence of chronic pain are of great importance in addressing quality of care and improved outcomes for patients with back pain. Strategies aimed at preventing injuries that cause initial back pain episodes and preventing CBP improve outcomes. The U.S. Preventive Services Task Force (USPSTF) and the COST B13 Working Group on European Guidelines for Prevention in LBP have synthesized the evidence for treatment and management of back pain. Of note, back belts that patients may commonly wear, especially in occupations with heavy lifting, have not been proven to prevent back injuries. An interprofessional approach to treating and managing back pain will improve outcomes. Patients have access to an enormous amount of information on the Internet about back pain treatments. HCPs must be ready to discuss evidence-based approaches to prevention, treatment, and management. In addition to physical therapy, massage and yoga therapy may be treatments patients inquire about and want to try. There is insufficient evidence to recommend for or against massage therapy for ALBP (Casazza, 2012). Yet, for chronic pain, it may be helpful. Moreover, one form of yoga has been shown to have benefit. A therapeutic form of yoga, Viniyoga, may provide relief to CBP. Research has shown that a 6-week course of yoga decreased medication use and provided more pain relief than exercise and self-care strategies for nonspecific back pain (Last & Hulbert, 2009). Clinicians who are aware of these and other therapies will help patients make informed decisions and engage them in shared decision making about their care.

Summary

The evaluation and treatment of back pain occurs along a continuum in most cases from the initial treatment aimed at alleviating the pain associated with an acute episode to improving pain and function with adequate pain care for patients experiencing CBP. It is important for HCPs in all settings to thoroughly assess patient's back pain even if the pain is chronic. There are a variety of causes of back pain and some may be serious requiring immediate intervention. It is also important to document and openly discuss patient expectations about pain care, self-care, alternative therapies, and return to their previous level of activity. Discussing and documenting goals and expectations at each encounter helps to provide continuity of care. HCPs must be vigilant in helping patients understand prevention strategies for back pain and how to recognize red flags that require urgent intervention.

Allen, A. R., & Hulbert, K. (2009). CLBP: Evaluation and management. *American Family Physician, 79*(12), 1067–1074.

Casazza, B. A. (2012). Diagnosis and treatment of ALBP. *American Academy of Family Physicians, 85*(4), 343–350.

Dowell, D., Haegerich, T. M., & Chou, R. (2016). CDC guideline for prescribing opioids for chronic pain—United States. *Journal of the American Medical Association, 315*(15), 1624. doi:10.1001/jama.2016.1464

Kincade, S. (2007). Evaluation and treatment of acute low back pain. *American Family Physician, 75*(8), 1181–1188.

Last, A. R., & Hulbert, K. (2009). CLBP: Evaluation and management. *American Family Physician, 79*(12), 1067–1074.

Ma, V. Y., Chan, L., & Carruthers, K. J. (2014). Incidence, prevalence, costs, and impact on disability of common conditions requiring rehabilitation in the United States: Stroke, spinal cord injury, traumatic brain injury, multiple sclerosis, osteoarthritis, rheumatoid arthritis, limb loss, and back pain. *Archives of Physical Medicine and Rehabilitation, 95*(5), 986–995. doi:10.1016/j.apmr.2013.10.032

Perina, D. G. (2017). Mechanical back pain. *Medscape.* Retrieved from http://emedicine.medscapre.com/article/822462-guidelines

Spector, L. R., Madigan, L., Rhyne, A., Darden, B., & Kim, D. (2008). Cauda equina syndrome. *Journal of the American Academy of Orthopaedic Surgeons, 16*(8), 471–479.

Stafford, M. A., Peng, P., & Hill, D. A. (2007). Sciatica: A review of history, epidemiology, pathogenesis, and the role of epidural steroid injection in management. *British Journal of Anaesthesia, 99*(4), 461–473. doi:10.1093/bja/aem238

Wheeler, A. H., & Berman, S. A. (2016). LBP and sciatica: Overview, pathophysiology, characteristics of pain-sensitive structures. *Medscape.* Retrieved from http://emedicine.medscape.com/article/1144130-overview

■ BURNS

Margaret Jean Carman

Overview

Burns is a traumatic tissue injury resulting from the application of thermal, electrical, chemical, or radiation sources to the body. The epithelial layers serve to promote temperature and fluid regulation, protect the body from infection, and provide ongoing sensory input from the environment. Significant injury results in a massive inflammatory response, with capillary leakage and fluid and electrolyte losses from the vascular space. Untreated hypovolemic shock and inhalation injuries often lead to an early death, whereas delayed deaths from burns occur chiefly because of infection. Nursing care of the individual with burn injuries extends across a trajectory from resuscitation to recovery and rehabilitation to promote a functional and emotionally secure future.

Background

Burn injuries lead to more than 3,000 deaths across the United States and 265,000 globally each year (American Burn Association [ABA], 2016; World Health Organization [WHO], 2016). The majority of fatalities result from residential fires, making primary prevention an important aspect of the nursing role. Sixty percent of the individuals requiring hospital admission are transferred to one of the 128 burn centers in the United States. Early identification of patients who meet the criteria for transfer is essential. Criteria include greater than 10% total body surface area (TBSA) burns in patients younger than 10 or older than 50 years of age, or more than 20% TBSA in people between 10 years and 50 years; full-thickness burns on more than 5% of the TBSA at any age; significant electrical burns, including lightning injuries; significant chemical burns; inhalation injuries, and burns occurring in an individual with significant comorbidities that may complicate treatment or recovery (ABA, 2016).

The vast majority of burn injuries involve thermal injury (77%), followed by chemical or contact (11%) and electrical (3%) etiologies (ABA, 2016). The acute phase of injury includes rapid assessment and initial resuscitation to prevent burn shock, although the ongoing care is focused on prevention and treatment of infection and promoting restoration of normal physiological function.

Burn injuries are a global problem. The risk of injury is greatest in underdeveloped countries, in populations of lower socioeconomic standing. Adult women and children aged 1 year to 9 years are most susceptible to injury, which can often be linked to environmental or behavioral factors. Open-fire cooking or lack of industrial standards in some countries increases the exposure to potential toxins or thermal hazards, increasing the risk of injury. Adequate supervision of children and injury prevention are key to decreasing the incidence of burns, particularly in middle and lower income countries (WHO, 2016). Behavioral factors, such as substance abuse, alcoholism, and tobacco abuse, are major contributors to the incidence of burns and may play a role in the mechanism of injury (WHO, 2016).

Clinical Aspects

Initial burn care includes actions to stop the burning process. For thermal injuries, cool water or moisten gauze saline should be used. Ice or cold water are avoided to prevent hypothermia or further damage to the injured tissue. Constricting items or those that may continue to convey heat should be immediately removed.

For patients with chemical or radiation injuries, consider consultation with a poison control center before decontamination. Chemicals remaining on the skin may compromise the safety of the providers and should be brushed off, as the use of water may activate the offending agent. Secure any information available on the substance and communicate this, to ensure that appropriate decontamination of chemical or radiation exposures can be executed.

ASSESSMENT

Rapid assessment, stabilization, and transfer to a designated burn center (if appropriate) are the initial priorities. The patient should be immediately assessed for associated trauma or inhalation injuries, which can cause rapid decompensation and loss of airway patency. Blast injuries or burns occurring in a confined space are at risk for inhalation injury; carbonaceous sputum or particles in the oropharynx, involvement of the face or neck, singed facial hair (including eyebrows and nasal hair), altered mentation, increased work of breathing, or hoarseness indicate airway compromise and the possible need for proactive intubation (American College of Surgeons Committee on Trauma).

Exposure to vaporized agents in the burning environment may result in carbon monoxide (CO) poisoning; clinical signs include a headache, nausea, and confusion. The classic finding of cherry-red skin discoloration is uncommon and not a reliable clinical indicator of CO poisoning; pulse oximetry is also unreliable, given that CO displaces oxygen from binding with the hemoglobin molecule, affecting saturation readings (Bozeman, Myers, & Barish, 1997). Other inhaled agents, such as cyanide, are commonly found in household items and should be considered for potential poisonous exposure.

Determination of the wound depth and TBSA burned are used to calculate fluid resuscitation and patient management. Superficial (first degree) burns affect two to three layers of the epidermis and are not included in the determination of TBSA. Superficial burns are painful and have pink or red coloration with no blistering. Partial-thickness (second degree) burns extend through the epidermis and into the dermal layer, affecting local vascular and nerve structures. These wounds may be further described as deep- partial-thickness burns and may result in the need for skin grafting. Partial-thickness burns result in the formation of blisters or bullae because of the leakage of plasma, swelling, and red discoloration, with severe pain. The remaining blood supply allows for blanching of the skin surface to pressure. Deep-partial-thickness injuries may progress to full thickness, particularly if the wound becomes infected. Secondary injury from tissue ischemia and the inflammatory response results in this further tissue loss.

Full-thickness injuries extend through the dermal layer, causing coagulation of blood vessels and destruction of deep structures, including hair follicles, sweat glands, and nerves. This increases the risk for thermal deregulation, infection, and massive fluid and electrolyte losses, leading to hypovolemic shock. Full-thickness injuries have a leathery, white, or waxy appearance because of the loss of vascularity, termed *eschar*. The wounds do not blanch to pressure, and while cutaneous sensation is lost, severe pain may be experienced because of inflammation in the adjacent, viable tissue. Circumferential injuries should be noted, as these may require fasciotomy to preserve circulation.

TBSA may be assessed using several well-validated tools, including the rule of nines or rule of palms. Although these tools provide an easy and rapid means for estimation, the Lund and Browder method provides increased accuracy and accounts for developmental age (Shariati & Mirhaghi, 2014). It is important to recognize that no tool provides an exact measurement. Digital, computer-based technologies will likely become the future standard of care to better determine the extent of the injury (Zuo, Medina, & Tredget, 2017).

NURSING INTERVENTIONS, MANAGEMENT, AND IMPLICATIONS

Fluid losses because of a burn injury can lead to massive dehydration, shock, and electrolyte abnormalities. Patients with more than 20% TBSA require fluid resuscitation over the first 24 hours post-injury (American College of Surgeons Committee on Trauma, 2008). The Parkland or modified Brooke formulas are most commonly used to calculate volume requirements, based on TBSA and patient weight. Crystalloid replacement is the initial standard for fluid resuscitation, with lactated Ringer's solution most commonly given to prevent metabolic acidosis. Albumin may be included in the resuscitation of certain patient populations and is often used to maintain colloidal pressures in the vascular space (ABA, 2011; Serio-Melvin et al., 2017; Wang et al., 2014).

Traditional methods for the estimation of fluid requirements can lead to overresuscitation or "fluid creep," resulting in increased morbidity and mortality from burn injuries. Complications include compartment syndromes, respiratory failure, and ocular hypertension (Pruitt, 2000; Saffle, 2016). Protocols for adjustment of fluid resuscitation are beneficial for prevention as compared to standard formulas (Cancio, Salinas, & Kramer, 2016). Urine output is an important measure of successful fluid replacement and is used to guide ongoing fluid administration. The standard goal for urine output is 0.5 to 1.0 mL/kg/hr, whereas evidence supports a more liberal target of 0.25 to 0.5 mL/kg/hr (Cancio et al., 2016).

The extent of electrical injuries may not be evident on assessment. Cardiac monitoring should be instituted, and the patient observed for cardiac dysrhythmias. Entrance and exit wounds may be visible as electrical current typically flows to the ground; the patient may display delayed appearance of tissue necrosis along this path. Rhabdomyolysis is common in burns, and more so with electrical injury (Coban, 2014).

Analgesia is critical to the nursing care of the burn patient. Intramuscular medications should be avoided initially to avoid sequestration in the peripheral tissues, because of impaired circulation and the risk for delayed mobilization, leading to potential overdose. Opioid medications are appropriate to treat acute pain, and nonsteroidal anti-inflammatory drugs are used for pain as well as limiting the severity of the inflammatory reaction.

Normal stress responses may lead to paralytic ileus or curling ulcer; gastrointestinal prophylaxis should be instituted for the critically ill, although adequate nutrition via enteral or parenteral routes should be considered early on to promote healing.

Infection is the most common cause of delayed death following a burn injury. Tetanus immunization status should be assessed early on (ABA, 2011). Wound management, including excision of eschar, skin grafting, or the use of biologic skin substitutes provides some degree of prevention (ABA, 2016; Israel, Greenhalgh, & Gibson, 2017). Antimicrobial dressings include silver or antibiotic-based preparations. Systemic antimicrobials are often required for bacterial or fungal infections. As recovery can be a long process in severe burns, the risk of developing antibiotic resistance is substantial.

Preservation or restoration of mobility and function through splinting and regular repositioning begin from the time of admission. Collaboration with physical and occupational therapy is the key. Compression devices, such as ACE wraps and customized garments to promote venous return and limit keloid formation can impact cosmetic appearance, lymphatic drainage, and range of motion.

Nursing care should include an ongoing assessment for signs of depression, posttraumatic stress disorder (PTSD), and other effects of altered body image. Patients experience a wide range of emotions ranging from depression to resilience (Kool, Geenen, Egberts, Wanders, & Van Loey, 2017). Attendance to the emotional aspects of burn injury and recovery can affect the patient's trajectory and quality of life for many years.

Summary

Burn injuries represent trauma to the largest and one of the most multifunctional organs of the body. Loss of skin integrity affects nearly every system in the body, rapidly leading to shock and death unless treated appropriately. Nursing care of the burn victim requires timely and effective intervention to maintain and restore thermal regulation, offer resistance from infection, attain fluid and electrolyte balance, and to address the physiological and emotional complications of injury. Although injury management is the most obvious role for nursing, primary prevention and community education should remain a priority for the professional nurse.

American Burn Association. (2011). Advanced burn life support (ABLS) provider course manual. Retrieved from https://evidencebasedpractice.osumc.edu/Documents/Guidelines/ABLSProviderManual_20101018.pdf

American College of Surgeons Committee on Trauma. (2008). *Advanced trauma life support for doctors: ATLS student course manual* (8th ed.). Chicago, IL: American College of Surgeons.

Bozeman, W. P., Myers, R. A., & Barish, R. A. (1997). Confirmation of the pulse oximetry gap in carbon monoxide poisoning. *Annals of Emergency Medicine, 30*(5), 608–611.

Cancio, L. C., Salinas, J., & Kramer, G. C. (2016). Protocolized resuscitation of burn patients. *Critical Care Clinics, 32*(4), 599–610.

Coban, Y. K. (2014). Rhabdomyolysis, compartment syndrome and thermal injury. *World Journal of Critical Care Medicine, 3*(1), 1–7.

Israel, J. S., Greenhalgh, D. G., & Gibson, A. L. (2017). Variations in burn excision and grafting: A survey of the American Burn Association. *Journal of Burn Care & Research, 38*(1), e125–e132.

Kool, M. B., Geenen, R., Egberts, M. R., Wanders, H., & Van Loey, N. E. (2017). Patients' perspectives on quality of life after burn. *Burns,* S0305–4179(16), 30497-1. doi:10.1016/j.burns.2016.11.016

Pruitt, B. A. (2000). Protection from excessive resuscitation: "Pushing the pendulum back." *Journal of Trauma, 49*(3), 567–568.

Saffle, J. (2016). Fluid creep and over-resuscitation. *Critical Care Clinics, 32*(4), 587–598. doi:10.1016/j.cc.c.2016.06.007

Serio-Melvin, M. L., Salinas, J., Chung, K. K., Collins, C., Graybill, J. C., Harrington, D. T., . . . Cancio, L. C. (2017). Burn shock and resuscitation: Proceedings of a symposium conducted at the meeting of the American Burn Association, Chicago, IL, 21 April 2015. *Journal of Burn Care & Research, 38*(1), e423–e431.

Shariati, S. M., & Mirhaghi, A. (2014). A comparison of burn size estimation methods' accuracy applied by medical students. *Future of Medical Education Journal, 8*(4), 36–40.

Wang, C. H., Hsieh, W. H., Chou, H. C., Huang, Y. S., Shen, J. H., Yeo, Y. H., . . . Lee, C. C. (2014). Liberal versus restricted fluid resuscitation strategies in trauma patients: A systematic review and meta-analysis of randomized controlled trials and observational studies. *Critical Care Medicine, 42*(4), 954–961.

World Health Organization. (2016). Burns. Retrieved from http://www.who.int/mediacentre/factsheets/fs365/en

Zuo, K. J., Medina, A., & Tredget, E. E. (2017). Important developments in burn care. *Plastic and Reconstructive Surgery, 139*(1), 120e–138e.

■ BURNS: CLASSIFICATION AND SEVERITY

Melanie Gibbons Hallman
Lamon Norton

Overview

Burns result from thermal, electrical, chemical, mechanical, or radioactive injury to tissues. The extent of burn depth varies from superficial, involving the epidermis, to deeper structures, including muscle, bone, and organs, particularly the lungs (Stavrou et al., 2014). The cardiovascular and nervous systems are significantly impacted by electrical and lightning insults, potentially resulting in immediate cardiac or respiratory arrest (Moore, 2015b). Each year, more than 265,000 deaths occur worldwide related to burns, producing life-altering changes for victims and their families (Zuo, Medina, & Tredget, 2017). Serious burns result in a cascade of physiological responses that can influence morbidity and mortality for affected patients (Jewo & Fadeyibi, 2015).

Background

Annually, more than 500,000 people in the United States are evaluated in emergency departments for burns. Forty thousand people are hospitalized and an estimated 3,400 victims die (Rowan et al., 2015). Burn risk is highest in children. Younger children are more likely to sustain scald burns, whereas children older than 6 years of age are more likely to experience burns from flames. The length of time that tissues are exposed to a burn source, the intensity of the source, and skin thickness determine the degree of burn (Rau, Spears, & Petruska, 2014).

The most common etiologies of burns are thermal (flame, steam, scalds), electrical (alternating current [AC] and direct current [DC], lightning), and chemical (alkaline and acid). Burns impart injury by damaging skin surfaces, by impairing airways and lungs via inhalation burns, and by ingesting chemicals or objects capable of causing mucosal burns. Multiple organs, tissues, and body systems are susceptible to burns as primary or secondary injuries. Complications of burn shock, infection, respiratory compromise, and multisystem organ failure may result in death (Stavrou et al., 2014). Prevention or rapid correction of these complications is essential to achieving desirable outcomes for burn victims.

Thermal burns may directly affect only the epidermis and dermis, or may involve deeper structures of fat, muscle, and bone. The extent of injury caused by electrical burns is determined by the type of electrical current, either low voltage (less than 1,000 volts) or high voltage (more than 1,000 volts). Severity is also determined by the length of time the victim is in contact with an electrical current. Lower voltage and less time exposed to the electrical source usually causes less severe injury (Moore, 2015b). Chemical burns require early identification and rapid decontamination and treatment. The concentration and acidity or alkalinity of a chemical, combined with the length of time the skin or mucosa is exposed to the agent, determine the significance of a chemical burn (Moore, 2015a).

Burn depth is categorized as first (superficial), second (partial thickness), and third degree (full thickness), with a deepest fourth degree category being possible (Zuo et al., 2017). First-degree burns commonly are superficial and involve the epidermis only, requiring little or no treatment. Second-degree burns include both superficial and deep partial-thickness burns. Superficial partial-thickness burns include injuries to the epidermis and the outermost dermis. Redness, swelling, and discomfort or pain accompany. Deep partial-thickness burns damage both the epidermal and dermal layers, causing necrosis and intercellular edema, resulting in blister formation. Second-degree burns are typically more painful than first-degree burns, with loss of skin integrity and subsequent fluid depletion. Full-thickness burns damage the epidermis, dermis, and subcutaneous tissue. Tissue necrosis evolves, producing eschar (leathery, sloughing, dead tissue) and leaving no protective barrier for remaining structures. Eschar increases the risk for bacterial infection in burns. Edema, inflammation, and vasodilation accompany this type of burn, and little or no sensation remains (Rau et al., 2014). Complications, including shock, infection, respiratory compromise, and multisystem organ failure, are common in burn injuries and evolve during the acute phase of injury (Stavrou et al., 2014).

Clinical Aspects

Determining the percentage of total body surface area (TBSA) and depth of burns is the first step in burn resuscitation (Stavrou et al., 2014). Selection of appropriate resuscitation fluid and the correct amount to infuse over the first 24 hours following burn injury directly affect burn wound healing and chances for survival (Cancio, 2014). There are multiple tools available to calculate the approximate area of burns in the prehospital and acute-phase settings. The rule of nines, modified Lund and Browder chart, and Parkland formula are among the most common measurement systems used for this purpose. More advanced methods for determining burn extent, such as laser Doppler imaging, may be initiated 2 to 5 days following preliminary burn resuscitation in order to avoid over-resuscitation with fluids, which poses an additional danger to patient outcomes (Martin, Lundy, & Rickard, 2014). The starting point for fluid resuscitation is typically between 2 and 4 mL/kg/TBSA/24 hr (Lundy et al., 2016).

Evaluation and definitive management of airway, breathing, circulation, and fluid resuscitation are the most crucial elements of care for burn patients with life-threatening injuries. Early intubation is imperative for patients sustaining airway burns. A detailed history of injury, including time; mechanism; voltage, if electrical source of injury; details of decontamination for chemical sources; a chemical safety data sheet if available; associated trauma; syncope; smoke exposure; abuse potential; and prehospital treatment should be obtained. Wet linens should be rapidly replaced with sterile dry linens. All jewelry and clothing should be removed, and careful evaluation of nonburn injuries should be done. Placement of urinary catheter and nasogastric tube should be accomplished during the reassessment phase of care (Cancio, 2014).

Multiple factors must be considered following the acute phase of burn resuscitation. Hypothermia is an early complication of burns. The greater the surface area burned, the more vulnerable the patient is to development of hypothermia. It is important that the patient be kept warm and dry in order to conserve energy expended from the postburn hypermetabolic state. Persistent hypermetabolism and muscle wasting in extensive burns requires early nutritional reinforcement, but balancing calories and the composition of nutrients must be individualized to avoid overconsumption and increased risk for hyperglycemia (Rowan et al., 2015). Pruritus (itching) is an unfortunate and very common result of burns. It occurs in almost every pediatric burn patient and in as much as 87% of affected adults. Itching may not respond favorably to anti-inflammatory drugs and other analgesics (Stavrou et al., 2014). Optimal management of pruritus should be addressed after patient stabilization during hospitalization and in discharge planning.

Contractures manifest related to loss of skin elasticity and pose great risk of loss of physical function. Mobilization of joints should begin as soon as possible during hospitalization. Essentially, every body system and organ can be affected following a significant burn injury. Duodenal ulcers, anemia, hypermetabolic syndrome, insulin resistance, and liver dysfunction may develop in response to injury. In addition, other common sequelae, including central nervous system inflammation, cardiac dysfunction, and respiratory compromise, may develop. Compartment syndrome from circumferential burns may develop acutely, necessitating escharotomy or fasciotomy in any area of the body. Kidneys may be damaged by lactic acidosis and urine myoglobin production (Rau et al., 2014). Elevation in urine myoglobin levels is commonly associated with rhabdomyolysis, an associated complication of significant burn injuries (Moore, 2015b). Monitoring urine output is important to guiding titration of fluid resuscitation. It is important that IV fluids for burn resuscitation be initiated early, and that fluid intake and output be accurately measured, recorded, and reported. The urine output goal for adults is 30 to 50 mL/hr, and for children, weighing 30 kg or less, 1 mL/kg/hr (Lundy et al., 2016).

Deep vein thrombosis (DVT) prevention strategies should begin immediately in burn patients, since these injuries result in a hypercoagulable state (Zuo et al., 2017). Nurses should anticipate initiation of anticoagulant prophylaxis therapy. Burn severity impacts the degree of pain that patients experience. Long-term pain and sensory dysfunction accompany more extensive burns. Acutely burned patients may experience pain in the form of many abnormal sensations, including burning, dullness, itching, and dysesthesia (Rau et al., 2014). Frequent pain assessment and response to specific medications are important to determine the most effective pain treatment options for individual patients.

Prevention of infection in burn patients is crucial to survival. Burn sepsis typically presents within the first week postinjury. The most common causes of burn sepsis include pneumonia, central vascular access devices, and burn-injured skin. It is essential that health care workers maintain sterile technique and adhere to strict infection control practices while caring for burn patients. Antibiotic selection is carefully determined by specimen cultures to avoid pathogen resistance (Zuo et al., 2017). Significant burn wounds often require wound debridement and advanced wound care. Skin grafting is necessary for almost all full-thickness burns. Aesthetic changes related to deeper burns can have lasting effects on mental, emotional, and social well-being. Anxiety and depression are common especially within the first year after injury. Symptoms of posttraumatic stress disorder may emerge during the recovery process (Stavrou et al., 2014). Psychosocial support is essential in provision of holistic patient care and to improve long-term outcomes.

Rapid communication with a regional burn center is advised by American Burn Association guidelines for patients with burn extent greater than 10% of total body surface area. Patients with inhalation injuries; burns associated with trauma; burns of the hands, feet, perineum, genitalia, or over major joints regardless of surface area burned; any third-degree burn; electrical, chemical, or lightning injuries; pediatric patients; and special needs patients, including those with social, emotional, or rehabilitation needs, require consultation with a burn center (Cancio, 2014).

Summary

Burn injuries pose significant challenges related to acute and long-term care. Nurses should remain current and knowledgeable regarding burn pathophysiology, assessment and treatment significant to this patient population. Awareness of the most current evidence-based care available to burn patients assists nurses in providing them relative and efficient care.

Cancio, L. C. (2014). Initial assessment and fluid resuscitation of burn patients. *Surgical Clinics of North America*, 94(4), 741–754.

Jewo, P. I., & Fadeyibi, I. O. (2015). Progress in burns research: A review of advances in burn pathophysiology. *Annals of Burns and Fire Disasters*, 28(2), 105.

Lundy, J. B., Chung, K. K., Pamplin, J. C., Ainsworth, C. R., Jeng, J. C., & Friedman, B. C. (2016). Update on severe burn management for the intensivist. *Journal of Intensive Care Medicine*, 31(8), 499–510.

Martin, N. A. J., Lundy, J. B., & Rickard, R. F. (2014). Lack of precision of burn surface area calculation by UK armed forces medical personnel. *Burns*, 40, 246–250.

Moore, K. (2015a). Hot topics: Chemical burns in the emergency department. *Journal of Emergency Nursing*, 41(4), 364–365.

Moore, K. (2015b). Hot topics: Electrical injuries in the emergency department. *Journal of Emergency Nursing*, 41(5), 455–456.

Rau, K. K., Spears, R. C., & Petruska, J. C. (2014). The prickly, stressful business of burn pain. *Experimental Neurology*, 261, 752–756.

Rowan, M. P., Cancio, L. C., Elster, E. A., Burmeister, D. M., Rose, L. F., Natesan, S., . . . Chung, K. K. (2015). Burn wound healing and treatment: Review and advancements. *Critical Care*, *19*(1), 243–255.

Stavrou, D., Weissman, O., Tessone, A., Zilinsky, I., Holloway, S., Boyd, J., & Haik, J. (2014). Health related quality of life in burn patients—a review of the literature. *Burns*, *40*(5), 788–796.

Zuo, K. J., Medina, A., & Tredget, E. E. (2017). Important developments in burn care. *Plastic and Reconstructive Surgery*, *139*(1), 120e–138e.

■ CHEST PAIN

Sharon R. Rainer

Overview

Chest pain is a common chief complaint that adult patients may present with across all clinical practice settings. In the absence of trauma, chest pain is a symptom of an underlying problem or condition that can range from life-threatening to benign. Nontraumatic chest pain is among the most common reasons patients seek medical attention, including calls to 9-1-1 to active emergency medical services (EMS) for suspected heart attacks. The evaluation of patients presenting with chest pain in all practice settings, including the emergency department, is challenging as there are several possible causes for the chest pain, some of which may prove fatal (Gupta & Munoz, 2016). In some cases, chest pain may be chronic; typically chest pain is an acute presenting symptom that necessitates rapid and careful assessment by the nurses and the health care team.

Background

Cardiovascular disease, including ischemic heart disease, is the leading cause of death for both men and women in the United States and worldwide (Kochanek, Murphy, Xu, & Arias, 2014). More than half of the deaths that occur as a result of heart disease are in men. *Heart disease* is a term used to describe several conditions, many of which are related to plaque buildup in the walls of the coronary arteries. Every year, approximately 2 million Americans have a heart attack or stroke and, as a result of these conditions, more than 600,000 die from cardiovascular disease (Kochanek et al., 2014). Due to the fact that chest pain is a common symptom of heart disease, acute chest pain must always be considered cardiovascular in nature until proven otherwise.

Chest pain generally falls into two broad categories: cardiac and noncardiac chest pain. Myocardial ischemia, injury, or infarct is the category in which an interruption in blood flow to the heart to some degree causes cardiac chest pain. It is synonymous with the condition angina pectoris and is a concern for all patients presenting with chest pain until there is a reasonable degree of clinical certainty established by a clinician that the chest pain is originating from a noncardiac source. Other cardiopulmonary causes of chest pain may include diseases of the aorta, pneumonia, pulmonary embolism, pleurisy, and pneumothorax and these conditions may be life-threatening and cause serious harm to patients if left undiagnosed and if a delay in treatment ensues. Underlying noncardiopulmonary conditions that may present with chest pain include gastrointestinal diseases; musculoskeletal problems; and psychological problems, including anxiety/panic attacks, depression, and cocaine use (Kontos, Diercks, & Kirk, 2010).

Acute coronary syndrome (ACS) is a constellation of clinical signs and symptoms encompassing myocardial ischemia, injury, and infarct. ACS includes unstable angina, non–ST-segment elevation myocardial infarctions (non-STEMI), and ST-segment elevation myocardial infarction (STEMI). Chest pain may be the presenting symptom of ACS. Angina is chest pain or discomfort caused when your heart muscle does not get enough oxygen-rich blood. ACS occurs when the patient has underlying coronary artery disease (CAD). CAD is defined as the formation of an atherosclerotic plaque in one or more of the coronary arteries that restricts flow of blood and oxygen delivery to the cardiac tissue.

ACS can result in reversible or irreversible cardiac injury or necrosis. Due to the high-risk nature of ACS, the American Heart Association (AHA) and the American College of Cardiology (ACC) recently updated practice guidelines and performance measure to help clinicians adhere to a standard of care for patients who present with symptoms of ACS (Amsterdam et al., 2014).

In addition, noncardiac chest pain may have similar presenting features as cardiac chest pain and also has multiple causes requiring careful evaluation. During the initial evaluation, the clinician may determine that ACS is less likely than other noncardiac causes of chest pain but should be considered. The mnemonic CHEST PAIN is often used to recall some of the common causes of noncardiac chest pain (Newberry, Barnett, & Ballard, 2005): C (costochondritis, cocaine abuse), H (herpes zoster, hyperventilation), E (esophagitis/esophageal spasm), S (aortic valve stenosis), T (trauma), P (pulmonary embolism, pneumonia, pneumothorax, pericarditis, pancreatitis), A (angina/aortic dissection/aortic aneurysm), I (infarction/intervertebral disk disease), N (neuropsychiatric disorders [i.e., anxiety, depression]).

Clinical Aspects

ASSESSMENT

A nurse's diagnostic accuracy requires careful attention to history, especially attributes of pain, to determine cardiac causes of pain. The use of the PQRST mnemonic helps shed light on symptoms that may indicate cardiac chest pain—provokes/palliates/precipitating factors; quality; region/radiation; severity/associated symptoms; time/temporal relations (Newberry et al., 2005). However, neither quality nor intensity of chest pain is ever a sufficient attribute to rule in or rule out an underlying cardiac cause. Typically, clinicians rely on a comprehensive history and physical examination of the patient with chest pain in order to develop a list of differential diagnoses that may include cardiac and noncardiac reasons for the symptom (McConaghy & Oza, 2013). In addition, clinicians will often apply a validated clinical decision rule to predict heart disease as a cause of chest pain.

Risk factors are important considerations when obtaining a patient's history. Several evidence-based tools exist to help clinicians identify and predict CAD as the cause of chest pain (McConaghy & Oza, 2013). The risk factors typically used to identify those with CAD are as follows: age/gender (55 years and older in men or 65 years or older in women); known CAD, occlusive vascular disease, or cerebrovascular disease; pain that is worse with exercise; pain not reproducible by palpation; and patient assumption that pain is of cardiac origin. A recent study identified that only 1% of those patients with none or one of these clinical features had CAD, whereas 63% of the patients with four or five of the features had CAD. The study further suggests that patients with chest pain and four or five of these components require urgent workups for chest pain and suspected ACS (McConaghy & Oza, 2013).

A nurse may be the first member of the health care team to identify and document risk factors associated with heart disease to help inform the history and physical exam done by clinicians. These risk factors are broadly categorized as medical conditions, behaviors, family history, and other factors (Kochanek, et al., 2014). Medical conditions include hypertension, hypercholesterolemia, and diabetes. Behaviors refer to those risk factors considered to be modifiable. These risk factors include diet, exercise, obesity, and tobacco and alcohol use. Family history, age, gender, and ethnicity are nonmodifiable, genetic characteristics that may predispose a patient to heart disease.

Therefore, it is important to determine those patients at risk for CAD who may be experiencing signs and symptoms of ACS. Chest pain may be the main symptom; however, it may not be present at all or may be vague in nature. Nurses should assess for other symptoms of ACS, including the following (O'Donnell, Mckee, O'Brien, Mooney, & Moser, 2012):

- Substernal pain that occurs with exertion and alleviates with rest
- Chest pain lasting for 20 minutes or longer
- Dull, heavy pressure in or on the chest
- Sensation of a heavy object on the chest
- Chest pain radiating to the back, neck, jaw, left arm, or shoulder, right arm, or back
- Chest pain affected by inspiration
- Chest pain not reproducible with chest palpation
- Accompanying diaphoresis
- Pain initiated by stress, exercise, large meals, sex, or any activity that increases the body's demand upon the heart for blood
- Fatigue
- Extreme fatigue or edema after exercise
- Shortness of breath
- Levine's sign: Chest discomfort described as a clenched fist over the sternum (the patient will clench his or her fist and rest it on or over his or her sternum)
- Angor animi: Fear of impending doom or death
- Pain high in the abdomen or chest, nausea and extreme fatigue after exercise, back pain, and edema can occur in anyone but are more common in women
- Nausea, lightheadedness, or dizziness

The 12-lead EKG is the test of choice in the initial evaluation of patients with chest pain (Hollander, Than, & Mueller, 2016; Overbaugh, 2009). ST-segment changes (elevation or depression), new-onset left bundle branch block, presence of Q waves, and new-onset T wave inversions increase the likelihood of ACS or acute MI. Nurses are not responsible for interpreting the EKG; however, rapid identification of ischemia, injury, and infarct is important so that treating clinicians or EMS can be rapidly alerted. The AHA/ACC recommends that patients presenting with acute chest pain symptom have a 12-lead EKG performed and interpreted by a health care provider within 10 minutes of the patient's arrival to the emergency department (Amsterdam et al., 2014).

NURSING INTERVENTIONS, MANAGEMENT, AND IMPLICATIONS

Providing nursing care to patients with chest pain can be challenging across all practice settings due to the broad range of underlying possible diseases that may exist. A nurse who obtains vital signs, including temperature, heart rate, blood pressure, respiration rate, oxygen saturation, and pain intensity, as close to the onset of chest pain as possible is making a significant contribution to the identification of a life- threatening emergency. A systematic approach is essential to determine whether the patient is stable or unstable. Tachycardia and hypotension are indicative of important hemodynamic changes that may be associated with an acute MI, cardiogenic shock, pulmonary embolism, pericarditis with tamponade, or tension pneumothorax. Acute aortic emergencies, such as aortic dissection, may present with severe hypertension but may be associated with hypotension when there is coronary arterial compromise or dissection into the pericardium. Tachycardia and hypoxia may indicate a pulmonary cause of the chest pain. The presence of low-grade fever is usually nonspecific but may be found in patients with acute MI and thromboembolism in addition to infection. Therefore, an accurate set of vital signs completed and documented in a timely manner is an important nursing intervention contributing to the workup of patients with chest pain (Overbaugh, 2009).

When a patient is diagnosed with angina, the nurse will carry out interventions to decrease damage to the heart muscle. Initial drug therapies that may be ordered include aspirin, oxygen, nitroglycerin, and morphine. Nurses often use the mnemonic MONA to recall these initial treatments, although MONA does not specify the correct order of administration. Patients with suspected ACS are often ordered 325 mg of aspirin by mouth as soon as possible after symptoms begin, unless contraindicated (Newberry et al., 2005; Overbaugh, 2009).

Signs and symptoms of ACS are not sufficient to make a clinical diagnosis, so clinicians rely on diagnostic testing. Identifying life-threatening ischemia, infarct, and injury is important in the initial evaluation of chest pain. Nurses are instrumental in facilitating the workup of chest pain patients. This may involve identifying risk factors and changes in symptoms. In addition, as the EKG and history and physical examination are often insufficient alone in diagnosing acute MI and ACS, clinicians in the acute setting will order blood tests to measure the concentration of cardiac troponin, a biomarker for cardiac injury and ischemia (Hollander et al., 2016).

Patient education focused on prevention of cardiovascular disease in all age groups is an important nursing intervention. By educating both the young and old on identifying and lowering modifiable risk factors related to cardiovascular disease, nurses promote health and prevent complications of heart disease. Interventions to help patients adhere to a cardiac-prudent diet, exercise, avoiding tobacco, managing stress, and controling diseases like hypertension and diabetes are part of a thorough intervention geared toward patients with chest pain and suspected CAD.

OUTCOMES

Chest pain represents a high-volume, high-risk clinical problem across all practice settings. Some 20 million patients in North America and Europe present to emergency departments annually with symptoms suggestive of ACS (Hollander et al., 2016). Rapid and careful early identification of those most at risk of dying from an acute MI or ACS is the goal of quality health care delivery. In order to save lives, nurses must be vigilant in identifying patients with chest pain and possible ACS as well as facilitate the workup of noncardiac reasons for chest pain. In some outpatient or community clinical settings, the nurse may need to activate the EMS for patients experiencing chest pain so that a thorough investigation into the cause can be conducted by an emergency clinician. In other clinical settings, such as in patient units or the emergency department, rapid prioritization of the patient with chest pain to ensure that vital signs and an EKG are safely and quickly obtained is imperative to facilitating the thorough assessment and treatment of the patient.

Summary

Chest pain is a common presenting symptom of patients who may be experiencing a host of underlying medical conditions. Although most patients presenting with chest pain are not having an acute MI, determining the cause of their chest pain warrants a careful medical and nursing evaluation. Given that the causes of chest pain can range from musculoskeletal disorders to life-threatening MI, and deadly aortic dissection or pulmonary embolism, nurses on the front lines must have a high level of suspicion about potentially life-threatening causes. Nurses are likely to be the first health care professional to encounter patients with chest pain. Therefore, the nurse must exercise vigilance and diligence in facilitating rapid clinical evaluation of all patients with chest pain in order to save lives and expedite the identification of the underlying cause.

Amsterdam, E. A., Wenger, N. K., Brindis, R. G., Casey, D. E., Ganiats, T. G., Holmes, D. R., . . . Zieman, S. J. (2014). 2014 AHA/ACC guideline for the management of patients with non-ST-elevation acute coronary syndromes: A report of the American College of Cardiology/American Heart Association Task Force on Practice Guidelines. *Circulation*, *130*(25), e344–e426. doi:10.1161/cir.0000000000000134

Gupta, R., & Munoz, R. (2016). Evaluation and management of chest pain in the elderly. *Emergency Medicine Clinics of North America*, *34*(3), 523–542. doi:10.1016/ j.emc.2016.04.006

Hollander, J. E., Than, M., & Mueller, C. (2016). State-of-the-art evaluation of emergency department patients presenting with potential acute coronary syndromes. *Circulation*, *134*(7), 547–564. doi:10.1161/circulationaha.116.021886

Kochanek K. D., Murphy S. L., Xu J., & Arias, E. (2014). *Mortality in the United States, 2013. NCHS data brief, no. 178.* Hyattsville, MD: National Center for Health Statistics, Centers for Disease Control and Prevention, U.S. Department of Health and Human Services.

Kontos, M. C., Diercks, D. B., & Kirk, J. D. (2010). Emergency department and office-based evaluation of patients with chest pain. *Mayo Clinic Proceedings, 85*(3), 284–299. doi:10.4065/mcp.2009.0560

McConaghy, J. R., & Oza, R. S. (2013). Outpatient diagnosis of acute chest pain in adults. *American Family Physician, 87*(3), 177–182.

Newberry, L., Barnett, G. K., & Ballard, N. (2005). A new mnemonic for chest pain assessment. *Journal of Emergency Nursing, 31*(1), 84–85. doi:10.1016/j.jen.2004.10.005

O'Donnell, S., McKee, G., O'Brien, F., Mooney, M., & Moser, D. K. (2012). Gendered symptom presentation in acute coronary syndrome: A cross sectional analysis. *International Journal of Nursing Studies, 49*(11), 1325–1332. doi:10.1016/j.ijnurstu.2012.06.002

Overbaugh, K. J. (2009). Acute coronary syndrome. *American Journal of Nursing, 109*(5), 42–52. doi:10.1097/01.naj.0000351508.39509.e2

■ CHILD ABUSE AND NEGLECT

Patricia M. Speck
Pamela Harris Bryant
Tedra S. Smith
Sherita K. Etheridge
Steadman McPeters

Overview

For a majority of states (46 out of 50), child abuse and neglect are serious public health problems. Among states contributing to a report published in 2014, there were 6.6 million children involved in 3.6 million reports of child abuse and neglect nationwide; authorities validated 2.2 million or 61%, with an incidence rate of 29 per 1,000 children (U.S. Department of Health and Human Services [HHS], 2016, p. ix). Professionals who have contact with children as part of their job are mandatory reporters responsible for over 45% of the reported cases (p. ix). Of the children evaluated, the majority had one report (83%), and some had two or more reports (16%; p. x). The children with validated experiences were neglected (75%) and physically abused (17%), but if the child experienced both, only one category counted toward maltreatment (p. x). Other types of maltreatment comprise the remaining percentage of validated reports. The mortality rate was 2.13 deaths per 100,000, or 1,546 fatalities (p. x). Boys had a higher fatality rate than girls (2.48 vs. 1.82 per 100,000), and Caucasians died more frequently (43%), followed by different minority populations of children (African American—30.3%; Hispanic—15.1%; p. x). The financial impact of abuse and neglect of children in 2008 was $124 billion (Fong, Brown, Florence, & Mercy, 2012). Perpetrators of child abuse and neglect were mostly women (54.1%), White (48.8%), mistreating two or more children (HHS, 2016, p. x).

Background

The Child Abuse Prevention and Treatment Act (CAPTA), with reauthorization, defined behaviors as acts of child abuse and neglect as:

> Any recent act or failure to act on the part of a parent or caretaker which results in death, serious physical or emotional harm, sexual abuse or exploitation; or an act or failure to act, which presents an imminent risk of serious harm. (p. viii)

Maltreatment includes psychological maltreatment (emotional abuse), neglect (including endangerment), and physical and sexual abuse (HHS, 2016). The Justice for Victims of Trafficking Act of 2015 (JVTA) requires states to report the number of identified sex-trafficked children younger than 18 years, allowing states to provide services and report identified victims up to age 24 years (Civic Impulse, 2017). Of the adults rescued at 18 years of age, overwhelmingly, their introduction to the industry began between the ages of 12 and 14 years. These legislative mandates at the national and state levels are helpful to the registered nurses responsible for evaluating injury in pediatric populations and reporting suspicions of abuse or neglect.

The children most at risk for child abuse and neglect are in chaotic or traumatized families, many experiencing social and personal environments not conducive to development or emotional health. Disparities and social determinants as risk factors diminish attainment of health outcomes. Social determinants include the environment and attitudes, exposure to crime and violence, disease and access to health care, and personal and support systems (Office of Disease Prevention and Health Promotion, 2017). Chronic stress in environments, whether from the individual's disease, the family, the community, or the system, increases hormonal dysregulation predisposing the child to increased risk of violence and disease (McEwen, 1998).

Building on the stress and adaptation theories of the 1990s, emerging science focuses on epigenetic transference of cellular environments that predisposes offspring to poor health outcomes (Whitman & Kondis, 2016). In fact, physically and sexually victimized children display at least one mental health disorder by age 18 (Silverman, Reinherz, & Giaconia, 1996), which passes on to their children, and is predictive of future victim experiences.

A tool to measure adverse childhood experiences (ACEs) validated that there is a connection between ACEs and health outcomes, including early death (Felitti et al., 1998). The research continues. Diseases, once thought to be a result of genetics, may be a result of physical changes following significant ACEs; in fact, the impact of ACEs affects all human body systems where earlier stress results in risk behaviors, chronic disease, and early death (Anda et al., 2009; Brown et al., 2009).

Pregnant women and their developing fetus(s), newborns, infants, and children exposed to violence experience elevated stress hormones and begin a quest to escape or calm the "fear" response. The neuroendocrine system creates the brainstem irritation response (fear) to a threat and the hormonal sequelae of several hormonal pathways, including the hypothalamic–pituitary–adrenal (HPA) axis (Malenka, Nestler, & Hyman, 2009). The resulting "fight-or-flight" response causes an elevation in stress hormones, cascading and triggering other hormones in the stressed environment of the body. The hormones in the stress response originate from the primitive emotional midbrain, stimulated by the brain stem in response to fear, resulting in a constellation of symptoms, called general adaptation syndrome (GAS; Selye, 1974). *The victim responds normally to abnormal stresses.* However, the stress hormones change end-organ function. Today, research documents change in response to chronic stress, for example, digestion, immune system, mood, anxiety, energy storage (fat), and other deleterious alterations, specifically in a child's brain architecture, affecting learning, behavior, and long-term health (Child Welfare Information Gateway, 2015). The child is handicapped socially and developmentally by the exposure, usually without sensitive identification and intervention to mitigate the normal response to serious stresses in the family. The health outcomes include behavioral aberrations, hypertension, obesity, autoimmune diseases, poor school performance, adoption of risk behaviors (with subsequent disease or injury), and others. Understanding the underlying physiology of stress and trauma in childhood prepares registered nurses to address obvious symptoms that lead to future poor health choices and outcomes.

Clinical Aspects

It is important that practicing registered nurses recognize that child abuse or neglect is caused by a parent (HHS, 2016). Each state defines child abuse differently, but all states follow federal legislation, so the practicing registered nurse must be familiar with state legislation related to reporting child maltreatment. If there is a suspicion of child abuse, the registered nurse (caring for a pediatric patient) is a mandatory reporter in every state and all U.S. territories (HHS, 2016; Parrish, 2016).

Nurses must receive *education* about abuse and neglect to successfully screen and document developmental milestones at all ages and developmental stages. The first requirement is to understand elements of abuse and neglect, which include emotional abuse, such as belittling the child to outright screaming obscenities; physical abuse, such as pinching, pushing, slapping, and shoving the child at any developmental age or chronologic age; and outcomes from the abuses, which include depression, self-injurious behavior, suicide, or homicide (HHS, 2016).

Screening for stresses and developmental milestones identifies at-risk children and gives the registered nurse an opportunity to provide anticipatory guidance and intervention (Larkin, Shields, & Anda, 2012), which may include reporting the event(s) to the state's child services agency. Registered nurses caring for pediatric populations need a strong institutional policy and procedure for the management of abused and neglected pediatric patients, as well as the skills to identify, mitigate, and prevent early relational stresses between the child and his or her primary parent or caretaker. The ACEs questions, when considered a vital sign and asked at every visit, provide the opportunity to intervene on multiple levels. The answers to the questions help the nurse monitor to prevent child abuse and neglect. The assessment domains for pediatric registered nurse providers include the areas of "language, literacy, and math," but also "interpersonal interaction and opportunities for self-expression" (Snow & Van Hemel, 2008, p. 22). Guidelines and validated tools for assessment at each developmental stage prepare the registered nurse provider to assist nonoffending parents with a comprehensive plan for intervention to mitigate the impact of abuse and neglect. Functional approaches for nurses require special training in the assessment of all children, including challenges and deficits in abilities. Parents from a variety of cultures, including minority and immigrant families, also positively respond to the anticipatory guidance provided by the registered nurses.

Using the totality of nursing education, the registered nurse as an expert in growth and development of children, incorporates Maslow's hierarchy of needs to include trusting one's environment at all developmental stages. When the closest caregiver (usually a parent) is unable or unwilling to provide the nurture, recognition is the first step to planning the necessary interventions to protect the safety of the child. Recommending prevention and parenting programs for at-risk families is a good first step, including home visitation or more frequent visits or phone calls to check on mother and child well-being. This is particularly important for the teen mother, who may be surviving a chaotic upbringing, experiencing the predictable high-risk behaviors of adolescence, and teen pregnancy.

All child assessments should be head to toe and include all mucous membrane areas (ears, eyes, nose, and throat and anogenital). The expectation with each visit is that the child evaluation includes behavior and skin injuries, asking about the manner and cause of the injury detected, and, if serious or inconsistent, reasons for delay in identification and treatment. The registered nurse assessment for child abuse or neglect is descriptive only, documenting objective information and monitoring activity between mother or caregiver and infant or child. If registered nurses are the first to suspect abuse or neglect, they are mandated reporters, regardless of other professionals' opinions. Not all injury or neglect is intentional, so the institutions designated to complete the comprehensive evaluation of the child, family, and social situation, while trying for all, are mandated to exercise legal authority over the child's safety. Throughout the process, the registered nurse's role is therapeutic and helpful, explaining the process of reporting and providing clarity to the process of the investigation. Nurses work with the institutional team to provide nursing care, assessment, and documentation, important for the safety and planning of the pediatric patient. In event of child removal from the home, the registered nurse's role is to comfort the nonoffending parent, provide community resources, and explain (to their ability) processes through anticipatory guidance.

Summary

Children depend on safe and secure environments created by their parent or caregiver to provide the love and support needed at all developmental stages and ages. Child abuse and neglect represent an inability of the responsible adult to nurture the child. During pregnancy, the stress of the mother transfers to the fetus and can result in spontaneous abortion; after delivery, lack of maternal nurture arrests the infant's development and changes the brain architecture, so the child is unable to navigate a learning environment. Stress creates anxiety in older children, which leads to the overproduction of stress hormones, crippling the capacity of the children to move through Maslow's basic hierarchical steps toward adulthood and independence.

Domestic violence, poverty, trafficking of human families, war, drug use (covered in other entries), neglect, and abuse by parent or caregivers create additional stress responses in the infant and child that doom the child to adopt risky behaviors beginning as young as 6 or 8 years of age. Registered nurses are in the position to recognize the child subjected to violence and the subsequent stress this causes. The developmental milestones provide clues for the pediatric registered nurses to begin the inquiry into ACEs, scales measuring depression and anxiety, and other validated methods for assessing mother and child. Recognition of the health signs of hypertension, obesity, risk behavior, mental health diagnoses, neglect, and other signs of fear in an infant or child provide the opportunity for all registered nurses to intervene, report, and participate in interprofessional team collaboration to create safe and secure environments for all children.

Anda, R. F., Dong, M., Brown, D. W., Felitti, V. J., Giles, W. H., Perry, G. S., . . . Dube, S. R. (2009). The relationship of adverse childhood experiences to a history of premature death of family members. *BMC Public Health*, *9*, 106. doi:10.1186/1471-2458-9-106

Brown, D. W., Anda, R. A., Tiemeier, H., Felitti, V. J., Edwards, V. J., Croft, J. B., & Giles, W. H. (2009). Adverse childhood experiences and the risk of premature mortality. *American Journal of Preventive Medicine 37*(5), 389–396. doi:10.1016/j.amepre.2009.06.021

Child Welfare Information Gateway. (2015). *Understanding the effects of maltreatment on brain development*. Washington, DC: U.S. Department of Health and Human Services, Children's Bureau.

Civic Impulse. (2017). H.R. 181—114th Congress: Justice for Victims of Trafficking Act of 2015. Retrieved from https://www.govtrack.us/congress/bills/114/hr181

Felitti, V. J., Anda, R. F., Nordenberg, D., Williamson, D. F., Spitz, A. M., Edwards, V., . . . Marks, J. S. (1998). Relationship of childhood abuse and household dysfunction to many of the leading causes of death in adults: The adverse childhood experiences (ACE) study. *American Journal of Preventive Medicine*, *14*, 245–258. doi:10.1016/S0749-3797(98)00017-8

Fang, X., Brown, D. S., Florence, C., & Mercy, J. A. (2012). The economic burden of child maltreatment in the United States and implications for prevention. *Child Abuse & Neglect*, *36*(2), 156–165. doi:10.1016/j.chiabu.2011.10.006

Larkin, H., Shields, J. J., & Anda, R. F. (2012). The health and social consequences of adverse childhood experiences (ACE) across the lifespan: An introduction to prevention and intervention in the community. *Journal of Prevention and Intervention in the Community*, *40*(4), 263–270. doi:10.1080/10852352.2012.707439

Malenka, R. C., Nestler, E. J., & Hyman, S. E. (2009). Neural and neuroendocrine control of the internal milieu. In A. Sydor & R. Y. Brown (Eds.), *Molecular neuropharmacology: A foundation for clinical neuroscience* (pp. 246, 248–259). New York, NY: McGraw-Hill Medical.

McEwen, B. S. (1998). Stress, adaptation, and disease: Alostasis and allostatic load. *Annals of the New York Academy of Sciences*, *840*, 33–44. doi:10.1111/j.1749-6632.1998.tb09546.x

Office of Disease Prevention and Health Promotion. (2017). Determinants of health. In *Healthy People 2020*. Retrieved from https://www.healthypeople.gov/2020/about/foundation-health-measures/Determinants-of-Health#social

Parrish, R. (2016). Legal system intervention in cases of child maltreatment. In A. P. Giardino, L. Shaw, P. M. Speck, & E. R. Giardino (Eds.), *Recognition of child abuse for the mandated reporter* (pp. 321–356). St. Louis, MO: STM Learning.

Selye, H. (1974). *Stress without distress*. Philadelphia, PA: Lippincott.

Silverman, A. B., Reinherz, H. Z., & Giaconia, R. M. (1996). The long-term sequelae of child and adolescent abuse: A longitudinal community study. *Child Abuse & Neglect*, *20*(8), 709–723.

Snow, C. E., & Van Hemel, S. B. (2008). *Early childhood assessment: Why, what, and how*. Washington, DC: National Research Council of the National Academies.

U.S. Department of Health & Human Services, Administration for Children and Families, Administration on Children, Youth and Families, Children's Bureau. (2016). Child maltreatment, 2014. Retrieved from http://www.acf.hhs.gov/programs/cb/research-data-technology/statistics-research/child-maltreatment

Whitman, B. V., & Kondis, J. (2016). Understanding the short-term and long-term effects of child abuse. In A. P. Giardino, L. Shaw, P. M. Speck, & E. R. Giardino (Eds.), *Recognition of child abuse for the mandated reporter* (pp. 165–178). St. Louis, MO: STM Learning.

■ *CLOSTRIDIUM DIFFICILE* INFECTION

Anita Sundaresh

Overview

Clostridium difficile, commonly referred to as *C. difficile* or *C. diff*, is an infectious pathogen that can result in life-threatening inflammation of the colon. The presence of symptoms, such as diarrhea and colonoscopic findings consistent with pseudomembranous colitis, or a positive stool specimen stool for *C. difficile* toxins or toxigenic C, establish a diagnosis of a *C. difficile* infection (Cohen et al., 2010). Early pharmacologic treatment and meticulous hand hygiene are essential components of nursing care for the patient with a *C. difficile* infection (CDI; Fernanda et al., 2015).

Background

C. difficile is a gram-positive anaerobic bacterium. It is transmitted from patients through the hands of health care personnel or in the environment by the ingestion of spores (Lessa, Gould, & Mc Donald, 2012). "Disruption of normal gut flora, typically by exposure to antimicrobials, allows *C. difficile* to proliferate, causing a broad spectrum of clinical manifestations that can range from asymptomatic carriage to diarrhea of varying severity to fulminant colitis and even death" (Lessa et al., 2012, p. 65). Fluid secretion, inflammation, and mucosal damage develop leading to diarrhea if the strain is toxigenic, namely, toxin A and B, resulting in a condition called *pseudomembranous colitis* (Barbut & Petit, 2001). The average incubation period for *C. difficile* is 1 to 20 days, and this pathogen is resistant to most disinfectants, heat, and some alcohol-based antiseptic agents. Therefore, the most effective strategy for *C. difficile* prevention is judicious and frequent handwashing with soap and water (Agha, 2010).

The mode of transmission of *C. difficile* is the fecal–oral route. Contributing factors to the development of CDI are broad-spectrum antibiotics, such as penicillin, penicillin associated with a beta-lactamase inhibitor, cephalosporin, and clindamycin, which alter the composition of the intestinal flora or gut microbiome (Barbut & Petit, 2001). Some other risk factors are medications and performance of nonsurgical gastrointestinal procedures such as a nasogastric tube, stool softeners, and antiulcer medications (Barbut & Petit, 2001).

Populations of individuals who are most at risk are patients in acute- or long-term care settings (Barbut & Petit, 2001). Patients with a CDI may present with unexplained leukocytosis and complain of abdominal pain. Owing to the toxigenic effects of the *C. difficile*, an innate immune response ensues, resulting in leukocytosis. As the severity of the infection worsens, patients may develop abdominal pain or distention related to a colonic ileus or toxic dilatation (Barbut & Petit, 2001). Complications of severe *C. difficile* colitis include dehydration, bowel perforation, hypotension, renal failure, systemic inflammatory response syndrome, sepsis, and death (Cohen et al., 2010). The risk of CDI is greater in the elderly population and disproportionately affects elderly females more frequently than their male counterparts (Agha, 2010).

A colectomy can be considered in patients who are severely ill. If surgical management is deemed necessary, then a subtotal colectomy preserving the rectum can be performed. The serum lactate levels have been shown to predict the perioperative mortality, in which higher serum lactate levels are associated with a high probability of death (Cohen et al., 2010). Having a subtotal colectomy can impact a patient's quality of life because CDI can be debilitating (Cohen et al., 2010). "*C. difficile* accounts for 20%–30% of cases of antibiotic-associated diarrhea and is the most commonly recognized cause of infectious diarrhea in health care settings" (Cohen et al., 2010, p. 435). The management of CDI cost $55.2 million and involved 55,380 inpatient hospital stays in Massachusetts from the years 1999 to 2003 (Cohen et al., 2010).

Clinical Aspects

ASSESSMENT

Assessing the patient with suspected or documented *C. difficile* begins with a health history and physical examination. The history should include number of bowel movements, color, odor, onset of changes, and any hospitalizations and recent medications, especially antibiotics. Stools should be collected for analysis and the number, color, consistency, and odor should also be documented.

NURSING INTERVENTIONS, MANAGEMENT, AND IMPLICATIONS

It is important for nurses to understand the diagnosis and treatment of CDI as it is the leading cause of hospital-associated illness affecting the health care system (Surawicz et al., 2013). Patients who are experiencing high-volume diarrhea with a recent history of antibiotic exposure should be presumed to have CDI. Stool specimens should be collected to verify the presence of the pathogen. Stringent contact precautions and hand hygiene should be implemented to prevent the transmission of the pathogen.

Hand hygiene is a critical aspect of the clinical care of a patient with a CDI that can mitigate transmission of the pathogen to others. It is important for nurses to perform hand hygiene to prevent *C. difficile* spores from reaching patients. Donning gowns and gloves before entering the patients' rooms can also be an effective barrier method. The use of disposable thermometers for patients who have CDI can reduce the spread of CDI (Rupnik, Wilcox, & Gerding, 2009).

Restrictive use of antibiotics should be the number one priority for preventing CDI. It is also important to wear vinyl gloves or to cohort patients with CDI to control outbreaks. "Control measures include strict antibiotic policy, a high degree of suspicion of *C. difficile*, prompt diagnosis, isolation, and treatment of infected patients, and implantation of enteric precautions" (Barbut & Petit, 2001, p. 409). It is important to maintain contact precautions until diarrhea has resolved (Cohen et al., 2010).

Nurses are encouraged to provide evidence-based supportive care for patients who are infected with *C. difficile*. Treatment should include intravenous fluid resuscitation, electrolyte replacement, and pharmacological venous thromboembolism prophylaxis. It is strongly recommended to discontinue use of any antimicrobial agent. Patients who have mild to moderate disease should be treated with metronidazole 500 mg orally three times a day for 10 days. Failure to respond to metronidazole in 5 to 7 days should prompt providers to switch treatment to vancomycin. Patients who are severely affected by CDI should be treated with vancomycin 125 mg four times a day for 10 days. Nurses should know the dosage recommendations to anticipate the medication needs of patients affected with CDI (Surawicz et al., 2013).

It is necessary to control and prevent the transmission of *C. difficile* in the hospital. The incidence of CDI can be decreased if hospitals institute a hospital-based infection control program. It is not recommended to routinely screen for CDIs to reduce the risk of the infection. Contact precautions should be initiated once a patient is confirmed to have a CDI. All health care workers and visitors should incorporate hand hygiene and use of gloves and gowns on entering the room of infected patients. It is also beneficial for nurses to use single-use disposable equipment to prevent the transmission of the disease. Disinfecting environmental surfaces with an Environmental Protective Agency (EPA)-recommended disinfectant can help to stop the spread of infection. Isolating the patients to a private room or combining patients with people who have *C. difficile* is recommended (Surawicz et al., 2013).

OUTCOMES

An early diagnosis of a CDI can significantly enhance a patient's mortality risk, and an effective use of contact precautions, as well as hand hygiene, can mitigate the likelihood of transmission of the pathogen to others. The adherence to evidence-based practice and clinical guidelines have also shown to minimize the transmission of *C. difficile*. Health care workers must comply with hand hygiene to prevent the transmission of the disease. It is necessary to maintain contact precautions until diarrhea is resolved. Given the variance in clinical manifestations of CDIs, nurses must be aware that the most judicious strategy to prevent a CDI is the appropriate administration of an antimicrobial therapy, and for patients with a CDI hand hygiene, contact precautions, and administration of the pathogen-specific antibiotic aid in reducing the patient's mortality risk (Cohen et al., 2010).

Summary

The delivery of nursing care must focus on reducing infections among the elderly and screening patients who are affected by CDI. Tools must be developed to identify virulence factors for CDIs, especially in the toxin-variant strains (Rupnik et al., 2009). Studies must also be conducted in populations that were previously considered at low risk, such as children and pregnant women. Separate studies must be conducted among patients who have mild and severe CDI. Further studies need to be done on the use of probiotics as a preventative measure for CDI. "Lack of standardization of preparations, including quality control to minimize variations in bacterial counts during storage, and the possibility of inducing bacteremia or fungaemia remain drawbacks of probiotic use" (Rupnik et al., 2009, p. 534).

Agha, M. (2012). Epidemiology and pathogenesis of *C. difficile* and MRSA in the light of current NHS control policies: A policy review. *Annals of Medicine and Surgery, 1,* 39–43.

Barbut, F., & Petit, J. C. (2001). Epidemiology of *Clostridium difficile*-associated infections. *Clinical Microbiology and Infection, 7*(8), 405–410.

Cohen, S. H., Gerding, D. N., Johnson, S., Kelly, C. P., Loo, V. G., McDonald, L. C., . . . Wilcox, M. H.; Society for Healthcare Epidemiology of America; Infectious Diseases Society of America. (2010). Clinical practice guidelines for *Clostridium difficile* infection in adults: 2010 update by the Society for Healthcare Epidemiology of America (SHEA) and the Infectious Diseases Society of America (IDSA). *Infection Control and Hospital Epidemiology, 31*(5), 431–455.

Fernanda, C. L., Yi, M., Wendy, M. B., Zintars, G., Ghinwa, K. D., John, R. D., . . . Clifford, L. M. (2015). Burden of Clostridium difficile infection in the United States. *New England Journal of Medicine, 372,* 825–834.

Lessa, F. C., Gould, C. V., & McDonald, L. C. (2012). Current status of *Clostridium difficile* infection epidemiology. *Clinical Infectious Diseases, 55*(Suppl. 2), S65–S70.

Rupnik, M., Wilcox, M. H., & Gerding, D. N. (2009). *Clostridium difficile* infection: New developments in epidemiology and pathogenesis. *Nature Reviews Microbiology, 7*(7), 526–536.

Surawicz, C. M., Brandt, L. J., Binion, D. G., Ananthakrishnan, A. N., Curry, S. R., Gilligan, P. H., . . . Zuckerbraun, B. S. (2013). Guidelines for diagnosis, treatment, and prevention of *Clostridium difficile* infections. *American Journal of Gastroenterology, 108*(4), 478–498; quiz 499.

■ CONTINUOUS VENO-VENOUS HEMOFILTRATION

Ian N. Saludares

Overview

Renal-replacement therapies (RRTs) represent a cornerstone in the management of severe acute kidney injury. This area of intensive care and nephrology has undergone significant improvement and evolution in recent years. Continuous RRTs have been a major focus of new technological and treatment strategies. RRT is being used increasingly in the intensive care unit (ICU), not only for renal indications but also for other organ-supportive strategies. Continuous veno-venous hemofiltration (CVVH) is one of the methods used in RRT. RRTs are an extracorporeal blood-purification therapy intended to compensate for impaired renal function over relatively short periods of time (Ronco et al., 2015).

This short-term treatment is used in ICU patients with acute or chronic renal failure. Usually, hemodialysis is typically done for patients with kidney failure. However, if the patient has low blood pressure or other contraindications for hemodialysis, CVVH may be a necessary alternative. Access to the circulation for CVVH is a large-bore dual-lumen central venous catheter designated for hemodialysis. CVVH is used in the critical care setting for patients with volume-overload, hemodynamically unstable conditions with azotemia or uremia (Astle, 2017).

Background

Acute kidney injury is associated with substantial morbidity and mortality (Bagshaw, George, & Bellomo, 2007) It is a common finding among patients in the ICU and is an independent predictor of mortality. Acute kidney injury that is severe enough to result in the use of renal-replacement therapy affects approximately 5% of the patients admitted to the ICU and is associated with a mortality rate of 60% (Uchino, 2005).

The optimal approach to RRT, as well as the optimal intensity and timing of such therapy in critically ill patients remains unclear. In one single-center, randomized, controlled study in which continuous RRT was the sole treatment approach, survival improved when the intensity of therapy was increased from an assigned effluent rate of 20 mL/kg of body weight per hour to either 35 or 45 mL/kg/hr (Bellomo, 2009).

CVVH was designed as an RRT for patients with acute renal failure. It is often chosen over intermittent hemodialysis when blood pressure instability is a problem, and CVVH is more efficient than peritoneal dialysis. CVVH is a technique characterized by a veno-venous circuit and a pump to perfuse the hemofilter. CVVH is suited to individualization of ultrafiltration and solute clearance in patients with acute renal failure and volume overload, specifically when there is impaired cardiovascular function or where arterial access is problematic.

RRTs are indicated in the following circumstances: patients with high-risk for hemodynamic instability who do not tolerate the rapid fluid shifts that occur with hemodialysis, in those who require large amounts of hourly intravenous (IV) fluids or parenteral nutrition, and in those who need more than the usual 3- to 4-hour hemodialysis treatment to correct the metabolic imbalances of acute renal failure. CVVH is used when patients primarily need excess fluid removed, whereas continuous veno-venous hemodialysis (CVVHD) is used when patients also need waste products removed because of uremia (Snyder, 2013).

In general, it appears that the decision to use RRT is affected by strongly held physician beliefs as well as a number of patient and organizational characteristics. Patient characteristics may include age, gender, race, illness acuity, and comorbidities. Organizational characteristics vary depending on the country, type of institution, type of ICU, type of physician or insurance provider, and the perceived cost of therapy. However, the strength of association of these characteristics with the decision to use RRT is not fully understood. Furthermore, large epidemiological studies are needed to establish the factors that are most important in determining practice patterns, and whether there are important access-to-care issues with this therapy (Ostermann et al., 2016).

Clinical Aspects

Basic knowledge is required to understand the principles of diffusion, ultrafiltration, osmosis, oncotic and hydrostatic pressures, and how they pertain to fluid and solute management during RRT (Astle, 2017). CVVH uses a hemofilter dialyzer that acts as an artificial kidney. This is a semipermeable membrane that creates two separate compartments: the blood compartment and the dialysis solution compartment.

ASSESSMENT

Patient assessment should include baseline vital signs, including hemodynamic parameters, weight, a review of current medications, laboratory values; assessments of neurological, vascular and nutritional status should also be conducted. The appraisal of the vascular access catheter insertion site for signs and symptoms of infection should also be included in the patient assessment. The insertion site can provide a portal entry for organisms, which may result in septicemia if unrecognized and treated. The patency of the vascular access catheter should also be assessed for adequate blood flow on aspiration and flushing, which is necessary during treatment to facilitate optimal fluid and solute removal. It is also important to note that the placement of the vascular access may compromise circulation to the distal parts of the access limb, which is why assessment of adequate circulation should also be completed.

NURSING INTERVENTIONS, MANAGEMENT, AND IMPLICATIONS

Continuous venovenous RRT is achieved with a pump system. The blood pump provides the pressure that drives the extracorporeal system. The most common sites used for vascular access catheters are the internal jugular, subclavian, and femoral veins. During continuous RRT, a dialysate, which is composed of water, a buffer usually lactate or bicarbonate, and various electrolytes, is used. Heparin citrate is often used during continuous RRT to prevent clotting of the extracorporeal circuit during treatment.

Some of the key parameters that should be documented during CVVH include (a) date and time of treatment initiation, mode of therapy, filter change; (b) condition of the vascular access regarding patency and quality of blood flow; (c) date and time of vascular access catheter insertion and dressing change; and (d) condition of insertion site and any signs or symptoms of infection. It is also very important to document vital signs and hemodynamic parameters before, during, and after the procedure. Status of pulse distal to vascular access site should also be noted. Most important, documentation of patient's response to treatment, hourly fluid balance calculation, daily weight, laboratory values before and after the treatment should be recorded.

OUTCOMES

CVVH is a temporary treatment for patients with acute renal failure who are unable to tolerate hemodialysis and are unstable. This is an extracorporeal blood purification therapy intended to substitute for impaired renal function over an extended period and is applied, or aimed at being applied, 24 hours per day. Although continuous RRT (CRRT) is a resource-intensive and expensive technology, it remains the default modality of support most frequently used for severely ill patients at high risk for death (Wald, 2014). CVVH uses the principles of ultrafiltration, hydrostatic pressure, and convection to remove both fluid and solutes from the patient. Owing to the large loss of fluid that occurs in this mode, the patient requires a replacement fluid to be programmed in the filter. The filter ensures that the amount programmed as the fluid replacement rate is the amount of fluid that is lost during hemofiltration, to ensure that the patient keeps an even balance.

Summary

The demand for CRRT is growing. The North American region is outpacing the global demand for CRRT. global demand for CRRT. The reason being the presence of a large number of major players in this area and the rising prevalence of kidney failure because of rising diabetes, cancer, and other chronic diseases ("Global Continuous Renal Replacement Therapy Market Insights," 2017).

Astle, S. M. (2017). Continuous renal replacement therapies. In D. L. Wiegand (Ed.), *AACN procedure manual for high acuity, progressive and critical care* (7th ed., pp. 1054–1055). St. Louis, MO: Elsevier.

Bagshaw, S. M., George, C., & Bellomo, R.; ANZICS Database Management Committee. (2007). Changes in the incidence and outcome for early acute kidney injury in a cohort of Australian intensive care units. *Critical Care, 11*(3), R68.

Bellomo, R. (2009). Intensity of continuous renal-replacement therapy. *New England Journal of Medicine, 361*, 1627–1638.

Global Continuous Renal Replacement Therapy Market Insights, Opportunity, Analysis, Market Shares and Forecast 2017–2023. (2017). Retrieved from http://www.research andmarkets.com/reports/3774875/global-continuous-renal-replacement -therapy#relb0

Ostermann, M., Joannidis, M., Pani, A., Floris, M., De Rosa, S., Kellum, J. A., & Ronco, C.; 17th Acute Disease Quality Initiative (ADQI) Consensus Group. (2016). Patient selection and timing of continuous renal replacement therapy. *Blood Purification, 42*(3), 224–237.

Ronco, C., Ricci, Z., De Backer, D., Kellum, J. A., Taccone, F. S., Joannidis, M., . . . Vincent, J. L. (2015). Renal replacement therapy in acute kidney injury: Controversy and consensus. *Critical Care, 19*, 146.

Snyder, A. C. (2013). Patient management: Renal system. In D. K. Patricia Gonce Morton (Ed.), *Critical care nursing: A holistic approach* (p. 646). Philadelphia, PA: Wolter Kluwer Health–Lippincott Williams & Wilkins.

Uchino, S, K. J. (2005). Acute renal failure in critically ill patients: A mulitnational, muli- center study. *Journal of the American Medical Association, 294*(7), 813–818.

Wald, R. S. S. (2014). The association between renal replacement therapy modality and long-term outcomes among critically ill adults with acute kidney injury. *Critical Care Medicine, 42*(4), 868–877.

■ DEFINITIONS OF EMERGENCY AND CRITICAL CARE NURSING

Nicole M. Hartman
Courtney Vose

Overview

Caring for critically ill patients, either emergently or over a period, requires advanced clinical knowledge, broader technical skills, and the ability to work calmly to manage crisis in an often-turbulent environment. In the emergency room, *crisis* refers to the immediate danger the patient experiences from either illness or injury. In the critical care setting, crisis refers to the complex care required to sustain life. In both situations, the registered nurses caring for these patients must possess the skills required to safely move the patient beyond the crisis. Knowledge of how the specialties of emergency room and critical nursing developed will enhance the skills of these crisis care clinicians.

Background

Emergency nursing is a specialty in which nurses are trained to care for patients in the critical time frame related to their illness or injury. A skill set these nurses must possess is the ability to quickly discern the criticality of the situation, as they are often the first clinicians to evaluate the patient. Emergency nurses must be comfortable functioning autonomously because they are at the front line and regularly start treatment. They are the ones who most frequently mobilize the care team emergently, urgently, or nonurgently. Physicians and providers rely on their judgment to determine the speed at which they need to respond in treatment arenas that are often overcrowded. The ability to appropriately triage patients is arguably the most crucial skill needed by all emergency nurses. In addition, these nurses provide vital support to the family and friends of their patients to help them work through the stress of loss, grief, or uncertainty. The importance of this skill set cannot be overemphasized.

Emergency nurses are best described as generalists, not specialists. They often provide emergent care for every age patient, from birth to death. They also must know about every specialty in order to assess, triage, and stabilize patients before they are transferred to specialty care areas like an intensive care unit. It is because of these diverse patient care experiences that emergency nursing attracts nurses from all specialties. It is no longer a perquisite to have critical care or prehospital experience.

Emergency nursing is a modern concept. Until the early 20th century, care was provided when the patient was injured or became ill and emergency departments (EDs) did not exist (Solheim, 2016). During World War II, the Korean War, and the Vietnam War, emergent care provided to soldiers demonstrated that rapid and acute care makes a difference in patient outcomes (Solheim, 2016). The success of these urgent-care venues led to growth of hospitals and emergency treatment spaces throughout the 20th century. These urgent-care spaces evolved from "rooms" to departments as the need for access to emergency and primary health care grew.

The postwar patient population was changing due to the development of EDs and the advent of medications, such as penicillin. Patients who used to die from critical illness were now able to survive, but required intensive care while in the hospital (Fairman & Lynaugh, 1998). Critical care nursing can trace its roots back to Florence Nightingale (1860), as she advocated for seriously ill patients to be grouped together in a quiet section of the hospital ward. This concept was more widely adopted by hospitals in the 1950s during extensive reorganization of hospital wards to allow for more efficient care of patient populations.

Changes in the 1960s and 1970s with health care technology increased the complexity of care patients received in the hospital. The number of hospitals with designated critical care areas was increasing and becoming the new standard of care. Nurses were now caring for patients recovering from open heart surgery, severe trauma, and various disease processes that used to end the patient's life. It became apparent that these complex patients required more focused one-on-one nursing care in addition to the medical technology support they were receiving (Fairman & Lynaugh, 1998).

The complexity of these critically ill patients' cases required more time, technology, and skill from their nurses and doctors. The idea of one nurse per patient was born of necessity. It simply took that much time for nurses to provide care and monitor these complex patients. The environment needed to be spacious enough for the equipment required to sustain life and for patients to be seen and treated (Fairman & Lynaugh, 1998). But grouping these patients together also presented new issues for nurses. The emotional toll that caring for the critically ill patients takes on the caregiver was a new concept. Nurses were often overwhelmed with the emotions they experienced more than the complexity of care they were providing (Fairman & Lynaugh, 1998).

The modern-day critical care unit owes much of its design and operation to the struggles of the 1950s and 1960s. Advancements were made of necessity and have become the evidence used to push the specialty of critical care nursing forward. The formation of the American Association of Critical-Care Nurses (AACN) in the 1960s has given this group of nurses a single voice to help shape the delivery of critical care.

Today, the AACN Synergy Model for Patient Care drives critical care nurses to deliver complex care that is focused on patients and families. This model focuses on the synergy that occurs when patient and family needs guide the formation of competencies for nursing care (Hardin & Kaplow, 2017). The characteristics of critically ill patients and families lead to skill development that will allow for optimal patient outcomes. It is this synergy between the nurses and the patients and their families that promotes healing in a safe environment (Hardin & Kaplow, 2017).

Clinical Aspects

The Emergency Nurses Association (ENA) is the only professional nursing association dedicated to defining the future of emergency nursing and emergency care through advocacy, expertise, innovation, and leadership (ENA, 2016). Emergency nursing was formally recognized as a specialty by the American Nurses Association (ANA) in partnership with the ENA in 2011. They wrote that

> emergency nursing was the care of individuals across their life span, which is episodic, typically short-term, and occurs in all settings.

Emergency nurses function in EDs, urgent care centers, and on advanced life support ambulances and helicopters most frequently. They also work in roles inclusive of entrepreneurs, forensic nurses, jobs with the federal government, cruise ship nurses, humanitarian nurses, disaster nurses, camp nurses, and on-set nurses (Solheim, 2016).

Advanced degrees and certifications are available for emergency nurses. They may advance their education and become clinical nurse specialists (CNSs) or nurse practitioners (NPs). Per the ENA (2016), these advanced practice nurses (APNs) are uniquely prepared to develop and apply theory, conduct research, educate health care providers and consumers, and develop standards of practice that contribute to optimum outcomes. The American Academy of Emergency Nurse Practitioners (AAENP) is an organization that represents emergency nurse practitioners (ENPs). The APNs practicing in the emergency setting care for patients autonomously and collaboratively providing assessment, diagnosis, interventions, evaluations, and interpretation of diagnostic studies.

There are currently two board certifications in emergency nursing: (a) certified emergency nurse (CEN) and (b) certified pediatric emergency nurse (CPEN). There are other certifications in subspecialties like certified flight registered nurse (CFRN) and certified transport registered nurse (CTRN). ENPs also have two routes to board certification. The American Nurses Credentialing Center offers board certification through professional portfolio, and the American Academy of Nurse Practitioners Certification Board offers board certification through examination.

Critical care nursing has transformed over history, not only in competencies for nurses, but also in the types of subspecialties that have developed. The AACN offers board certification as critical care registered nurse (CCRN) adult, pediatric, and neonatal. There are also certifications specific to various subspecialties, such as cardiac and progressive care. The role of the nurse has changed in the critical care setting, but direct care nurse is still the most common role. This includes providing care for patients in various subspecialties, such as cardiac, neurological, surgical, pediatric, and neonatal intensive care units (Urden, 2016).

The CNS has emerged as a predominate APN in the critical care setting. The CNS serves as an educator providing clinical teaching, research development, leadership, and consultative skills to nurses in the numerous intensive care settings. The CNS is often designated by specialty, such as neurology CNS. In addition, a CNS can serve as a case manager for specific critical care populations, such as stroke patients (Urden, 2016).

Another common role for APNs in the critical care setting is the NP. These nurses receive specialized training to manage the care of designated patients, including diagnosis and treatment. They may have prescriptive authority based on the state's nurse practice laws. The NPs are often a consistent presence for many patients and families, as they interact with the patient throughout all aspects of care (Urden, 2016). These roles demonstrate the need for highly skilled, specialized nurses caring for critically ill patients.

Summary

EDs and critical care units require nurses with special education, enhanced skills, and behavioral characteristics that allow them to work calmly under stress to care for complex patient populations. The significant improvements made in health care technology are allowing sicker patients to be treated and to live longer. Nurses caring for critically ill patients accept the challenges these patients present and develop a critical care specialty. In addition, the role of the APN allows nurses to provide care in different ways, such as a CNS or NP. These advancements in nursing for emergent and critically ill patients are truly life-changing.

American Nurses Association & Emergency Nurses Association. (2011). American Nurses Association recognizes emergency nursing as specialty practice. Retrieved from http://www.nursingworld.org/FunctionalMenuCategories/MediaResources/PressReleases/2011-PR/ANA-Recognizes-Emergency-Nursing-Specialty-Practice.pdf

Emergency Nurses Association. (2016). Retrieved from https://www.ena.org/Pages/default.aspx

Fairman, J., & Lynaugh, J. (1998). *Critical care nursing: A history.* Philadelphia: University of Pennsylvania Press.

Hardin, S. R., & Kaplow, R. (2017). *Synergy for clinical excellence: The AACN synergy model for patient care* (2nd ed.). Burlington, MA: Jones & Bartlett.

Nightingale, F. (1860). *Notes on nursing: What it is, and what it is not.* Philadelphia, PA: Wilder Publications.

Solheim, J. (2016). *Emergency nursing: The profession, the pathway, the practice.* Indianapolis, IN: Sigma Theta Tau International.

Urden, L. D. (2016). Caring for the critically ill patient. In L. D. Urden, K. M. Stacy, & M. E. Lough (Eds.), *Priorities in critical care nursing* (7th ed., pp. 1–9). St. Louis, MO: Elsevier Mosby.

■ DENTAL EMERGENCIES

Melanie Gibbons Hallman
Lamon Norton

Overview

Common dental injuries include chipped or fractured teeth, luxation, and tooth avulsion affecting primary and permanent teeth. Approximately 33% of adults and 25% of school-age children experience dental trauma (DiAngelis et al., 2012). A systematic approach to evaluation of dental injury, correct diagnosis, and determination of urgency of care are important to tooth survival (Keels et al., 2014). Mouth cellulitis, including dental abscesses are a common reason for patients to seek emergency care (Allareddy, Rampa, Lee, Allareddy, & Nalliah, 2014). Nurses play an important role in triage and history acquisition, assessment, provision of care, and education for patients experiencing dental trauma and infections.

Background

Dental conditions typically seen in emergency departments include trauma related to accidents, athletics, and violence. Treatment is determined by degree of severity, type of injury, and dental location (American Association of Endodontists, 2017). Most oral injuries arise before age 10 and occur less frequently after age 30. Dental injuries are seen in young males more than females, possibly related to higher risk-taking behavior. The anterior teeth are at highest risk of injury. Dental trauma can be costly not only financially but also in time lost at work and school and in health care manpower and expenses (Andersson, 2013).

Preschool children are prone to falls, often resulting in oral injuries. In school-age children, sports and direct contusions are the common causes of dental injury. Child abuse may be a factor in dental injuries sustained by children (Hicks, Green, & Van Wicklin, 2016). Motor vehicle accidents and assaults are common causes of dental injuries in adolescents and young adults. Studies reveal that alcohol contributes to injuries experienced in these age groups, most often occurring during leisure time and on weekends (Andersson, 2013).

Injury to permanent dentition requires professional attention. Dental avulsion occurs when a tooth is displaced from the socket, usually due to trauma. This condition affects dental ligament cells, nerves, and blood supply, as well as the bone and gingiva (Hicks et al., 2016). Survival of an avulsed tooth is time-dependent. Dental concussion is caused by contusion and results in tooth tenderness. Increased mobility and bleeding at the tooth/gum interface are not associated with this injury. Dental fractures may affect the crown, root, or dental alveoli (sockets). Individual tooth or group tooth mobility raises suspicion for fracture. Luxation may present with abnormal tooth mobility or as a tooth locked into a displaced position. The tooth may be partially avulsed, or impacted into the alveolus with bleeding usually present. Injuries to primary dentition typically require minimal or no treatment (Keels et al., 2014), whereas permanent teeth often require treatment. Failure to appropriately address dental injuries and abscesses can result in physical, psychological, and financial detriment to patients, which may be lifelong (DiAngelis et al., 2012). A periodontal abscess consists of localized pockets of infection that form around a tooth causing erythema and pain, often accompanied by palpable swelling. The tooth itself may be healthy. Patients with dental abscesses are commonly afebrile and if the abscess is left untreated, a local infection may progress to cellulitis and possibly a systemic infection (Hodgdon, 2013; Veerasathpurush, Rampa, Lee, Allaerddy, & Malliah, 2014).

Clinical Aspects

ASSESSMENT

A concise medical and dental history, including tetanus status, current medications, and medication allergies, should be acquired. The mechanism of injury is important to determining potential associated head injury or physical abuse. It is crucial to inquire whether the patient experienced loss of consciousness, headache, dizziness, nausea, or vomiting. These symptoms may indicate a concussion or other brain insult. If head injury is suspected, the patient's cervical spine should be assessed and protected until evaluated and cleared by a provider. If tooth or mouth contamination is suspected, the need for tetanus booster and antibiotic prophylaxis should be considered (Keels et al., 2014). Rapid assessment and treatment are crucial to tooth survival in avulsion injuries affecting permanent teeth.

NURSING INTERVENTIONS, MANAGEMENT, AND IMPLICATIONS

Care should focus on keeping patients calm and comfortable and determining whether the affected tooth is primary or permanent. Do not touch the root of the tooth; only handle by the crown (the white end of the tooth) wearing gloves and using gauze. Determine how long the tooth has been out of socket. If the tooth remains dry greater than 1 hour before being replanted or placed in a physiologic transport medium such as milk, saliva, saline, tissue culture medium, or Hank's balanced storage solution (HBSS), the tooth is considered likely nonviable. Never rub the tooth to get it clean. Immediately notify a provider if an avulsed tooth is still potentially viable in order to expedite its care and remain within the 1-hour window. Place the avulsed tooth in available physiologic medium if this has not already been initiated, even if it is more than 1 hour out of socket. If an avulsed tooth was replanted before arrival at the emergency department, the patient may gently bite down on a gauze pad to maintain stability if he or she is alert and mature enough to follow instructions. The patient should remain upright. Replantation does not guarantee long-term tooth survival (Andersson et al.,

2012). Tooth avulsion injuries are common in children. Completely avulsed primary teeth should not be replanted. The nurse should inquire whether the tooth was found. If not found, radiographs should be ordered to ensure that the tooth was not inhaled, swallowed, or impacted (Keels et al., 2014).

Dental concussions of primary and permanent teeth do not require immediate treatment. The patient or caregiver should be informed to observe for darkening of an injured tooth over a period of days to months following injury. This would indicate possible pulpal necrosis and require immediate dental evaluation. Dental crown fractures require early referral to a dentist, especially if the pulp is exposed. Many fractures require dental splinting, which must be managed by a dental professional. The less mature the permanent tooth, the worse the prognosis (Keels et al., 2014).

Luxation injuries are categorized by the direction in which the tooth is displaced. Mild luxation may not require treatment, but notable displacement may require gentle repositioning by a medical or dental provider. The tooth is usually tender to touch or to tapping and presents with varying degrees of increased mobility. Increased tooth sensitivity is common. Bleeding at the tooth/gum interface is often seen (DiAngelis et al., 2012).

Injuries to primary dentition in children are common. The roots of primary teeth are closely approximated to evolving permanent teeth. An impaction injury to a primary tooth can pose a risk of injury to the adjacent evolving permanent tooth. Patients sustaining primary tooth impaction should be urgently referred to a dental provider for evaluation. Some luxation injuries to primary teeth often heal spontaneously (Malmgren et al., 2012).

Dental injuries and abscesses commonly result in patient anxiety and pain. Frequently assess the patient's airway patency and maintain bleeding control. Calm the patient and make him or her as comfortable as possible. Reassure him or her and keep him or her informed of activities and the ongoing plan of care. Assessment of pain status is a key component of care for the patient experiencing a dental injury or infection. Nonaspirin analgesics may provide substantial relief of dental pain (Hicks et al., 2016). Request pain medication when indicated, ensuring no allergy exists. Notify the medical provider if the patient's pain intervention is not effective. Ice pack application may be painful related to dental nerve injury. A heat pack may serve to be more soothing for pain. Anticipate antibiotic administration in cases of dental fracture, tooth avulsion, and dental abscess. Absent or decreased pain, reduction of swelling and bleeding, and decreased anxiety are desirable outcomes following dental trauma.

Summary

Patients sustaining dental injuries and abscesses often seek care in emergency departments. Nurses play a vital role in assessment, care, and treatment for these patients. Providing discharge instructions that are understandable and individualized to patient and caregiver literacy level is crucial to achieving desirable outcomes for these patients. Providing resource options for timely dental follow-up care is necessary.

Allareddy, V., Rampa, S., Lee, M. K., Allareddy, V., & Nalliah, R. P. (2014). Hospital-based emergency department visits involving dental conditions: Profile and predictors of poor outcomes and resource utilization. *Journal of the American Dental Association, 145*(4), 331–337.

American Association of Endodontists. (2016). Traumatic dental injuries. Retrieved from http://www.aae.org/patients/treatments-and-procedures/traumatic-dental-injuries .aspx

Andersson, L. (2013). Epidemiology of traumatic dental injuries. *Journal of endodontics, 39*(3), S2–S5.

Andersson, L., Andreasen, J. O., Day, P., Heithersay, G., Trope, M., DiAngelis, A. J., & Hicks, M. L. (2012). International Association of Dental Traumatology guidelines for the management of traumatic dental injuries: 2. Avulsion of permanent teeth. *Dental Traumatology, 28*(2), 88–96.

DiAngelis, A. J., Andreasen, J. O., Ebeleseder, K. A., Kenny, D. J., Trope, M., Sigurdsson, A., . . . Lenzi, A. R. (2012). International Association of Dental Traumatology guidelines for the management of traumatic dental injuries: 1. Fractures and luxations of permanent teeth. *Dental Traumatology, 28*(1), 2–12.

Hicks, R. W., Green, R., & Van Wicklin, S. A. (2016). Dental avulsions: Review and recommendations. *Nurse Practitioner, 41*(6), 58–62.

Hodgdon, A. (2013). Dental and related infections. *Emergency Medicine Clinics of North America, 31*(2), 465–480.

Keels, M. A., Segura, A., Boulter, S., Clark, M., Gereige, R., Krol, D., & Slayton, R. (2014). Management of dental trauma in a primary care setting. *Pediatrics, 133*(2), e466–e476.

Malmgren, B., Andreasen, J. O., Flores, M. T., Robertson, A., DiAngelis, A. J., Andersson, L., . . . Malmgren, O. (2012). International Association of Dental Traumatology guidelines for the management of traumatic dental injuries: 3. Injuries in the primary dentition. *Dental Traumatology, 28*(3), 174–182.

Veerasathpurush, A., Rampa, S., Lee, M. K., Allaerddy, V., & Malliah, R. (2014). Hospital-based emergency department visits involving dental conditions. *Journal of the American Dental Association, 145*(5), 331–337.

■ DISASTER RESPONSE

Darlie Simerson

Overview

Disaster response in the emergency department (ED) begins with disaster preparedness in partnership with the community. The Department of Homeland Security (DHS) developed the National Response Framework to facilitate national preparedness for any events deemed to pose the greatest risk to our nation. Four phases identified were mitigation, preparedness, response, and recovery (DHS, 2016). These phases start at the community level and extend into the ED, the entry point of care to the hospital. Emphasis is placed on preparation for the hazards that each community is most at risk of experiencing. The ED and community resources, including first responders and public health departments, rely heavily on each other to function efficiently and effectively. Our nation has been through several recent natural disasters and terrorist events in which lessons have been learned on best practices to use in handling disasters. Issues specific to the ED include disaster triage, personnel safety, symptom surveillance, patient surge capacity, throughput, and clinical management preparedness for all potential hazards (Emergency Nurses Association [ENA], 2013).

Background

Disasters are catastrophic events that may cause injury or loss of life. There are both man-made and natural disasters that include environmental, chemical, biological, and nuclear incidences. When humans are adversely affected, the ED is customarily the desired point of care. Often disasters cause a disruption of services within the ED, which necessitates careful allocation of resources with essential functions taking priority. An emergency operations plan (EOP) is mandated by The Joint Commission (TJC) for all hospitals and is activated to accommodate a surge in patient numbers in the ED. Disaster training drills are the recommended modality for members of the community and ED to interact and take part in disaster simulations. This allows for all members of the team to become familiar with their role in the EOP. These drills also provide an opportunity for identification of training needs and for assessment of the level of preparedness (TJC, 2014).

It is important that ED nurses are prepared to anticipate many of the possible disaster scenarios. Prior training in the management of all hazards is necessary to prevent the ED from becoming overwhelmed in a sudden event. Nurses in the ED play a pivotal role in symptom surveillance, triage, and patient surge management during a disaster response. They are often the first member of the ED team to encounter the patient and the first to discover a hazard exposure. Nurses must take on a leadership role in implementing the EOP. It is important that they are prepared for this role by being familiar with the plan and how to access specific hazard information. Personnel safety is paramount to prevent more casualties from being added to the already heavy burden caused by the disaster. Use of personal protective equipment (PPE) and making PPE available to others when necessary is the first priority. The need for patient isolation and decontamination must be quickly recognized and initiated.

Clinical Aspects

Specific hazards of concern in the ED include injuries secondary to natural disasters and chemical contamination as well as illness secondary to biological exposures. The first priority is to protect others, including the nurse, from injury or contamination. PPE should be readily available and training should be provided to the nurses before the incident. Isolation and contamination needs should be identified in triage if at all possible to prevent further spread throughout the ED. Resources, such as safety data sheets, must be easily accessible at the point of initial contact so that nurses can quickly acquire treatment guidelines for chemical and other known exposures. Some other important resources are the Centers for Disease Control and Prevention (CDC) and the local public health department.

ASSESSMENT

Disaster triage for mass casualties determines resource requirements such as ED staffing numbers and bed availability. This is an assignment for nurses experienced in triage procedures. The EOP includes guidelines that are implemented to aid in identification of the patient level of severity and the appropriate location for treatment. This is particularly true of trauma-related disasters in which isolation and decontamination are not necessary. It is of paramount importance that prior preparation, through EOP drills, has occurred so that ED staff are able to handle a surge in patient numbers in a sudden disaster. Additional ED nurse responsibilities include surge discharge of noncritical patients and increased throughput of stabilized patients to other hospital treatment areas in order to increase ED bed availability.

Anticipatory training is recommended for ED nurses in preparation for those hazards most likely to be seen in the ED. It is impossible to know everything about all hazards but the ED nurses should know where to quickly access information. Types of disasters with the potential to result in a large influx of ED patients include bioterrorism, chemical emergencies, radiation emergencies, natural disasters or severe weather, and infectious outbreaks. In addition, particular attention is directed to vulnerable populations such as children, elderly, chronically ill, and mentally ill (ENA, 2013).

Although not all inclusive, anthrax, botulism, plague, and smallpox are considered to be the most likely encountered bioterrorism agents. The CDC provides specific information regarding management of infection or exposure. It is important that ED nurses recognize an unusual increase in patients with the same symptoms, especially fever, respiratory, or gastrointestinal complaints. An unusual pattern or uncharacteristic timing to the symptoms should be noted (CDC, 2016).

Chemical emergencies can result from a vast number of sources. When these are hazmat events, there is customarily communication from first responders indicating the type of exposure. The CDC and regional poison control centers are excellent resources for management information. Decontamination may be dry or wet depending on the chemical and is sometimes carried out at the scene of the exposure. Identification of the type of chemical is key to the treatment needed.

Radiation emergencies have the potential to quickly overwhelm the ED. Use of PPE is essential for nurses and other ED staff. Decontamination is necessary to lessen the risk of acute skin injury, to lower the risk of internal contamination, and to reduce the risk of contamination to health care providers. Removal of all clothing can reduce contamination on the patient up to 90% (U.S. Department of Health and Human Services, 2016). Further decontamination occurs by washing the patient. Contaminated water collected afterward must be properly disposed of as in dedicated ED decontamination showers.

Natural disasters or severe weather may include hurricanes, tornados, and flooding. These may result in mass casualties from trauma. Events such as these have the potential to cause a sudden surge in patients arriving in the ED with a large variety of injuries. Again, ED nurses must rely on previous training and the EOP to manage resource availability. The sequela of these events may be a rapid failure in health care areas that are less prepared for disasters such as nursing homes, clinics, and dialysis centers. The ED may be the only available resource for care following a catastrophic event.

Last of all are the infectious outbreaks. Surveillance is an important aspect of ED nursing as mentioned in the bioterrorism section. ED nurses are in a unique position to recognize reoccurring symptoms presenting to the ED. In recent years, an Ebola outbreak in West Africa has raised our awareness of the potential for an epidemic and the need to screen patients for possible exposure. Recent travel information has become a familiar part of initial information obtained on all patients entering the ED. Use of PPE for personnel protection and proper use of isolation techniques are the mainstays of infection management.

Summary

Disaster response in the ED can be determined by a vast number of potential agents. Although impossible to have in-depth knowledge regarding each, it is important for ED nurses to recognize the need to protect personnel and act quickly to address immediate patient needs to lessen sequelae. It is the responsibility of ED nurses to participate in preparedness exercises and continuing education in anticipation of taking a leadership role in the event of a disaster.

Centers for Disease Control and Prevention. (2016). Emergency preparedness and response. Retrieved from https://emergency.cdc.gov/hazards-specific.asp

Department of Homeland Security. (2016). *National response framework* (3rd ed.). Retrieved from https://www.fema.gov/media-library/assets/documents/117791

Emergency Nurses Association. (2013). Position statement: Disaster and emergency preparedness for all hazards. Retrieved from https://www.ena.org/SiteCollection Documents/Position%20Statements/AllHazards.pdf

The Joint Commission. (2014). Emergency management resources: New and revised requirements. Retrieved from https://www.jointcommission.org/emergency_ management.aspx

United States Department of Health and Human Services. (2016). Radiation emergency medical management. Retrieved from https://www.remm.nlm.gov/ext_contami nation.htm

■ DISSEMINATED INTRAVASCULAR COAGULATION

Joyce E. Higgins

Overview

Disseminated intravascular coagulation (DIC) is a secondary syndrome resulting in the activation of clotting and thrombolytic systems that impair tissue perfusion and result in devastating end-organ damage (Wada, Matsumoto, & Yamashita, 2014). The extent of organ destruction related to the imbalances in the coagulation and fibrin activity that result in DIC and the primary etiologic mechanism, such as an infection (Asakura, 2014). Although there are many causes, sepsis in combination with DIC has a higher mortality rate and can be very difficult to manage in the critically ill adult (Ishikura et al., 2014).

Background

According to the Scientific Standards Committee (SSC) formed in the International Society on Thrombosis and Hemostasis (ISTH; 2001), DIC is defined as an acquired syndrome, characterized by the intravascular activation of coagulation and the loss of localization coming from different causes. It can originate from and cause damage to the microvasculature that, if sufficiently severe, can produce organ dysfunction (Taylor, Toh, Hoots, Wada, & Levi, 2001).

Organ dysfunction is a latent characteristic of systemic inflammatory response syndrome (SIRS) and sepsis. The inflammatory response causes circulatory instability throughout the body. When SIRS is not a locally managed inflammation in the body, it is referred to as *sepsis*. Sepsis is identified as a failure of two or more body systems that can lead to organ failure. Sepsis in the adult can increase in severity when combined with the coagulopathy disorders of DIC (Davis, Miller-Dorey, & Jenne, 2016; Ishikura et al., 2014; Okamoto, Tamura, & Sawatsubashi, 2016). Early detection and management of DIC with sepsis can help decrease client mortality.

Several studies use the British Committee for Standards in Haematology (BCSH), Japanese Society of Thrombosis and Hemostasis (JSTH), Italian Society for Thrombosis and Hemostasis (SISET), and the ISTH/SSC as collaborative guideline recommendations for diagnosis and treatment plans in DIC (Wada et al., 2013). As DIC is not a primary condition, a combination of tests and treatments are needed to achieve a successful outcome. The use of a scoring system and treatment of the underlying disease process is highly recommended across all guidelines to assist in the treatment and a decrease in mortality (Wada et al., 2013, 2014). The severity of the clients' ailments can be scored using the Sequential Organ Failure Assessment (SOFA), Acute Physiological and Chronic Health Evaluation (APACHE II), or Japanese Association for Acute Medicine as in a study by Ishikura et al. (2014), which identified sepsis-induced DIC in classifications of mild, moderate, and severe. Each classification had more complications and brought on higher mortality.

There are different types of DIC, such as bleeding, massive bleeding, fibrin growth related to tumors, and organ failure. Each type presents with different characteristics, bleeding is a slow or constant leaking from coagulation; massive uncontrolled bleeding as occurs in surgery, ruptured placenta, or aortic aneurysms; hyperfibrinolysis from tumor growth as seen in leukemia; and hypercoagulation or hyperfibrinolysis as found in organ failure with sepsis (Wada et al., 2014). Sepsis is the decompensation of two or more organ systems that can be difficult to overcome, especially with the presentation of DIC.

Sepsis is diagnosed based on the cellular inflammatory response in the body increasing the tissue factor (TF) and preventing fibrinolysis because of an accumulation of plasminogen activator inhibitor type-1 (PAI-1). This causes a growth of fibrin in capillaries and small vessels called *microemboli* or *clots* that destroy cell structures. The destruction of cells leads to organ failure, and multiple organ failures can lead to death (Ishikura et al., 2014; Wada et al., 2014).

The clients in intensive care units (ICUs) are more susceptible to the development of DIC because of SIRS. The underlying disease process of some of these diagnoses are an infection, burn surgeries, hepatitis, acute pancreatitis, and rhabdomyolysis (Asakura, 2014). The inflammatory response releases neutrophils, histones, cathepsin G, and neutrophil extracellular traps (NETs) that bind together to defeat the infection. This adds to the activation of the coagulation cascade causing a buildup of cells in the vasculature (Davis et al., 2016). According to Okamoto et al. (2016), DIC in sepsis is defined by escalation of the inflammation and its collection of released responses along with the coagulation pathways. The coagulation complication in combination with thrombocytopenia increases the risk of intracranial hemorrhage by 88%, further increasing mortality (Levi & Hunt, 2015).

Clinical Aspects

The treatment of DIC is divided as mentioned previously by the SSC of the ISTH. The SSC recommendations are for a collaboration of tests and treatment of the underlying cause. As DIC is a secondary syndrome, the nurse needs to be alert for changes that can arise both gradually and suddenly.

ASSESSMENT

Constant monitoring of vital signs and assessment requires ICU admission. Overt signs of bleeding can be hematuria, hemoptysis, bleeding from old puncture sites, and change in the level of consciousness (LOC). Signs of alteration in coagulation causing an embolic development can include but are not limited to purpura, petechiae, cyanosis, gangrene, chest pain, acute myocardial infarction, respiratory distress, abdominal pain and/or distention, constipation, and change of LOC. Frequent clinical and laboratory measurements are required for a proper evaluation of DIC (Levi & Hunt, 2015).

Laboratory markers of low platelets, increased prothrombin time (PT), increased activated partial thromboplastin time (a PTT), prolonged fibrinogen, and fibrin degradation products (D-dimer) vary in the reliability to diagnose DIC (Levi, 2014). Each test is reflective of other disease processes and not specific to DIC. Other laboratory studies, such as thromboelastography (TEG), can be used to assess coagulation factor function, as well as platelet function, clot strength, and fibrinolysis. The use of TEG can help the health care team determine the pharmacologic interventions that might be most beneficial to patients with DIC (Levi & Hunt, 2015).

NURSING INTERVENTIONS, MANAGEMENT, AND IMPLICATIONS

Treatment using heparin is useful for both the inflammatory response of platelets, histones, and the NETs, as well as, altering the thrombin of the clotting factors (Davis et al., 2016). The anticoagulated agent heparin has a short acting half-life making it easier to adjust in high-risk clients who are more likely to bleed. Several ongoing studies have shown to have beneficial responses using both low-dose heparin and molecular weight-based dosing for treatment of sepsis and DIC-related sepsis (Davis et al., 2016; Okamoto et al., 2016).

Additional treatments include transfusion of clotting factors, such as platelet concentration (PC), fresh frozen plasma (FFP), and fibrinogen as cryoprecipitate. Not all the guidelines recommend blood product infusion, although doing so helps with patients who have active bleeding and also replenishes the diminishing factors in the clotting cascade (Davis et al., 2016). Red blood cell (RBC) transfusion is used with massive blood loss related to trauma, surgery, and in DIC if necessary (Davis et al., 2016).

Antithrombin (AT) is a glycoprotein made in the liver inhibiting thrombin activity and clotting cascade factors (Davis et al., 2016). The AT is significantly depleted in DIC. Japan reflects several studies of DIC using AT treatment. Okamoto et al.'s (2016) randomized multicenter control trial with treatment using moderate AT dosing ranges showed a decrease in DIC scores and faster recovery. Not all guidelines recommend the use of AT administration for the treatment of DIC, although in Japan, Tagami, Matsui, Horiguchi, Fushimi, and Yasunaga (2014) showed a decrease in the 28-day mortality with AT dosage in severe pneumonia and DIC.

Current and future studies are ongoing to validate treatment and diagnostics for DIC. The guideline recommendations of ISTH/SSC, SISET, BCSH, and JSTH and scoring systems can assist with building strategies for future comparison in trials to benefit clients.

OUTCOMES

Prevention of DIC is the priority nursing outcome. It is imperative to institute early and rapid interventions to correct the underlying offender and prevent further damage. DIC can be devastating and is truly life-threatening. Evaluating the patient for early signs is key in preventing this disorder.

Summary

DIC is a diversely complicated secondary disease. The diagnosis and treatment can be a long process. All experts do not agree on the treatment modalities. However, they do concur that it is more beneficial to the high-risk clients of the ICU to diagnose and treat early-onset symptoms and underlying causes of DIC. No single laboratory measurement identifies DIC. It takes a combination of assessment, skill, and diagnostic testing to identify and treat DIC. Nursing personnel can continue to stay abreast of the clinical changes in the client that may trigger DIC. They can collaborate to treat the inflammatory response system and replace the products of the coagulation pathway as needed to decrease severity and mortality of the client.

Asakura, H. (2014). Classifying types of disseminated intravascular coagulation: Clinical and animal models. *Journal of Intensive Care, 2*(1), 20.

Davis, R. P., Miller-Dorey, S., & Jenne, C. N. (2016). Platelets and coagulation in infection. *Clinical & Translational Immunology, 5*(7), e89.

Ishikura, H., Nishida, T., Murai, A., Nakamura, Y., Irie, Y., Tanaka, J., & Umemura, T. (2014). New diagnostic strategy for sepsis-induced disseminated intravascular coagulation: A prospective single-center observational study. *Critical Care, 18*(1), R19.

Levi, M. (2014). Diagnosis and treatment of disseminated intravascular coagulation. *International Journal of Laboratory Hematology, 36*(3), 228–236.

Levi, M., & Hunt, B. J. (2015). A critical appraisal of point-of-care coagulation testing in critically ill patients. *Journal of Thrombosis and Haemostasis, 13*(11), 1960–1967.

Okamoto, K., Tamura, T., & Sawatsibashi, Y. (2016). Sepsis and disseminated intravascular coagulation. *Journal of Intensive Care, 4*, 4–23. doi:10.1186/s40560-016-0149-0

Tagami, T., Matsui, H., Horiguchi, H., Fushimi, K., & Yasunaga, H. (2014). Antithrombin and mortality in severe pneumonia patients with sepsis-associated disseminated intravascular coagulation: An observational nationwide study. *Journal of Thrombosis and Haemostasis, 12*(9), 1470–1479.

Taylor, F. B., Toh, C. H., Hoots, W. K., Wada, H., & Levi, M.; Scientific Subcommittee on Disseminated Intravascular Coagulation of the International Society on Thrombosis and Haemostasis. (2001). Towards definition, clinical and laboratory criteria, and a scoring system for disseminated intravascular coagulation. *Thrombosis and Haemostasis, 86*(5), 1327–1330.

Wada, H., Matsumoto, T., & Yamashita, Y. (2014). Diagnosis and treatment of disseminated intravascular coagulation (DIC) according to four DIC guidelines. *Journal of Intensive Care, 2*(1), 15.

Wada, H., Thachil, J., Di Nisio, M., Mathew, P., Kurosawa, S., Gando, S., . . . Toh, C. H. (2013). Guidance for diagnosis and treatment of disseminated intravascular coagulation from harmonization of the recommendations from three guidelines. *Journal of Thrombosis and Haemostasis, 11*, 761–767. doi:10.1111/jth.12155

■ DOMESTIC VIOLENCE

Patricia M. Speck
Diana K. Faugno
Rachell A. Ekroos
Melanie Gibbons Hallman
Gwendolyn D. Childs
Tedra S. Smith
Stacey A. Mitchell

Overview

Domestic violence (DV), also known as *family* or *intimate partner violence*, is obvious in the Code of Hammurabi (1780 BCE), ancient laws designed to guide male heads of household in the infliction of punishment to control members of their family and property (King, 2008). Legal thinking evolved, and in the 1700s, a legal decision curtailed carte blanche violence against wives, apprentices, and children by defining the "Rule of Thumb," which was a common law limiting penalties to a whip or stick size—no bigger than the man's thumb! In 1871, first to deny Great Britain's custom of wife beating, the State of Alabama prosecuted a husband for assault and battery, codifying the wife's citizen rights and protections under the U.S. Constitution (Supreme Court of Alabama, 1871, p. 3). Although greater society believes that DV is a "family matter," legislation passed since the 1970s squarely identifies DV behavior as assault, warranting criminal justice intervention (Erez, 2002). Important to nurses referring victims, DV legislation guarantees victims access to community support programs funded by the Family Violence Prevention and Services Act (Family Violence Prevention and Services Programs, 2016).

Background

There is a demonstrated association between DV and immediate and long-term health, social, and economic consequences (DuMonthier & Dusenbery, 2016) taking the form of "physical assault, psychological abuse, social abuse, financial abuse, or sexual assault" (Kaur & Garg, 2008, p.74). The economic impact in the United States is between $4 billion and $9 billion, with $6.3 billion in direct medical and mental health care costs (Breiding et al., 2014; Hughes & Brush, 2015). For RNs charged with the evaluation and referral of patients at risk for DV, the evidence is mixed, and further study is needed about the cost-benefit of identification and the effectiveness of referral (O'Doherty et al., 2015). No one factor contributes to DV, but there are linkages for male and female offenders with a history of DV, depression, social isolation, antisocial behavior, and substance abuse (Capaldi, Knoble, Shortt, & Kim, 2012), in which single lifestyle and separation from partner create vulnerability, and marriage is protective of women. Nursing practice is fundamental in the prevention of DV, where there is clear understanding of the contributing factors and coordinating resources necessary for change in communities.

Estimating the incidence of DV is difficult as victims do not report and when they do, recording of the event reflects community language, not consistent with national data terms (Fernandes-Alcantara, 2014). Victims also may fear the law enforcement response, particularly in small communities where everyone is known, there is shame, or they experience fear of increasing abuse after disclosure. Research demonstrates that DV is very common, both men and women experience victimization (sexual, physical, and psychological), but women are victimized more often than men, and minority women more than nonminority women (Breiding et al., 2014).

DV creates chaos in traumatized families whereby offenders isolate and economically deprive the partner of employment, financial decisions, and control of funds (DuMonthier & Dusenbery, 2016). The children of victims of DV are most at risk for child abuse and neglect, many experiencing personal environments of social isolation, not conducive to normal development or emotional health (Bair-Merritt, Blackstone, & Feudtner, 2006). Disparities and social determinants create complex risk factors in DV environments that diminish attainment of health. Those environments and attitudes include exposure to crime and violence, disease, and lack of access to health care and personal and support systems (Braveman & Gottlieb, 2014; Chung et al., 2016), with isolation and lack of social support (Capaldi et al., 2012).

Building on the stress and adaptation theories of the 1990s, chronic stress in DV environments increases hormonal dysregulation predisposing the family members to increased risk of violence and disease, and early death (Felitti et al., 1998; McEwen, 1998). Pregnant women and their developing fetus(s), newborns, infants, and children exposed to DV experience elevated stress hormones and begin a quest to escape or calm the "fear" response (a comprehensive explanation of the biophysiology appears in the Child Abuse and Neglect entry). For the adolescent and adult subjected to DV, similar biological responses increase risk of aberrant and risk-taking behaviors (Hyman, Malenka, & Nestler, 2006; McEwen & Seeman, 1999). Understanding the underlying biophysiology of stress and trauma responses of the adolescent or adult DV victims prepares the RN to address obvious anxiety, mood, and depression symptoms that lead to poor health choices and outcomes (Felitti et al., 1998; McEwen, 1998).

Clinical Aspects

The incidence and prevalence of DV ensures that nurses will care for patients in a DV situation, because half the women they serve experience psychological aggression by an intimate partner, and a third experience physical aggression (Breiding et al., 2014). However, there are many challenges to obtaining a history of DV from patients. The social beliefs are barriers, particularly when communities believe it is a "family" matter. Other barriers to asking about or disclosing DV information is that it is a sensitive topic, reflecting personal shame and self-blame in victims, and where providers lack training about how to ask and what to do (Campbell, Sharps, Sachs, & Yam, 2003; Connor, Nouer, Speck, Mackey, & Tipton, 2013; O'Doherty et al., 2015). There is an economic and emotional dependency in patients, and for some, insecurity reflects their inability to support their families (Gutmanis, Beynon, Tutty, Wathen, & MacMillan, 2007). Nurses need to recognize DV's mental and physical health outcomes, which are directly related to the biology of trauma and include depression, anxiety, posttraumatic stress disorder, psychosis, inability to trust others, self-harm, and a host of psychosomatic conditions (Stewart & Vigod, 2017), as well as heart disease, obesity, hypertension, obstructive lung diseases, and stroke (Felitti et al., 1998; McEwen, 1998).

Nurses receiving concept-based education about forensic nursing might experience a simulation using DV as an exemplar. There are eight concepts in a routine nursing inquiry, which include "preparedness, self-confidence, professional supports, abuse inquiry, practitioner consequences of asking, comfort following disclosure, practitioner lack of control, and practice pressures" (Gutmanis et al., 2007, p. 4). When interviewed, DV victims acknowledged wanting health care professionals who were "nonjudgmental, nondirective, and individually tailored, with an appreciation of the complexity of partner violence" and health care providers who were able to listen, express concern, empathy, and support (Feder, Hutson, Ramsay, & Taket, 2006, p. 34). Women's perceptions of health care provider interactions depended on the woman's readiness to address the issue and trust of a health care provider (Feder et al., 2006). With didactic and simulation preparation, variability in health care practices diminishes and the identification, plans for intervention with trauma-informed and patient-centered care improves, all necessary support DV victims and their families throughout disclosure (Gutmanis et al., 2007).

ASSESSMENT

A number of screening tools exist and include Abuse Assessment Screen/Abuse Assessment Screen-Disability (AAS/AASD); Humiliation, Afraid, Rape, and Kick (HARK); Hurt, Insulted, Threatened, or Screamed Questionnaire (HITS); Partner Abuse Interview; Partner Violence Screen; Suicide Assessment Five-step Evaluation (SAFE-T); STaT; Women Abuse Screening Tool (WAST); WAST Short Form; and Women's Experience with Battering Scale. However, of these, only three are validated to assess all three areas of abuse—physical, sexual, and psychological—and they are AAS, HARK, and WAST (Arkins, Begley, & Higgins, 2016). These tools are useful for nurses in many settings, including emergency departments, surgical areas, perinatal care, and mental health. It is suspected that other practice areas are amenable to screening, but need validated tools in their populations that are reliable and "screen for all three types of abuse" (Arkins et al., 2016, p. 233). The tools noted are not generalizable, therefore testing in unique communities and cultures is recommended. Lethality assessments are sensitive and provide a tool to first responders estimating the risk of near lethal and deadly violence (Campbell et al., 2003; Campbell, Webster, & Glass, 2009). The lethality scales do not predict who will die from DV; therefore, consider their use in health care practices carefully.

NURSING INTERVENTIONS, MANAGEMENT, AND IMPLICATIONS

The RN is in a position to speak frankly and comfortably with the patient about all health risks, including DV. When suspected, the nurse should therapeutically explore the possibility of the patient's vulnerability to DV, past experiences, and current situation. If the patient does disclose, the nurse should advise the patient about options to reporting. If he or she does not disclose, anticipatory guidance about community resources is warranted. For both the discloser and nondiscloser, the nurse should strongly advise the escape/elopement from the abuser to be secret and deliberate. Unfortunately, when victims threaten to leave the abuser or announce they will leave the abuser or they leave, the abuser is at greatest risk to commit murder of the partner, their children, other family members, and animals.

The RN and the institutional team provide trauma-informed and patient-centered care, assessment, and documentation, important for the safety and postencounter planning of the patient and family. If the RN is the first to suspect DV, he or she should consider counseling the patient to connect with DV community resources while the patient is with him or her. The nurse alerts hospital social workers and community collaborators, who have experience with DV and institutional relationships through memorandum. The RN assessment for DV or other forensic nursing presentations is descriptive only, documenting objective information and addressing anxiety and fear through the creation of a safe environment. Throughout the process, the RN role is therapeutic and helpful, explaining each step in the process and providing clarity to the legal investigation.

OUTCOMES

The patient should be cautioned to work with the community resources to plan and prepare, leaving the relationship only when the first opportunity presents, without fanfare, fights, or threats, which raise the lethality index. Of note, if the offender is aware of the plans to leave, all providers at the institution and in the community are at risk; there is also an increased risk of partner and family harm. Institutions need safety policies and procedure plans, where active shooter training applies to DV offenders, especially when the victim prepares to elope from the relationship. Of course, when the victim requires urgent or emergent care, procedures that deidentify the name and location are prudent.

Summary

Safety is a human desire, and families depend on health care providers to supply information about their health and welfare. In DV, chaos ensues with physical, sexual, and psychological stresses unknown to those outside the relationship. During the relationship-building phases that trap victims, the time between events and apologies keep some people with their partners. Others are trapped in slave-like conditions, never experiencing pleasant times, instead experiencing toxic trauma bonding with a boyfriend trafficker. The continuum of violence creates stress and health outcomes contributing to economic deprivation and insecurity, fear for DV victims themselves and their families, and eventually for their survival. The nurse is positioned to begin a conversation about violence and its impact on health, as well as options that patients may accept from a comprehensive community response, with reassurance and anticipatory guidance for the victims perceived and real dangers. For nurses, it is wise to recognize the importance of existing danger for the care provider and coworkers who facilitate elopement, where vicarious trauma and structural change require attention to ensure trauma-informed and patient-centered care. Finally, recognize that adults have liberties to return to the abuser (see the Child Abuse and Neglect entry if you suspect children are at risk); it is to be hoped that there will be another opportunity to influence the victim's decision to escape.

Arkins, B., Begley, C., & Higgins, A. (2016). Measures for screening for intimate partner violence: A systematic review. *Journal of Psychiatric and Mental Health Nursing, 23*(3–4), 217–235. doi:10.1111/jpm.12289

Bair-Merritt, M. H., Blackstone, M., & Feudtner, C. (2006). Physical health outcomes of childhood exposure to intimate partner violence: A systematic review. *Pediatrics, 117*(2), 278–290. doi:10.1542/peds.2005-1473

Braveman, P., & Gottlieb, L. (2014). The social determinants of health: It's time to consider the causes of the causes. *Public Health Reports, 129*(Suppl. 2), 19–31.

Breiding, M. J., Smith, S. G., Basile, K. C., Walters, M. L., Chen, J., & Merrick, M. T. (2014). Prevalence and characteristics of sexual violence, stalking, and intimate partner violence victimization—National Intimate Partner and Sexual Violence Survey, United States, 2011. Retrieved from https://www.cdc.gov/mmwr/pdf/ss/ss6308.pdf

Campbell, J. C., Sharps, P. W., Sachs, C., & Yam, M. L. (2003). Medical lethality assessment and safety planning in domestic violence cases. *Clinics in Family Practice, 5*(1), 101–112.

Campbell, J. C., Webster, D. W., & Glass, N. (2009). The danger assessment: Validation of a lethality risk assessment instrument for intimate partner femicide. *Journal of Interpersonal Violence, 24*(4), 653–674. doi:10.1177/0886260508317180

Capaldi, D. M., Knoble, N. B., Shortt, J. W., & Kim, H. K. (2012). A systematic review of risk factors for intimate partner violence. *Partner Abuse, 3*(2), 231–280. doi:10.1891/1946-6560.3.2.231

Chung, E. K., Siegel, B. S., Garg, A., Conroy, K., Gross, R. S., Long, D. A., . . .Fierman, A. H. (2016). Screening for social determinants of health among children and families living in poverty: A guide for clinicians. *Current Problems in Pediatric and Adolescent Health Care, 46*(5), 135–153. doi:10.1016/j.cppeds.2016.02.004

Connor, P. D., Nouer, S. S., Speck, P. M., Mackey, S. N., & Tipton, N. G. (2013). Nursing students and intimate partner violence education: Improving and integrating knowledge into health care curricula. *Journal of Professional Nursing, 29*(4), 233–239. doi:10.1016/j.profnurs.2012.05.011

DuMonthier, A., & Dusenbery, M. (2016). Intersections of domestic violence and economic security. Retrieved from https://iwpr.org/wp-content/uploads/2017/01/B362-Domestic-Violence-and-Economic-Security-1.pdf

Erez, E. (2002). Domestic violence and the criminal justice system: An overview. *Online Journal of Issues in Nursing, 7*(1), 4.

Family Violence Prevention and Services Programs. (2016). Final rule. *Federal Register, 81*(212), 76446–76480.

Feder, G. S., Hutson, M., Ramsay, J., & Taket, A. R. (2006). Women exposed to intimate partner violence: Expectations and experiences when they encounter health care professionals: A meta-analysis of qualitative studies. *Archives of Internal Medicine, 166*(1), 22–37. doi:10.1001/archinte.166.1.22

Felitti, V. J., Anda, R. F., Nordenberg, D., Williamson, D. F., Spitz, A. M., Edwards, V., . . . Marks, J. S. (1998). Relationship of childhood abuse and household dysfunction to many of the leading causes of death in adults. The Adverse Childhood Experiences (ACE) Study. *American Journal of Preventive Medicine, 14*(4), 245–258.

Fernandes-Alcantara, A. L. (2014). Family Violence Prevention and Services Act (FVPSA): Background and funding. Retrieved from https://fas.org/sgp/crs/misc/R42838.pdf

Gutmanis, I., Beynon, C., Tutty, L., Wathen, C. N., & MacMillan, H. L. (2007). Factors influencing identification of and response to intimate partner violence: A survey of physicians and nurses. *BMC Public Health, 7*, 12. doi:10.1186/1471-2458-7-12

Hughes, M. M., & Brush, L. D. (2015). The price of protection. *American Sociological Review, 80*(1), 140–165. doi:10.1177/0003122414561117

Hyman, S. E., Malenka, R. C., & Nestler, E. J. (2006). Neural mechanisms of addiction: The role of reward-related learning and memory. *Annual Review of Neuroscience, 29*, 565–598. doi:10.1146/annurev.neuro.29.051605.113009

Kaur, R., & Garg, S. (2008). Addressing domestic violence against women: An unfinished agenda. *Indian Journal of Community Medicine, 33*(2), 73–76. doi:10.4103/0970-0218.40871

King, L. W. (2008). The Code of Hammurabi. Retrieved from http://avalon.law.yale.edu/ancient/hamframe.asp

McEwen, B. S. (1998). Stress, adaptation, and disease: Allostasis and allostatic load. *Annals of the New York Academy of Sciences, 840*, 33–44. doi:10.1111/j.1749-6632.1998.5b09546.x

McEwen, B. S., & Seeman, T. (1999). Protective and damaging effects of mediators of stress. Elaborating and testing the concepts of allostasis and allostatic load. *Annals of the New York Academy of Sciences, 896*, 30–47.

O'Doherty, L., Hegarty, K., Ramsay, J., Davidson, L. L., Feder, G., & Taft, A. (2015). Screening women for intimate partner violence in healthcare settings. *Cochrane*

Database of Systematic Reviews, *2015*(7), CD007007. doi:10.1002/14651858 .CD007007.pub3

Stewart, D. E., & Vigod, S. N. (2017). Mental health aspects of intimate partner violence. *Psychiatric Clinics of North America*, *40*(2), 321–334. doi:10.1016/j.psc.2017.01.009

Supreme Court of Alabama. (1871). Fulgham v. The State Ala. 1871. Retrieved from http://faculty.law.miami.edu/zfenton/documents/Fulghamv.State.pdf

■ EAR, NOSE, AND THROAT EMERGENCIES

Kathleen Bradbury-Golas

Overview

Ear, nose, and throat (ENT) disorders are common daily occurrences seen in the emergency department. Most of these disorders are primary care conditions, ranging from foreign objects, trauma, to infection and are usually non–life-threatening. Emergency care for ENT disorders, regardless of age, is focused on an accurate assessment of the complaint, associated symptoms, and priority management of airway and breathing patterns.

ENT disorders can occur separately or in combination with one or more other organ systems. For example, the common cold may include nasal congestion and sinus pressure, sore throat, and ear popping or pain, whereas bacterial pharyngitis may include only a sore throat and fever. All are capable of leading to more dangerous complications (i.e., pneumonia) when not treated accordingly.

Background

Ear, nose, and throat problems are one of the most common causes for which a person seeks medical care. These problems are more common in children than adults, due to their wider and more horizontal Eustachian tubes and an under-developed immunity (Surapaneni & Sisodia, 2016). Otitis media (middle/inner ear infection) remains one of the most common infections in children, affecting up to 75% of children at least once between the ages of 5 and 11 years (Liese et al., 2015). The occurrence of otitis media decreases markedly after age 6, with other head, face, and sinus conditions causing secondary otalgia in adults (Dains, Baumann, & Scheibel, 2016).

ENT disease can be caused by a variety of microorganisms with rhinoviruses as the leading cause of the common cold in all age groups. Acute pharyngitis, sinusitis, and otitis media are mainly associated with respiratory viruses and common bacteria. The most common bacterial agent for pharyngitis is *Group A beta-hemolytic Streptococcus* (GABS), accounting for 20% to 40% of cases in children, but only 10% of cases in adults (Cohen, Bertille, Cohen, & Chalumeau, 2016). Unfortunately, overuse of antibiotics for viral infections has led to antibiotic resistance, especially with *Streptococcus pneumoniae*, thereby complicating treatment. According to the Centers for Disease Control and Prevention (CDC; 2015), antibiotic adverse drug events are responsible for one out of five emergency department visits and over half of antibiotics prescribed for acute respiratory infections are inappropriate. In 2009, the United States spent $10.7 billion on combined inpatient and outpatient antibiotic use (CDC, 2015).

In addition to common upper respiratory infections, foreign object removal is often a common reason for visiting the emergency department. The nostrils and ears are prime locations for a foreign object to be found, with luck, before infection has taken place. A ruptured tympanic membrane (eardrum) can occur from either excessive fluid behind the ear due to infection or trauma from foreign objects (i.e., cotton swabs). The ear is the organ of hearing as well as equilibrium, therefore loss of hearing or vertigo and dizziness are also signs of possible issues within this system. Due to the vastness of symptomology within the many different disorders, a thorough nursing assessment is the starting point for differentiation of the cause of clinical manifestations.

Clinical Aspects

ASSESSMENT

Completing an accurate history and assessment is a critical component of nursing care and begins the process of clinical reasoning and triage. Utilizing the acronym OLDCART will assist the nurse in determining the onset and duration of the illness; major system affected; characteristics, including associated symptoms; activities that might make it worse; factors that have helped relieve the symptoms; and when during the day the symptoms are worse or better (Bickley, 2017). OLDCART stands for onset, location, duration, characteristics, alleviating factors, relieving factors, and timing. Specific medical history for comorbid conditions that increase complication risk and social history, such as immunization status, tobacco and alcohol use, and exposure to childcare/preschool, will be necessary to obtain. Many studies in developing countries have reported that socioeconomic status, especially poor living conditions, poor nutrition, and overcrowding increase the incidence of acute respiratory infections in the pediatric population, which in turn increases mortality risk (Chen, Williams, & Kirk, 2014; Ide & Uchenwa-Onyenegecha, 2015). In addition to determining complication risk, history will also help determine treatment modalities and additional teaching/health promotion needs.

The ears are complex sensory organs of hearing and balance. When assessing "ear pain" or otalgia, note that the pain can be primary (coming from the ear itself) or secondary (from other regions). Causes of primary otalgia include infections, inflammation, or foreign body, whereas causes of secondary otalgia include jaw, dental, and periodontal problems, along with infections of the nasopharyngeal areas. Otitis media (infection of the middle/inner ear) and otitis externa (infection of the ear canal or "swimmer's ear") are two examples of primary otalgia. Otitis media usually presents with a sharp pain, fever, feeling of fullness, and possible hearing loss. Children will often be irritable and pull on the affected ear. Otitis externa presents with pain upon movement of the tragus or jawline, purulent discharge from the ear canal, and possible hearing loss.

When assessing hearing loss or dizziness and vertigo, the nurse should note how the onset has occurred—sudden or gradual. Dizziness or vertigo is second only to back pain of adults seeking medical help (Rhoads & Petersen, 2014). Disorders, such as cerumen impaction, foreign body, labyrinthitis (inflammation of the inner ear), ruptured tympanic membrane, and Ménière's disease, should be considered.

The nose and sinuses are responsible for filtering/warming the air, primary site for inspiration and expiration, and the sense of smell and speech sounds. Nasal congestion, discharge, and sinus pressure or pain are the most common complaints offered. However, appetite and taste are also often disrupted with nasal disorders. It is essential for the nurse to assess for nasal discharge (rhinorrhea) including thickness, color, duration, and another other associated symptoms. Nasal discharge and sinus pressure are often primary symptoms of the common cold. Sinusitis is a sinus inflammation, with many possible causes, including infection, chemical irritants, cocaine use, and dental abscesses. Sinus pain, purulent nasal drainage, and fever are the most common symptoms. Allergic rhinitis (nasal membrane inflammation) is an allergic response to an environmental allergen (i.e., dust, pollen) and exhibits watery nasal drainage, congestion, sneezing, and sore throat. Foreign bodies in the nose occur most often in the pediatric population and aspiration of the object is a major concern. Other pediatric considerations should include careful assessment of the respiratory status as children may present with difficulty breathing and stridor. Epistaxis (nose bleed or hemorrhage) can occur from many different reasons, including but not limited to nose picking, nasal trauma (such as nasal fracture), hypertension and anticoagulant and inhalant use. Herbal therapies contribute to epistaxis as items such as ginkgo biloba increase the risk of bleeding through antiplatelet activity.

The mouth and oropharynx aid in speech, provide taste sensation, act as a passageway for air, and pass food into the esophagus. The most common complaint within the oropharyngeal area is a sore throat or pharyngitis. Again, assessing for other associated symptoms will assist in differentiating possible causes. Sore throats caused by bacterial infections usually occur suddenly; viral infections are more gradual in onset. The most common bacterial cause of pharyngitis is *group A beta-hemolytic Streptococcus* infection. Along with a sore throat, the patient will present with fever, hoarseness, enlarged lymph nodes, halitosis, and malaise. A "rapid strep" or throat culture may be indicated for these patients. If an abscess forms around the tonsil area (peritonsillar abscess), it must be treated immediately to prevent airway obstruction.

NURSING, INTERVENTIONS, MANAGEMENT, AND IMPLICATIONS

During triage, it is essential for the nurse to complete a full history and begin the clinical reasoning process to differentiate the possible causes of the illness/complaint. At this time, the nurse will be instrumental in determining the acuity level of each patient, ensuring that patients are treated accordingly. In the case of foreign object removal, the nurse should prepare for removal through suction, irrigation, alligator forceps, or ear curette. If the health care provider is unable to remove the object, an ENT specialist may need to be consulted. Cerumen impaction removal requires irrigation with warm water and peroxide. Epistaxis will require direct pressure to the bridge of nose, ice application, and possible nasal packing and cauterization. For all procedures, the emergency department nurse should be knowledgeable of the procedure and protocol.

Most ENT infections are treated using a variety of prescribed and over-the-counter medications. Therapeutic interventions include decongestants, antipyretics, pain medication, and antibiotic therapy, when indicated. Decongestants are contraindicated for all patients with hypertension and heart disease due to their vasoconstriction effect.

Antibiotic therapy can be either systemic or topical (Emergency Nurses Association, 2013). Penicillin is the standard systemic antibiotic prescribed, with macrolides (i.e., erythromycin) being prescribed if the patient has a penicillin allergy. Accurate dosing, especially with the pediatric patient, is necessary; therefore, the nurse needs to double check the amount/dose to ensure patient safety. For topical antibiotic administration, as with ear infections and the use of otic antibiotics, the nurse should make sure the drops are warm before administration. In instances when the ear canal is extremely edematous, an ear wick may be used to facilitate delivery of topical medications into the medial canal. For inflammatory reactions, as with seasonal allergies, antihistamines may be prescribed. These medications can also be administered either systemically or topically.

Patient and family education is essential for maximizing outcomes. Instructing the patient and family on completing the full antibiotic course; side effects of any of the medications; proper medication techniques; gargling with warm salt water; keeping ear (s) dry through use of plug(s); using steam, warm compresses, or humidifiers to loosen secretions; good handwashing; and increasing fluid intake should all be addressed upon discharge (Emergency Nurses Association, 2013).

OUTCOMES

The overall goal of therapy for most ENT disorders is resolution of symptoms within 7 to 14 days. Should symptoms continue past that time period, the patient may need a referral to ENT specialist. Chronic sinusitis occurs when the sinus ostia is remodeled leading to changes in the clearance mechanisms of the nares. Though rare now in the United States, *Streptococcal* pharyngitis may develop into a more serious complication, such as acute glomerulonephritis or rheumatic fever. Acute otitis media or blockage of the Eustachian tube can lead to a persistently draining perforation of the tympanic membrane (chronic otitis media). Once treatment has been initiated in the emergency department, the patient should be referred to his or her primary care provider for follow-up evaluation.

Summary

ENT disorders are common everyday occurrences. Most can be effectively treated with early intervention. In rare circumstances, when not detected or treated early, diseases, such as cancer or systemic infections, can cause death.

Good history taking and differentiation of symptoms, subsequent nursing care, prescribed pharmacotherapy, and discharge education are essential elements of patient care management and health promotion.

Bickley, L. S. (2017). *Bates' guide to physical examination and history taking* (12th ed.). Philadelphia, PA: Lippincott.

Centers for Disease Control and Prevention. (2015). Fast facts about antibiotic resistance. Retrieved from http://www.cdc.gov/getsmart/community/about/fast-facts.html

Chen, Y., Williams, E., & Kirk, M. (2014). Risk factors for acute respiratory infection in the Australian community. *PLOS ONE, 9*(7), e101440. doi:10.1371/journal.pone.0101440

Cohen, J., Bertille, N. Cohen, R., & Chalumeau, M. (2016). Rapid antigen detection test for group A streptococcus in children with pharyngitis. *Cochrane Database of Systematic Reviews, 2016*, CD010502. doi:10.1002/14651858.CD010502.pub2

Dains, J., Baumann, L., & Scheibel, P. (2016). *Advanced health assessment and clinical diagnosis in primary care* (5th ed.). St. Louis, MO: Elsevier.

Emergency Nurses Association. (2013). *Sheehy's manual of emergency care* (7th ed.). St. Louis, MO: Mosby

Ide, L., & Uchenwa-Onyenegecha, T. (2015). Burden of acute respiratory tract infections as seen in University of Port Harcourt Teaching Hospital Nigeria. *Journal of US–China Medical Science, 12*, 158–162. doi:10.17265/1548-6648/2015.04.003

Liese, J. G., Giaquinto C., Carmona A., Larcombe J. H., Garcia-Sicilia, J., . . . Rosenlund, M. R. (2015). Incidence and clinical presentation of acute otitis media in children aged <6 years in European medical practices. *Epidemiologic Infection, 142*(8), 1778–1788.

Rhoads, J., & Petersen, S. (2014). *Advanced health assessment and diagnostic reasoning* (2nd ed.). Burlington, MA: Jones & Bartlett.

Surapaneni, H., & Sisodia, S. (2016). Incidence of ear, nose and throat disorders in children: A study in a teaching hospital in Telangana. *International Journal of Otorhinolaryngology and Head and Neck Surgery, 2*(1), 26–29.

■ ELDER ABUSE AND NEGLECT

Patricia M. Speck
Richard Taylor
Stacey A. Mitchell
Diana K. Faugno
Rita A. Jablonski-Jaudon

Overview

In 1900, those 65 years and older were one in 25 (3.1 million) persons in the United States and by 2060, one in four (98.2 million) persons in the United States will be older than 65 years (National Criminal Justice Reference Service, 2017; U.S. Census Bureau, 2017), and the oldest old, who are aged 85 and older, will be 25% of all elders 65 years and older and 5% of the total U.S. population in 2013 (U.S. Census Bureau, 2011, 2017). In the elderly population, women outnumber men, with approximately 10% of elders 65 to 74 years, residing in institutions; by age 85 to 100, 50% reside in nursing homes (U.S. Census Bureau, 2011). Emotional elder abuse by care staff (40%; Pillemer & Moore, 1989) and physical abuse (40%) by nonresidents are prevalent (Bloemen, Rosen, Clark, Nash, & Mielenz, 2015). With the gradual increase in elder parent placement in institutions, increasing numbers of dependent elders foretell that most practicing nurses in 2030 will care for older persons. An unknown portion of their patients will be targeted for or will experience neglect, abuse, and/or exploitation (Alzheimer's Association, 2017; National Clearinghouse of Abuse in Later Life, 2013).

Background

The lack of a universal definition of elder abuse has diminished the accuracy in reporting the incidence and prevalence of this public health problem (J. Hall, Karch, & Crosby, 2016). Many definitions are descriptions of behaviors by offenders, matching legal definitions of the crimes. The Centers for Disease Control and Prevention's Violence Division defines *elder abuse* as:

■ *Physical Abuse:* The intentional use of physical force that results in acute or chronic illness, bodily injury, physical pain, functional impairment, distress, or death.
■ *Sexual Abuse or Abusive Sexual Contact:* Forced or unwanted sexual interaction (touching and nontouching acts) of any kind with an older adult [including incapacitated older adult].
■ *Emotional or Psychological Abuse:* Verbal or nonverbal behavior that results in the infliction of anguish, mental pain, fear, or distress.
■ *Neglect:* Failure by a caregiver or other responsible person to protect an elder from harm, or the failure to meet needs for essential medical care, nutrition, hydration, hygiene, clothing, basic activities of daily living or shelter, which results in a serious risk of compromised health and safety.

■ *Financial Abuse or Exploitation*: The illegal, unauthorized, or improper use of an older individual's resources by a caregiver or other person in a trusting relationship, for the benefit of someone other than the older individual.(Centers for Disease Control and Prevention, 2016, paras 2, 3, 4, 5, 6)

The incidence and prevalence of elder neglect, abuse, and exploitation is unknown (National Institute of Justice, 2015). The reporting incidence and prevalence is divided into community-residing older persons and older persons in residential care facilities where 11% reported an experience of emotional, physical, sexual abuse, or neglect in the past year. In residential care facilities, caretakers primarily abuse older persons with critical remarks and humiliation; however, recent research highlighted resident-to-resident abuse and the need for training of care providers to mitigate or diminish future events (J. Hall et al., 2016; National Institute of Justice, 2015). Physical and mental health change in an older person creates vulnerability to neglect, abuses, and exploitation (National Institute of Justice, 2015). Abuse may include intentional isolation or abandonment, food insecurity, financial exploitation, emotional and psychological abuses, as well as physical and sexual assaults (National Council on Aging, n.d.). In persons with dementia, the elder person may resist care because dementia's neurodegeneration heightens perception of threats (Jablonski, Therrien, & Kolanowski, 2011; Jablonski, Therrien, Mahoney, et al., 2011). Care-resistant behavior increases exponentially as the dementia worsens (Jablonski, Therrien, & Kolanowski, 2011; Jablonski, Therrien, Mahoney, et al., 2011). In holistic palliative care (PC), elders, declining due to end-of-life factors, are at significantly higher risk of victimization by caregiver perpetrators of abuse (Jayawardena & Liao, 2006). For the dependent older person recently enrolled in PC, instead of improved quality of life and a "good death" (which is the intention of PC), abusive relationships in a private home are now serendipitously observed by RNs (Fisher, 2003), who are mandated reporters.

Calculating incidence and prevalence in a population of diverse elderly is complex. A sample of community-dwelling older persons nationally ($N = 5777$) found 11.4% ($n = 589$) experienced mistreatment in the past year, including "neglect and emotional, physical, and sexual abuse" (Acierno et al., 2010, p. 293), providing an opportunity for nursing to raise awareness and develop prevention interventions, particularly in high-risk racial and ethnic minorities (Beach, Schulz, Castle, & Rosen, 2010; DeLiema, Gassoumis, Homeier, & Wilber, 2012). *The Crimes Against the Elderly*, 2003–2013 (Morgan & Mason, 2014), reports a nonfatal violent crime rate of 3.6 per 1,000 and property crime rate of 72.3 per 1,000 for this 10-year period, providing opportunity for anticipatory guidance from RNs with safety concerns for community-dwelling elders.

Older persons have U.S. constitutional guarantees, including a right to self-determination (J. Hall, 2016, p. 37), including the right to self-neglect. This right to self-determination is more complex when dementia is present; for instance, family and formal caregivers may misinterpret the perception of threat as an exercise in autonomy (J. A. Adams, Bailey, Anderson, & Docherty, 2011).

RNs behaviors may also contribute to failure to administer necessary treatments or medications because the person with dementia "refused," when in fact, the nurses' approaches triggered the care-refusal behavior (Jablonski, Kolanowski, Winstead, Jones-Townsend, & Azuero, 2016).

Disparities and social determinants as risk factors diminish attainment of health. Social determinants include the environment and attitudes, exposure to crime and violence, disease and access to health care, financial and food security, and personal and caregiver support systems (Leff, Kao, & Ritchie, 2015; National Criminal Justice Reference Service, 2017). Chronic stress in environments increases allostatic load risk, in which situational elevations in the allostatic load following abuse are also responsible for an increase in mortality following trauma in the elderly (Lachs, Williams, O'Brien, Pillemer, & Charlson, 1998) and contribute to the estimated additional $5.3 billion health expenditures, not to mention the prosecution, law enforcement, corrections, and other ongoing expenses in pursuit of justice (A. Hall et al., 2016).

Epigenetics is gaining favor as the explanation for intergenerational poor health outcomes, in which brain trauma from emotional or physical abuse or violence by intimates and family may predict future generation's diseases and focal dementias in older persons (Klengel, Pape, Binder, & Mehta, 2014).

Adverse childhood experience (ACE) scores are recommended as a routine vital sign, and provide insight about life experiences and health states (Felitti et al., 1998; Lachs et al., 1998), where ACEs correlate with all human body system diseases. ACEs explain the impact of a history of abuses in a population of persons in PC who report increased distress and anxiety (Probst, Wells-DiGregorio, & Marks, 2013) and experience somatic and mental health disorders, chronic disease, and early death (Probst et al., 2013). For example, elderly Holocaust survivors reexperience memories as dementia progresses (La Ganga, 2007) and Hurricane Katrina spiked elder death rates for several years (V. Adams, Kaufman, Van Hattum, & Moody, 2011).

The victims of elder neglect, abuse, or exploitation initially respond in a normal fashion to psychological stressors or traumatic events. However, the neuro-endocrine system creates a sudden brainstem irritation response (fear) activating the hypothalamic–pituitary–adrenal axis, and when high hormonal levels cooccur with comorbid disease states in older persons, internal crisis of disease and stress leads to death (Christakis & Allison, 2006; Elwert & Christakis, 2008; Selye, 1974). Understanding the underlying physiology of stress and trauma prepares the RNs to recognize maladaptive and negative symptoms in chronically victimized elderly (Selye, 1956, 1974) and intercede with evidence-based interventions (Schneiderman, Ironson, & Siegel, 2005).

Clinical Aspects

ASSESSMENT

Screening the older person identifies at-risk elders and provides RNs an opportunity for anticipatory guidance and intervention (The Hartford Institute for

Geriatric Nursing, 2017). The RNs caring for elder populations need a strong institutional policy and procedure reflecting the domains in geriatric care, which include skills in screening, identification, and management of abused and neglected older patients, and an interprofessional comprehensive plan to establish a safe environment for the older person to mitigate the impact of abuse and neglect (National Research Council, 2008, p. 22).

A nursing assessment includes the physical examination and emotional aspects of an older person's behavior with his or her caregiver, capacity to understand what happened, and a head-to-toe physical examination, which includes all skin and mucous membrane areas. The RNs consider other causes of injury, including bleeding diseases, medication side effects, falls, or previous assaults (including rape and domestic violence). The RNs document the assessment for elder neglect, abuse, or exploitation using descriptive terms only, such as color, size, and location. If the RNs are the first to suspect abuse or neglect, they are mandated reporters, regardless of others' opinions (Falk, Baigis, & Kopac, 2012; A. Hall et al., 2016). The RNs who objectively and comprehensively document the history and physical findings will fare well as "fact" witnesses in any criminal trial. Not all neglect or injury is intentional, so anticipating and educating family caregivers can prevent future neglect or injury. Throughout the assessment process, the RN role is therapeutic and supportive, mitigating mental health exacerbations (anger, depression, anxiety; Brown, 2012; Y. H. Chen, Lin, Chuang, & Chen, 2017).

NURSING INTERVENTIONS, MANAGEMENT, AND IMPLICATIONS

Nursing management after identification of elder abuse or neglect includes understanding that older persons have a lifetime of experiences with effective methods for integrating new information (Y. Chen & Blanchard-Fields, 1997). The RNs explain the process of reporting and provide clarity to the organizational processes such as mandating reporting. The RNs work with the institutional team to provide nursing care, assessment, and documentation, which are important for the safety and planning for the elder patient. When the closest caregiver (usually a child) is unable or unwilling to provide nurture and safety, recommending prevention or respite programs for at-risk families is a good first step, including more frequent home visitations or phone calls to check on the older persons and their caretaker's well-being (Bomba, 2006; Shugarman, Fries, Wolf, & Morris, 2003; Stark, 2012). The RNs understand that chaotic upbringing and/or abuses create hostility, which may result in self-injury, depression, or suicide or death (Johnson, 2016; Schulz & Sherwood, 2008). In the event the elder is deemed unable to return to his or her home, the RN's role is to comfort the older person, allow the older person to vent his or her feelings, and provide community resources to the family.

Elder abuse is defined differently by state laws, but all states follow federal legislation of the Elder Justice Act (2010), so the practicing RNs must be familiar with their state laws related to reporting elder neglect, abuse, or exploitation. If there is a suspicion of elder abuse, the RNs are obligated by law in most states to report to adult protective services and local law enforcement, which will address the criminal aspects of the case (Burgess, 2006).

Summary

Elder persons depend on safe and secure environments to live out their years. Elder neglect, abuse, and exploitation represent intentional crimes against them, primarily by family members, acquaintances, and other caretakers. Rarely do strangers gain access to older persons. Domestic violence, poverty, trafficking of human persons, war, drug use (covered in other entries), as well as neglect, abuse, and exploitation by family or caregivers create additional stress. Stress response following neglect, abuse, and exploitation creates a burden on the elder's existing disease states through overproduction of stress hormones. The stress hormones cripple the elder's capacity to overcome the trauma reaction, and sometimes the elders die before they can process the trauma.

RNs are in the position to recognize the elder subjected to violence and identify the subsequent stress reactions by using the nursing process. The RNs practicing with older persons should have serial vital signs in the elder's health record, including historical ACEs, scales measuring depression and anxiety, cognitive assessments, and other validated methods for assessing the older persons and their caretaker. The RNs ask the questions related to life events, important to the older person desiring nostalgia. Recognition of stress responses, including uncontrolled hypertension, diabetes, mental health exacerbation while on medication, neglect, and other signs of fear in the older person provide the opportunity for all RNs to intervene, report, and participate in interprofessional team collaboration to create safe, supportive, and secure environments for all older persons and their caretakers (Dong et al., 2011).

Acierno, R., Hernandez, M. A., Amstadter, A. B., Resnick, H. S., Steve, K., Muzzy, W., & Kilpatrick, D. G. (2010). Prevalence and correlates of emotional, physical, sexual, and financial abuse and potential neglect in the United States: The National Elder Mistreatment Study. *American Journal of Public Health*, *100*(2), 292–297. doi:10.2105/AJPH.2009.163089

Adams, J. A., Bailey, D. E., Anderson, R. A., & Docherty, S. L. (2011). Nursing roles and strategies in end-of-life decision making in acute care: A systematic review of the literature. *Nursing Research and Practice*. doi:10.1155/2011/527834

Adams, V., Kaufman, S. R., Van Hattum, T., & Moody, S. (2011). Aging disaster: Mortality, vulnerability, and long-term recovery among Katrina survivors. *Medical Anthropology*, *30*(3), 247–270. doi:10.1080/01459740.2011.560777

Alzheimer's Association. (2017). 2017—Alzheimer's disease, facts, and figures. *Alzheimers Dementia*, *13*, 325–373.

Beach, S. R., Schulz, R., Castle, N. G., & Rosen, J. (2010). Financial exploitation and psychological mistreatment among older adults: Differences between African Americans and non-African Americans in a population-based survey. *The Gerontologist*, *50*(6), 744–757. doi: 10.1093/geront/gnq053

Bloemen, E. M., Rosen, T., Clark, S., Nash, D., & Mielenz, T. J. (2015). Trends in reporting of abuse and neglect to long term care ombudsmen: Data from the National Ombudsman Reporting System from 2006 to 2013. *Geriatric Nursing*, *36*(4), 281–283. doi:10.1016/j.gerinurse.2015.03.002

Bomba, P. A. (2006). Use of a single page elder abuse assessment and management tool: A practical clinician's approach to identifying elder mistreatment. *Journal of Gerontological Social Work*, *46*(3–4), 103–122. doi:10.1300/J083v46n03_06

Brown, L. (2012). *Assessing, intervening, and treating traumatized older adults.* Paper presented at the Biennial Trauma Conference: Addressing Trauma across the Lifespan: Integration of Family, Community, and Organizational Approaches, Florida.

Burgess, A. W. (2006). *Elderly victims of sexual abuse and their offenders* (p. 157). Boston College, Boston, MA: National Institutes of Justice Office of Justice Programs.

Centers for Disease Control and Prevention. (2016). Elder abuse: Definitions. Retrieved from https://www.cdc.gov/violenceprevention/elderabuse/definitions.html

Chen, Y., & Blanchard-Fields, F. (1997). Age differences in states of attributional processing. *Psychology and Aging*, *12*(4), 694–703. doi:10.1037/0882-7974.12.4.694

Chen, Y.-H., Lin, L.-C., Chuang, L.-L., & Chen, M.-L. (2017). The relationship of physiopsychosocial factors and spiritual well-being in elderly residents: Implications for evidence-based practice. *Worldviews on Evidence-Based Nursing*. Advance online publication. doi:10.1111/wvn.12243

Christakis, N. A., & Allison, P. D. (2006). Mortality after the hospitalization of a spouse. *New England Journal of Medicine*, *354*(7), 719–730. doi:10.1056/NEJMsa050196

DeLiema, M., Gassoumis, Z. D., Homeier, D. C., & Wilber, K. H. (2012). Determining prevalence and correlates of elder abuse using promotores: Low-income immigrant Latinos report high rates of abuse and neglect. *Journal of the American Geriatrics Society*, *60*(7), 1333–1339. doi:10.1111/j.1532-5415.2012.04025.x

Dong, X. Q., Simon, M. A., Beck, T. T., Farran, C., McCann, J. J., Mendes de Leon, C. F., . . . Evans, D. A. (2011). Elder abuse and mortality: The role of psychological and social wellbeing. *Gerontology*, *57*(6), 549–558.

Elwert, F., & Christakis, N. A. (2008). Variation in the effect of widowhood on mortality by the causes of death of both spouses. *American Journal of Public Health*, *98*(11), 2092. doi:10.2105/AJPH.2007.114348

Falk, N. L., Baigis, J., & Kopac, C. (2012, August 14). Elder mistreatment and the Elder Justice Act. *Online Journal of Issues in Nursing*, *17*(3), 7. doi:10.3912/OJIN .Vol17No03PPT01

Felitti, V. J., Anda, R. F., Nordenberg, D., Williamson, D. F., Spitz, A. M., Edwards, V., . . . Marks, J. S. (1998). Relationship of childhood abuse and household dysfunction to many of the leading causes of death in adults. The Adverse Childhood Experiences (ACE) Study. *American Journal of Preventive Medicine*, *14*(4), 245–258.

Fisher, C. (2003). The invisible dimension: Abuse in palliative care families. *Journal of Palliative Medicine*, *6*(2), 257–264.

Hall, A., McKenna, B., Dearie, V., Maguire, T., Charleston, R., & Furness, T. (2016). Educating emergency department nurses about trauma informed care for people presenting with mental health crisis: A pilot study. *BMC Nursing*, *15*(1), 21. doi:10.1186/s12912-016-0141-y

Hall, J., Karch, D. L., & Crosby, A. (2016). Elder abuse surveillance: Uniform definitions and recommended core data elements. Retrieved from https://www.cdc.gov/violenceprevention/pdf/EA_Book_Revised_2016.pdf

The Hartford Institute for Geriatric Nursing (Producer). (2017, May 1). Elder mistreatment training manual and protocol. Retrieved from https://consultgeri.org/education-training/e-learning-resources/elder-mistreatment-training-manual-and-protocol

Jablonski, R. A., Kolanowski, A., Winstead, V., Jones-Townsend, C., & Azuero, A. (2016). Maturation of the MOUTh intervention: From reducing threat to relationship-centered care. *Journal of Gerontological Nursing*, *42*(3), 15–23.

Jablonski, R. A., Therrien, B., & Kolanowski, A. (2011). No more fighting and biting during mouth care: Applying the theoretical constructs of threat perception to clinical practice. *Research and Theory for Nursing Practice*, *25*(3), 163–175.

Jablonski, R. A., Therrien, B., Mahoney, E. K., Kolanowski, A., Gabello, M., & Brock, A. (2011). An intervention to reduce care-resistant behavior in persons with dementia during oral hygiene: A pilot study. *Special Care in Dentistry*, *31*(3), 77–87.

Jayawardena, K. M., & Liao, S. (2006). Elder abuse at end of life. *Journal of Palliative Medicine*, *9*(1), 127–136.

Johnson, L. (2016). Pushed to the edge: Caregivers who kill. Retrieved from https://www.agingcare.com/articles/caregivers-kill-parents-commit-suicide-150336.htm

Klengel, T., Pape, J., Binder, E. B., & Mehta, D. (2014). The role of DNA methylation in stress-related psychiatric disorders. *Neuropharmacology*, *80*, 115–132. doi:10.1016/j.neuropharm.2014.01.013

Lachs, M. S., Williams, C. S., O'Brien, S., Pillemer, K. A., & Charlson, M. E. (1998). The mortality of elder mistreatment. *Journal of the American Medical Association*, *280*(5), 428–432.

La Ganga, M. (2007). Fearing the Nazis again. *Los Angeles Times*, August 23. Retrieved from http://articles.latimes.com/2007/aug/23/local/me-rachel23

Leff, B., Kao, H., & Ritchie, C. (2015). How the principles of geriatric care can be used to improve care for medicare patients. *Journal of the American Society on Aging*, *39*(7), 99–105.

Morgan, R., & Mason, B. (2014). Crimes against the elderly, 2003–2013: Special Report, U.S. Department of Justice, Bureau of Justice Statistics. November. Retrieved from https://www.bjs.gov/content/pub/pdf/cae0313.pdf

National Clearinghouse of Abuse in Later Life. (2013). An overview of elder abuse: A growing problem. Retrieved from http://www.ncdsv.org/images/NCALL_Overview-of-elder-abuse-a-growing-problem_2013.pdf

National Council on Aging. (n.d.). Elder abuse facts. Retrieved from https://www.ncoa.org/public-policy-action/elder-justice/elder-abuse-facts

National Criminal Justice Reference Service. (2017). Special feature: Elder abuse. Retrieved from https://www.ncjrs.gov/elderabuse

National Institute of Justice. (2015). Extent of elder abuse victimization. Retrieved from https://www.nij.gov/topics/crime/elder-abuse/Pages/extent.aspx

National Research Council. (2008). Early childhood assessment: Why, what, and how? In Committee on Developmental Outcomes and Assessments for Young Children, C. E. Snow, & S. B. Van Hemel (Eds.), *Board on children, youth and families, board on testing and assessment, division of behavioral and social sciences and education.* Washington, DC: National Academies Press.

Pillemer, K., & Moore, D. W. (1989). Abuse of patients in nursing homes: Findings from a survey of staff. *The Gerontologist, 29*(3), 314–320.

Probst, D. R., Wells-Di Gregorio, S., & Marks, D. R. (2013). Suffering compounded: The relationship between abuse history and distress in five palliative care domains. *Journal of Palliative Medicine, 16*(10), 1242–1248. Retrieved from https://doi.org/10.1089/jpm.2012.0619

Rhodes, J., Chan, C., Paxson, C., Rouse, C. E., Waters, M., & Fussell, E. (2010). The impact of hurricane Katrina on the mental and physical health of low-income parents in New Orleans. *American Journal of Orthopsychiatry, 80*(2), 237–247. doi:10.1111/j.1939-0025.2010.01027.x

Schneiderman, N., Ironson, G., & Siegel, S. D. (2005). Stress and health: Psychological, behavioral, and biological determinants. *Annual Review of Clinical Psychology, 1,* 607–628. doi:10.1146/annurev.clinpsy.1.102803.144141

Schulz, R., & Sherwood, P. R. (2008). Physical and mental health effects of family caregiving. *American Journal of Nursing, 108*(Suppl. 9), 23–27. doi:10.1097/01.NAJ.0000336406.45248.4c

Selye, H. (1956). *The stress of life.* New York, NY: McGraw-Hill.

Selye, H. (1974). *Stress without distress.* Philadelphia, PA: Lippincott.

Shugarman, L. R., Fries, B. E., Wolf, R. S., & Morris, J. N. (2003). Identifying older people at risk of abuse during routine screening practices. *Journal of the American Geriatrics Society, 51*(1), 24–31.

Stark, S. (2012). Elder abuse: Screening, intervention, and prevention. *Nursing, 42*(10), 24–29; quiz 29–30. doi:10.1097/01.nurse.0000419426.05524.45

U.S. Census Bureau. (2011). Sixty-five plus in the United States. Retrieved from https://www.census.gov/population/socdemo/statbriefs/agebrief.html

U.S. Census Bureau. (2017). Older Americans month: May 2017. Retrieved from https://www.census.gov/content/dam/Census/newsroom/facts-for-features/2017/cb17-ff08.pdf

■ ENCEPHALOPATHY

Deborah Vinesky

Overview

Encephalopathy is a general term that means brain disease, damage, or malfunction; the defining characteristic is an altered mental state. Encephalopathy most often occurs as a secondary complication of a primary neurological problem. Neurological problems can result from infections, trauma and physical injuries, genetics, environmental influences, and nutrition-related causes. Early treatment of most causes can decrease, eliminate, or stop the symptoms related to encephalopathy (Davis, 2015). The development of effective therapies that prevent and treat encephalopathy requires an understanding of its pathologic and physiologic processes (Williams, 2013).

Background

The National Institute of Neurological Disorders and Stroke (NINDS, 2017) defines encephalopathy as:

> Encephalopathy is a term for any diffuse disease of the brain that alters brain function or structure. Encephalopathy may be caused by infectious agent (bacteria, virus, or prion), metabolic or mitochondrial dysfunction, brain tumor or increased pressure in the skull, prolonged exposure to toxic elements (including solvents, drugs, radiation, paints, industrial chemicals, and certain metals), chronic progressive trauma, poor nutrition, or lack of oxygen, or blood flow to the brain. Care of the patient with encephalopathy presents unique challenges because generally it is manifested by an altered state accompanied by physical manifestations. (NINDS, 2017)

There are two distinct categories of encephalopathy: acute and chronic. The chronic encephalopathies are characterized by chronic mental status change that are slowly and insidiously progressive. In addition, they usually result from permanent and usually irreversible structural changes in the brain itself. In contrast, acute encephalopathy is characterized by a functional alteration of mental status due to systemic factors. It may be reversible when the abnormalities are corrected, and a full return to baseline mental status is expected. Acute encephalopathy can be further described as toxic, metabolic, or toxic-metabolic (Pinson, 2015).

Toxic encephalopathy can occur following exposure to acute or chronic neurotoxins. Neurotoxins include chemical compounds of chemotherapy, heavy metals, pesticides, and industrial and cleaning solvents. Exposure to toxins can lead to a variety of neurological symptoms, characterized by memory loss, visual disturbances, and an altered mental status. Metabolic encephalopathy, or toxic-metabolic encephalopathy, is a category of encephalopathy describing abnormalities related to water, electrolytes, vitamins, and other chemicals that have the potential to adversely affect brain function. Neurotoxins are chemical agents affecting the transmission of chemical signals between neurons, at any step in neural transmission.

"Delirium" and "acute encephalopathy" are virtually two different terms that essentially represent the same condition. Delirium describes the mental manifestation, whereas encephalopathy is the underlying pathophysiologic process. Manifestations of delirium include reduced awareness of the environment, cognitive impairment, emotional disturbances, and changes in behavior. Changes in behavior include hallucinations, restlessness, agitation or combative behavior, lethargy, and disturbed sleep patterns. The *Diagnostic and Statistical Manual of Mental Disorders*, Fifth Edition (DSM-5; American Psychiatric Association, 2013), does not use encephalopathy in its definition and classification of delirium (Pinson, 2015). Historically, delirium has been considered a manifestation of generalized cerebral metabolic insufficiency and may result in a combination of abnormal blood flow, abnormal energy metabolism, abnormal neurotransmission, and abnormal cellular maintenance processes (Williams, 2013).

Clinical Aspects

ASSESSMENT

Care of the patient will vary depending on the etiology of the encephalopathy. Altered mental status is the hallmark of encephalopathy; the initial approach should be systematic and should focus on stabilization. In many patients, particularly the elderly, there exists some preexisting degree of chronic and ongoing cognitive impairment, dementia, or psychiatric illness. Various infections, including bacteria, viruses, prions, and parasites, can cause temporary or permanent brain damage leading to encephalopathy. Restricted oxygen supply to the brain, alcohol abuse, metabolic disease, tumors, prolonged inhalation of toxic chemicals, exposure to radiation, and drug abuse can lead to encephalopathy.

The most important part of the workup will be the history and physical examination, including vital signs. If the patient is alert and cooperative, and/or there are family members present, information should be obtained, including current medical illness, medications (recent and present), or possible ingestion of toxins. Data are obtained that will aid in ruling out causes that have the potential to harm the patient, and those that are correctable. Acute change in mental status is a symptom and must be monitored for and documented appropriately. Once the patient is stabilized, an assessment based on a systems approach should be conducted, utilizing previously gained information related to the patient's history (Parmley & Neeley, 2017).

NURSING INTERVENTIONS, MANAGEMENT, AND IMPLICATIONS

Hospitalized patients suffering from encephalopathy have complex nursing needs. These same patients are susceptible to poor quality of care that has the potential to affect their quality of life. Nursing is challenged with recognizing and addressing the unique needs of this special population. Misinterpretation of the needs of this vulnerable population may result in the patients receiving suboptimal care with further decline in cognitive functioning (Joosse, Palmer, & Lang, 2013).

OUTCOMES

The primary outcome of evidence-based strategies is to minimize the patient's risk and exposure to toxins that may contribute to manifestation of encephalopathy. Nursing care should focus on the assessment of patient's mental status and change in behaviors, which include aimless wandering, agitation, impaired balance and gait, and interrupted sleep and rest. Given the altered mental status, a central clinical symptom of encephalopathy, nursing care should be also focused on maintaining a safe environment of care for patients with this medical condition.

To aid the nurse in providing quality care, it is necessary to be able to synthesize and translate evidence-based practice into best practices to be used at the bedside. Early assessment and preventive measures are useful in maintaining function and preventing decline. Functional impairment and behavioral symptoms include inability to initiate meaningful activity, disorientation and anxiety, apathy, repetitive vocalization, resistiveness, combativeness, and dietary issues like food refusal; all interfere with nursing care (Joosse et al., 2013). Electronic support services provide clinical support for patient care services. These services promote evidence-based early recognition, risk assessment, identification of problems, and selection of appropriate nursing interventions and outcomes (Joosse et al., 2013).

Summary

Encephalopathy most often occurs secondary to a complication of a primary neurological problem. Care of the patient with encephalopathy is dependent upon its etiology. Hospitalized patients suffering from acute and chronic encephalopathy have complex nursing needs requiring astute assessment skills, based on a systems approach once the patient is stabilized. Recognizing and addressing the unique needs of this population will promote optimal quality of care. With a focus on promoting independence and controlling risk factors, a decline in cognitive functioning will be prevented. Safety is of the utmost importance in this population, as is early assessment and instituting preventive measures.

American Psychiatric Association. (2013). *Diagnostic and statistical manual of mental disorders* (5th ed.). Arlington, VA: American Psychiatric Publishing.

Davis, C. P. (2015). Encephalopathy. Retrieved from http://www.medicinenet.com/encephalopathy/article.htm

Joosse, L. L., Palmer, D., & Lang, N. (2013). Caring for elderly patients with dementia: Nursing interventions. *Nursing Research and Reviews, 3,* 107–117.

National Institute of Neurological Disorders and Stroke. (2017). Encephalopathy information page. Retrieved from https://www.ninds.nih.gov/Disorders/All-Disorders/Encephalopathy-Information-Page

Parmley, C. L., & Neeley, R. (2017). Acute altered mental status, mental status changes, depressed mental status, lethargic, obtunded, altered level of consciousness. *Clinical Reviews, 27*(2).

Pinson, R. (2015). Encephalopathy. American College of Physicians Hospitalist. Retrieved from https://acphospi talist.org/archives/2015/01/coding.htm

Williams, S. (2013). Pathophysiology of encephalopathy and delirium. *Journal of Clinical Neurophysiology, 30*(5), 435–437.

■ ENDOCRINE EMERGENCIES

Diane Fuller Switzer

Overview

Endocrine emergencies are life-threatening conditions that require early and prompt identification, assessment, and aggressive pharmacologic and nursing interventions to prevent adverse consequences such as death. The endocrine system is very complex and although integrated, individual organ dysfunction has a unique presentation and requires specialized pharmacologic and nursing management to correct the imbalance as it impacts all the body systems.

Although the endocrine system consists of the hypothalamus, pituitary, thyroid, parathyroid, adrenals, pancreas, testes, and ovaries, this chapter focus on specific emergencies and nursing management related to the pancreas, thyroid, and adrenal glands. These emergencies include diabetic ketoacidosis (DKA), hyperosmolar hyperglycemia syndrome (HHS), hypoglycemia, thyrotoxicosis, and adrenal crisis.

Background

Diabetes mellitus is a complex, chronic condition identified by hyperglycemia resulting in macrovascular, microvascular, and neuropathic complications. Although the disease affects 29 million or 9.3% of the U.S. population, 8.1 million are unaware that they have the disease (Centers for Diseases Control and Prevention [CDC], 2012; Sease & Shealy, 2016). This disease is caused by a defect in insulin whereby the body does not make enough of it or is unable to use it, resulting in hyperglycemia. There are four classifications: type 1 an autoimmune disorder, type 2 insulin resistance or impaired insulin release, gestational, and secondary (genetic defects, drug induced, infections; Clutter, 2016; Sease & Shealy, 2016). The incidence of type 2 diabetes mellitus (T2DM), which accounts for 90% of diabetes mellitus, is expected to increase with an aging population, sedentary lifestyle, and rising obesity. In 2012, T2DM affected 11.2 million people aged 65 years or older, and 34.9% of the U.S. population were diagnosed with obesity (CDC, 2012; Sease & Shealy, 2016).

DKA is defined as a manifestation of severe insulin deficiency, often associated with stress and activation of counterregulatory hormones, resulting in hyperglycemia, dehydration, and electrolyte abnormalities resulting in a metabolic acidosis, which can lead to life-threatening metabolic derangements, myocardial depression, hypotension, coma, and death (Clutter, 2016; Sanuth, Bidlencik, & Volk, 2014; Sease & Shealy, 2016; Westerberg, 2013). Although DKA tends to affect younger populations with type 1 diabetes mellitus (T1DM), it may occur in individuals with T2DM who have ketosis-prone diabetes. In an individual with undiagnosed diabetes mellitus, DKA may be the presenting symptom. The most common causes of DKA are an infection, new-onset diabetes mellitus, and an interruption of insulin therapy, trauma, myocardial infarction (MI), and physiologic stressors (Clutter, 2016; Lenahan & Holloway, 2015; Sanuth et al., 2014; Sease & Shealy, 2016; Westerberg, 2013). It is listed as a primary diagnosis in approximately 7 patients per 1,000 hospital discharges, associated with an average length of stay of 3.4 days, with an annual expenditure estimated at $2.4 billion, and the incidence continues to rise (American Diabetes Association [ADA], 2016; CDC, 2012; Gosmanov, Gosmanova, & Kitabchi, 2015).

HHS is a life-threatening condition similar to DKA with hyperglycemia and dehydration but without acidosis or ketonuria. This condition occurs more often in older adults with T2DM and is expected to increase in incidence (Gosmanov et al., 2015; Lenahan & Holloway, 2015). Often, patients are unaware they have T2DM as they have not been diagnosed with it. The common causes of HHS include disease states such as infection (pneumonia), silent MI, cerebral vascular accident (CVA), and medications such as steroids, or thiazide diuretics (Clutter, 2016; Gosmanov et al., 2015; Lenahan & Holloway, 2015).

DKA and HHS share similar symptoms such as malaise, fatigue, recent illness or infections, but DKA is differentiated from HHS in that the onset of symptoms occurs across several days with nausea, vomiting, diffuse abdominal pain, increase in thirst, and sweet smelly breath (acetone). As DKA worsens, Kussmaul respirations (deep breaths because of an anion gap metabolic acidosis with respiratory compensation) may develop and confusion and drowsiness may be present. Lab results demonstrate an elevated glucose level less than 600, and positive ketones in urine. HHS has a gradual onset over several days to weeks and may present with dehydration, stupor, coma, elevated glucose more than 600, but without ketones in the urine. DKA is more common, usually with (T1DM), in a younger population (aged 20–29 years) with mortality of 5% to 10%. HHS is less common, usually occurs with T2DM, but can be T1DM, more severe illness with an older population (aged 57–70 years) and a higher mortality of 10% to 20% (ADA, 2016; Clutter, 2016; Gosmanov et al., 2015; Lenahan & Holloway, 2015).

Hypoglycemia occurs when the blood glucose level is 60 to 70 mg/dL or lower, usually affects patients with T1DM, but can occur with or without diabetes as a result of too much insulin or hypoglycemic medications, a delay or decrease in food intake, increase in exercise, alcohol, chronic kidney disease, liver failure, or sepsis. Hypoglycemia is common. In 2014, there were a total of 14.2 million emergency department visits for hypoglycemia; 245,000 (CDC, 2017) in the hospital setting are associated with a higher mortality rate (ADA, 2016; Clutter, 2016; Lenahan & Holloway, 2015; Westerberg, 2013). Hypoglycemia should be considered with any individual who has risk factors and who presents or develops symptoms of hypoglycemia such as a headache, confusion, shakiness, anxiety, sweating, tachycardia, irritability, drowsiness, or unresponsiveness.

Thyrotoxicosis is caused by excess thyroid hormone released from the thyroid gland, with clinical presentations of autonomic hyperactivity such as nervousness, tremor, palpitations, tachycardia, irritability, and increased perspiration. Graves' disease is the most common cause (60%–80%), with clinical features of exophthalmos, eyelid retraction, periorbital edema, proptosis, and diffuse thyroid enlargement. Thyrotoxicosis in the elderly usually occurs from toxic thyroid nodules or multinodular goiter. If left untreated, it can progress to an acute life-threatening condition called *thyroid storm* that is evidenced by a high fever, tachycardia, tachypnea, dehydration, delirium, and coma (Katz, 2016).

Adrenal crisis, or acute adrenal insufficiency, occurs when the body is unable to respond to excessive physiologic stress with an increase of endogenous cortisol (Dang, Chen, Pucino, & Calis, 2016). Adrenal crisis can occur in patients who have chronic adrenal insufficiency and do not receive sufficient glucocorticoid replacement in times of stress, in patients who have bilateral adrenal infarction, and in the critically ill, especially those in septic shock. Abrupt discontinuation or rapid tapering of glucocorticoid steroids can precipitate an adrenal crisis as well. These patients progress to circulatory collapse without immediate glucocorticoid replacement, and require volume resuscitation, correction of electrolyte abnormalities, and search for a precipitant such as an infection (Dang et al., 2016).

Clinical Aspects

ASSESSMENT

When caring for the patient with DKA, a detailed history from the individual or family member regarding the onset of symptoms, if onset is acute or gradual, type of symptoms (malaise, fatigue, anorexia, fever, chills, nausea, vomiting, abdominal pain, chest pain, increase in thirst [polydipsia], and/or urination [polyuria], weight loss, recent illnesses, stressors [surgery/infection/MI], medications [noncompliance], substance abuse, alcohol intake, comorbid conditions, living conditions, and history of previous or similar episodes) is necessary to determine the type of endocrine emergency the individual may be experiencing.

Frequent assessment of cardiovascular status (blood pressure, heart rate, temperature, color, volume status or perfusion as assessed by skin turgor, color, extremity pulses, warmth, and capillary refill) is necessary to prevent hypotension and maintain organ and tissue perfusion. The initial respiratory assessment must be performed to observe for Kussmaul respirations, tachypnea, shortness of breath, and oxygen saturation. Auscultation of the lungs can identify adventitious or absent breath sounds, which may be an indication of pneumonia or fluid overload. A chest x-ray can confirm whether an infectious process or fluid overload is present in the cardiopulmonary system. A renal system assessment is necessary to monitor for urine output following fluid resuscitation and correction of electrolyte abnormalities (hyperglycemia, hypokalemia), and nonanion gap metabolic acidosis. The neurological system is assessed for mental status changes that may indicate cerebral edema. The integumentary system should be assessed for signs of dehydration, infection, perfusion, color, and warmth.

The treatment of DKA requires large amounts of fluid resuscitation, insulin infusion, potassium replacement, and closure of the anion gap metabolic acidosis. Close attention to the potassium shift with insulin administration, prevention of hypoglycemia, hypokalemia, and complications associated with these electrolyte abnormalities (altered mental status, cerebral edema, EKG changes) are dependent on frequent nursing assessments and nursing interventions to correct the abnormalities.

HHS is similar to DKA with hyperglycemia, dehydration, and electrolyte losses, but without acidosis or ketonuria. As with DKA, the treatment and nursing care are similar with intravenous fluid resuscitation, cardiac monitoring, frequent electrolyte and serum glucose checks with electrolyte replacement, and to prevent a rapid reduction in serum glucose reduction, which may precipitate cerebral edema.

Hypoglycemia can occur with or without diabetes. Any patient who presents with an altered mental status or unresponsiveness, or develops mental status changes during hospitalization, requires immediate evaluation and nursing intervention to correct the hypoglycemia. Frequent nursing assessments of patients at risk, and providing patient education regarding diet, exercise, and frequent blood sugar monitoring to increase awareness of hypoglycemia triggers and symptoms help prevent complications.

NURSING INTERVENTIONS, MANAGEMENT, AND IMPLICATIONS

Successful management of endocrine emergencies is dependent on early and frequent nursing assessments to search for precipitating events such as infection, medications, and stressors. As these presentations may mimic neurologic, psychiatric, or substance abuse disorders, it is important that the nurse perform an accurate assessment, including history, physical exam, and response to nursing interventions, to determine the underlying cause for the alteration in a mental and physical presentation. Priority nursing-related problems include confusing presentations, so the nurse must search for and treat the precipitating event. This involves correction of volume deficits with fluid resuscitation and monitoring fluid status with frequent vital signs, including blood pressure, heart rate, respiratory rate, temperature, and urine output. Electrolyte abnormalities need to be corrected to promote fluid and acid–base balance. Frequent assessment of mental status is the key to determine whether a worsening condition is developing or if the patient is not responding to the current therapy. The administration of pharmacologic interventions requires close attention to maintain hemodynamic stability ensuring oxygenation and perfusion of organs and tissues.

OUTCOMES

The expected outcomes of evidence-based nursing care for endocrine emergencies are to prevent complications that may lead to adverse outcomes with an increase in morbidity and mortality. Structured order sets for the management of these conditions employ "best practice" and high-quality, evidence-based, safe patient care, so that these individuals can be stabilized safely and quickly, have a short hospital stay, and receive patient education to prevent future hospitalizations.

Summary

Adults with endocrine emergencies present with metabolic derangements in fluid and acid–base balance with unstable hemodynamics and altered mental status, which can progress to coma and death. Complications can be prevented with frequent nursing assessments and initiation of aggressive evidence-based nursing interventions. Adherence to hospital protocol-based treatment algorithms may prevent adverse outcomes.

American Diabetes Association. (2016). Standards of medical care in diabetes—2016. *Diabetes Care, 38*(Suppl. 1), S4–S93. Retrieved from http://care.diabetesjournals .org/content/suppl/2015/12/21/39.Supplement_1.DC2/2016-Standards-of-Care.pdf

Centers for Diseases Control and Prevention. (2017). Diabetes, data, and trends. Retrieved from https://www.cdc.gov/diabetes/pdfs/data/statistics/national-diabetes -statistics-report.pdf

Clutter, W. E. (2016). Endocrine diseases. In P. Bhat, A. Dretler, M. Gdowski, R. Ramgopal, & D. Williams (Eds.), *The Washington manual of medical therapeutics* (35th ed., pp. 758–778). Philadephia, PA: Wolters Kluwer/Lippincott Williams & Wilkins.

Dang, D. K., Chen, J. T., Pucino, Jr. F., & Calis, K. A. (2016). Chapter 45: Adrenal gland disorders. In M. A. Chisholm-Burns, T. L. Schwinghammer, & B. G. Wells (Eds.), *Pharmacotherapy, principles, and practice* (4th ed., pp. 695–710). New York, NY: McGraw-Hill.

Gosmanov, A. R., Gosmanova, E. O., & Kitabchi, A. E. (2015). Hyperglycemic crises: Diabetic ketoacidosis (DKA), and hyperglycemic hyperosmolar state (HHS). In L. J. De Groot, G. Chrousos, K. Dungan, K. R. Feingold, A. Grossman, J. M. Hershman . . . A. Vinik (Eds.), *Endotext* [Internet]. South Dartmouth, MA: MDText. com. Retrieved from https://www.ncbi.nlm.nih.gov/books/NBK279052

Katz, M. D. (2016). Thyroid disorders. In M. A. Chisholm-Burns, T. L. Schwinghammer, & B. G. Wells (Eds.), *Pharmacotherapy, principles, and practice* (4th ed., pp. 679–694). New York, NY: McGraw-Hill.

Lenahan, C. M., & Holloway, B. (2015). Differentiating between DKA and HHS. *Journal of Emergency Nursing, 41*(3), 201–207. Retrieved from http://www.jenonline .org

Sanuth, B., Bidlencik, A., & Volk, A. (2014). Management of acute hyperglycemic emergencies: Focus on diabetic ketoacidosis. *AACN Advanced Critical Care, 25*(3), 197–202. Retrieved from http://aacn.org

Sease, J., & Shealy, K. (2016). Diabetes mellitus. In M. A. Chisholm-Burns, T. L. Schwinghammer, & B. G. Wells (Eds.), *Pharmacotherapy, principles, and practice* (4th ed., pp. 651–678). New York, NY: McGraw-Hill.

Westerberg, D. (2013). Diabetic ketoacidosis: Evaluation and treatment. *American Family Physician, 87*(5). Retrieved from http://www.aafp.org/afp

■ ENVIRONMENTAL EMERGENCIES

Brittany Newberry

Overview

Environmental emergencies are common reasons for patients to seek care in the emergency department (ED) and the risk of becoming ill or injured during travel or recreation depends on many factors (Brunette, 2016). These injuries can happen at home, work, or recreational settings. Environmental injuries and emergencies are varied and require the clinician to have a high index of suspicion and focused history taking and assessment skills. Patients who experience environmental emergencies may have differing levels of prehospital care and may have additional complications such as exposure, heavily contaminated wounds, and/or prolonged extrication times (Lipman et al., 2014).

Environmental emergencies include, but are not limited to, envenomation and poisoning injuries, high altitude and decompression illnesses, and thermoregulation injuries. Prevention is an important aspect of reducing the morbidity and mortality associated with environmental emergencies. Environmental emergencies can also include day-to-day illnesses that can occur in the wilderness such as abdominal pain, stroke, and myocardial infarction.

Background

There are many types of environmental emergencies and the types of injuries/illnesses seen often depend on the area of practice. Some environmental injuries are more common in certain areas, such as envenomation, high altitude and decompression illnesses, and thermoregulation injuries, and clinical staff should be aware of emergencies that are common to their geographic area. Other emergencies, such as poisoning, occur in more widespread geographic areas.

Envenomation injuries can occur anywhere and are not uncommon events. Physical response to an envenomation may vary from a mild local reaction to severe systemic and/or anaphylactic reactions (Ittyachen, Abdulla, Anwarsha, & Kumar, 2015). Clinicians need to be familiar with venomous animals in their geographic area to rapidly recognize and treat these potential life-threatening injuries. Envenomation injuries can occur from spiders, scorpions, insects, snakes, marine animals, bees, or wasps. Each vector contains a unique toxin that requires rapid identification and potential specific treatment. A thorough history is important for these patients.

Poisoning injuries can be accidental or intentional. Oftentimes these injuries are the result of substance abuse by patients for recreational purposes (Vallersnes, Jacobsen, Ekeberg, & Brekke, 2016). However, children and adults can also be the victim of unintentional poisoning because of ingestion or exposure. Suicide attempts should generally be considered for these patients. A thorough history from the patient and any knowledgeable friends or family members are essential. The clinician should not hesitate to contact poison control to ensure that proper treatment is being initiated.

High altitude and decompression illnesses: More than 100 million people visit altitudes greater than 8,000 feet every year. Acute mountain sickness (AMS) can occur in unsuspecting healthy people and is usually a benign illness. However, at times, AMS may progress to life-threatening events such as high altitude cerebral edema (HACE) or high altitude pulmonary edema (HAPE; Netzer, Strohl, Faulhaber, Gatterer, & Burtscher, 2013). Clinicians working in potential exposure areas need to have astute assessment skills to recognize subtle changes or deterioration in condition for these patients.

Decompression illnesses consist of decompression sickness (DCS) and pulmonary overinflation syndrome (POIS). These illnesses occur when divers ascend too rapidly without giving time for carbon dioxide to properly off-gas from the blood. POIS has the additional complication of causing ruptured alveoli in the lungs, which then causes the extravasation of air bubbles into the tissues (Hall, 2014). Decompression illnesses are most commonly seen in coastal areas where diving is a popular recreational or occupational activity.

Thermoregulation injuries include the two extremes of hypothermia and hyperthermia. Each is a deviation from the body's ability to maintain homeostasis of temperature because of environmental or metabolic factors. Acute hypothermia can result from exposure or metabolic derangement and requires normalization. Severe hypothermia can lead to coagulopathy, cardiac arrest, and even death (Katrancha & Gonzalez, 2014).

Heat-related illnesses can be exercise induced or result from exposure to extreme temperatures or certain medications (Canel, Zisimopoulou, Besson, & Nendaz, 2016). Exertional heat illness (EHI) includes heat edema, heat cramps, heat syncope, and heat exhaustion and can lead to exertional heat stroke (EHS), which is a medical emergency (Pryor, Bennett, O'Connor, Young, & Asplund, 2015). EHS can lead to rhabdomyolysis, electrolyte imbalances, organ failure, and death if not treated.

Clinical Aspects

ASSESSMENT

Any envenomation injury or poisoning patient should have his or her vital signs monitored carefully and assessed for any signs of allergic reaction or anaphylaxis.

Poisoning patients from substance abuse should be assessed for any evidence of self-harm and receive appropriate monitoring and counseling if required. In addition, patients should be screened for substance abuse and potential withdrawal symptoms. High-altitude and decompression illnesses: Signs of AMS may include a headache, dizziness, vomiting, anorexia, fatigue, and/or insomnia, which usually occurs between 6 and 36 hours of high-altitude exposure.

NURSING INTERVENTIONS, MANAGEMENT, AND IMPLICATIONS

Envenomation injury or poisoning need rapid identification of the vector or substance, which is important to help guide treatment. Depending on the injury, treatment may consist of cold compresses, antihistamines, steroids, fluid resuscitation, antivenom, surgical intervention, and/or pain medications. A great number of insects, snakes, and other animals are venomous and can create complex and even fatal manifestations (Haddad, Amorim, Haddad, & Costa- Cardoza, 2015). Ensure that poison control has been contacted and that treatment recommendations are followed.

Rapid assessment and identification of potential substances are important to determine the best treatment. However, any life-threatening situations should be treated emergently. Patients should have the vital signs consistently monitored and airway, breathing, and circulation (ABCs) continuously assessed. These patients may be discharged home, transferred to another facility, observed, or admitted depending on the severity of their symptoms. Patient and/or parent education is an important facet of discharging poisoning patients, as prevention is paramount.

The treatment for AMS is descent. Signs, such as ataxia, hallucinations, confusion, vomiting, decreased activity, or severeunbearable headache, should cause the clinician to consider HACE. Ataxia is the hallmark sign of HACE. HAPE symptoms include dyspnea at rest, cough, weakness, and chest tightness. The patient may also have central cyanosis, frothy sputum, and crackles/wheezing in at least one lung field, tachypnea, and tachycardia. HAPE is most often misdiagnosed as pneumonia pointing to the importance of taking a thorough history (Netzer et al., 2013). Mild AMS can be treated with cessation of ascension and symptomatic treatment until the symptoms are resolved. HAPE and HACE should be treated with immediate descent and evacuation, oxygen therapy, and appropriate medications depending on the symptoms and severity.

Decompression illnesses (DCS and POIS) are best prevented with the regulated and monitored ascent to the water surface. Greater depth and longer dive times put divers at greater risk for decompression illness. Symptoms of DCS include joint pain (particularly in the shoulder) that is not worsened with the range of motion. POIS manifestations can include arterial gas embolism (AGE), pneumothorax, mediastinal emphysema, and/or subcutaneous emphysema. All of these symptoms result from overdistention and rupture of lung alveoli from expanding gases during ascent (Hall, 2014). Treatment primarily entails hyperbaric oxygen therapy but may require additional respiratory support for severe barotrauma.

Patients who experience acute nontherapeutic hypothermia should be rewarmed even in the absence of vital signs. Patients with a core body temperature of less than 32°C should have active rewarming via heated blankets, heating pads, radiant heat, warm baths, or forced warm air (Giesbrecht, 2000). During rewarming, monitor patients, as removal from the cold environment may result in peripheral vasodilation potentially leading to hypotension, inadequate coronary perfusion, and/or ventricular fibrillation (Brown, Brugger, Boyd, & Paal, 2012).

Patients who experience frostbite should have the affected areas rapidly rewarmed in warm water with the temperatures ranging from 37°C to 39°C (Nygaard et al., 2017). During rewarming, be prepared to assess the patient for and treat pain.

People who have had EHI in the past are more prone to experience heat-related illnesses and complications at subsequent exposures (Pryor et al., 2015). The classic triad of EHS is core body temperature more than 105°F, central nervous system dysfunction, and hot skin (often with anhidrosis). Other signs may include tachycardia, hypotension, tachypnea, rales, nausea, vomiting, diarrhea, cutaneous vasodilation, renal failure because of rhabdomyolysis, and coagulopathy. Immediate treatment for EHS is removal from the heat stressor and ABCs, rapid cooling for body temperature more than 105°F, aggressive fluid administration for any blood pressure (BP) less than 90/60, rehydration with isotonic fluids, and correction of electrolyte imbalances. Laboratory studies should be monitored carefully until the patient returns to baseline. Patients who experience EHS need thorough education about their illness, when to return to the ED, and how to prevent heat-related illnesses in the future.

OUTCOMES

Patients who are exposed to environmental emergency require immediate and deliberate care. Nurses working in emergency settings should first assess the patient to begin to differentiate a probable source of the injury. Because patients exposed to an environmental emergency can rapidly decompensate, it is critical that patients, family members, and emergency medical technicians be queried to gain information about the patient's condition. Stabilization and definitive care is needed to attenuate the progression of the injury.

Summary

Environmental injuries are common reasons for patients to seek care in the ED setting. Clinicians must have a high index of suspicion and initiate a thorough history and assessment. In addition, the clinician should be familiar with common environmental injuries in their geographic area to facilitate the rapid recognition and treatment of these injuries. All injuries should begin with the rapid assessment and treatment of ABCs and the recognition and treatment of associated life- or limb-threatening conditions such as anaphylaxis, neurovascular compromise, and hemorrhage.

Brown, D. J., Brugger, H., Boyd, J., & Paal, P. (2012). Accidental hypothermia. *New England Journal of Medicine, 367*(20), 1930–1938.

Brunette, G. W. (2016). *CDC health information for international travel.* New York, NY: Oxford University Press.

Canel, L., Zisimopoulou, S., Besson, M., & Nendaz, M. (2016). Topiramate-induced severe heatstroke in an adult patient: A case report. *Journal of Medical Case Reports, 10*, 95.

Giesbrecht, G. G. (2000). Cold stress, near drowning and accidental hypothermia: A review. *Aviation, Space, and Environmental Medicine, 71*(7), 733–752.

Haddad, V., Amorim, P. C., Haddad, W. T., & Cardoso, J. L. (2015). Venomous and poisonous arthropods: Identification, clinical manifestations of envenomation, and treatments used in human injuries. *Revista da Sociedade Brasileira de Medicina Tropical, 48*(6), 650–657.

Hall, J. (2014). The risks of scuba diving: A focus on decompression illness. *Hawai'i Journal of Medicine & Public Health, 73*(11, Suppl. 2), 13–16.

Ittyachen, A. M., Abdulla, S., Anwarsha, R. F., & Kumar, B. S. (2015). Multi-organ dysfunction secondary to severe wasp envenomation. *International Journal of Emergency Medicine, 8*, 6.

Katrancha, E. D., & Gonzalez, L. S. (2014). Trauma-induced coagulopathy. *Critical Care Nurse, 34*(4), 54–63.

Lipman, G. S., Weichenthal, L., Stuart Harris, N., McIntosh, S. E., Cushing, T., Caudell, M. J., . . . Auerbach, P. S. (2014). Core content for wilderness medicine fellowship training of emergency medicine graduates. *Academic Emergency Medicine, 21*(2), 204–207.

Netzer, N., Strohl, K., Faulhaber, M., Gatterer, H., & Burtscher, M. (2013). Hypoxia-related altitude illnesses. *Journal of Travel Medicine, 20*(4), 247–255.

Nygaard, R. M., Lacey, A. M., Lemere, A., Dole, M., Gayken, J. R., Lambert Wagner, A. L., & Fey, R. M. (2017). Time matters in severe frostbite: Assessment of limb/digit salvage on the individual patient level. *Journal of Burn Care & Research, 38*(1), 53–59.

Pryor, R. R., Bennett, B. L., O'Connor, F. G., Young, J. M., & Asplund, C. A. (2015). Medical evaluation for exposure extremes: Heat. *Wilderness & Environmental Medicine, 26*(4, Suppl), S69–S75.

Vallersnes, O. M., Jacobsen, D., Ekeberg, Ø., & Brekke, M. (2016). Outpatient treatment of acute poisoning by substances of abuse: A prospective observational cohort study. *Scandinavian Journal of Trauma, Resuscitation and Emergency Medicine, 24*, 76.

■ EXTRACORPOREAL LIFE SUPPORT

Grant Pignatiello
Katherine Hornack
Julie E. Herzog

Overview

Extracorporeal life support (ECLS) is a variation of cardiopulmonary bypass that provides support to the lungs and/or heart for patients in the intensive care unit (ICU) (Gaffney, Wildhirt, Griffin, Annich, & Radomski, 2010). According to the most recent data available from the Extracorporeal Life Support Organization (ELSO) registry, approximately 86,000 individuals have received ECLS, with 30% of these individuals being adults (ELSO, 2017). ECLS is a complex treatment modality for individuals experiencing severe critical illness; thus, the nursing care of this unique cohort entails rigorous monitoring of physiological parameters, thorough analysis of the clinical situation, and adapt management and advocacy of the family's psychosocial experience.

Background

ECLS, an expansion of the commonly known extracorporeal membrane oxygenation (ECMO), describes all extracorporeal, life support treatments (e.g., oxygenation, carbon dioxide removal, and hemodynamic support) that are used in the management of the critically ill patient suffering from severe pulmonary or cardiorespiratory failure. Broadly, there are two main categories of ECLS: venous–venous (VV) and venous–arterial (VA; Gaffney et al., 2010; Makdisi & Wang, 2015). VV ECLS is used as an advanced respiratory support modality that is indicated when the lungs' oxygenation capabilities are impaired as a result of physiologic insult (e.g., acute respiratory distress syndrome, pulmonary contusion, inhalation injury, lung transplantation, and status asthmaticus). VV ECLS consists of the implantation of a large catheter into a large vein (femoral or internal jugular) and the superior vena cava or right atrium; deoxygenated blood is then pulled from one of the catheters, cycled through an oxygenator, and returned to the patient through the right atrium.

Conversely, VA ECLS provides both respiratory and hemodynamic support. Indicated in situations in which the heart is unable to provide sufficient cardiac output despite inotropic and afterload-reducing support (e.g., cardiogenic shock, pulmonary embolism, cardiomyopathy, acute coronary syndrome, etc.), VA ECLS functions similarly to VV ECLS, except the oxygenated blood is returned to the arterial system through the femoral, axillary, carotid, or ascending aortic arteries—not relying on the left side of the heart to circulate independently.

ECLS is indicated for the critically ill patient who demonstrates profound respiratory and/or cardiac insufficiency that is refractory to other clinical treatments. Thus, ECLS is available to critically ill patients of all ages—from neonates to adults. However, a review of the available data suggests ECLS demonstrates the greatest effectiveness when implemented in neonatal and pediatric populations. According to the ECLS Organization (ELSO) registry, ECLS is used 3.5 and 2.5 times more often in neonatal populations than pediatric and adult populations, respectively (ELSO, 2017). In neonatal populations, VV and VA ECLS mortality is approximately 15% and 36%, respectively with 73% of VV and 40% of VA surviving to hospital discharge or transfer from the ICU. Mortality rates do not appear to differ in pediatric populations, as approximately 70% of pediatric patients survive ECLS treatment, regardless of ECLS type (i.e., VV or VA); however, pediatric patients who receive VV ECLS are more likely to survive to be discharged (57% vs. 50%; ELSO, 2017).

In adults, ECLS associated-mortality depends on the indication of ECLS initiation. Like the pediatric and neonatal population, survival rates are higher in adults who receive VV ECLS when compared to adults who receive VA ECLS (66% vs. 56%; ELSO, 2017). However, the use of VA ECLS for severe cardiogenic shock or cardiac arrest demonstrates more discouraging outcomes, with survival rates ranging from 20% to 30% (Makdisi & Wang, 2015). Furthermore, the complications associated with ECLS therapy are numerous, with end-organ system damage and infection being a common risk (Zangrillo et al., 2013). Therefore, it is consensually noted that before ECLS is initiated, the full clinical perspective of the patient be taken into perspective, as ECLS is a costly and resource-intensive treatment modality often necessitating a prolonged ICU length of stay (Aubron et al., 2013; Gaffney et al., 2010; Munshi, Telesnicki, Walkey, & Fan, 2014). Furthermore, the complications associated with ECLS initiation and management potentiate the risk of chronic critical illness—which is associated with its unique array of management complexities and increased morbidity and mortality.

Clinical Aspects

ASSESSMENT

A team approach is essential in managing patients who require ECLS. Most ECLS care is provided in tertiary-level ICUs with specially trained health care personnel, including critical care physicians, perfusion clinicians, advanced practice clinicians, nurses, respiratory therapists, and surgeons (Williams, 2013). A large portion of the nursing care is evaluating for complications. Complications associated with a patient on ECLS are cannula dislodgement, bleeding, intracranial bleeding, sepsis, air emboli, renal injury, disseminated intravascular coagulation, vascular complications, and decubitus ulcers (Gay, Ankney, Cochran, & Highland, n.d.). Thus, goals of nursing care are multifaceted in nature and require thorough assessment skills.

The incidence of neurological injury is approximately 16% in neonatal patients and 10% among adult and pediatric populations. The injury is precipitated by the nature of the underlying pathology, which commonly includes hypoxia and hypoperfusion, as well as coagulopathies related to anticoagulation therapy. Types of neurological injury include seizure, hemorrhage, infarction, and brain death (Mehta & Ibsen, 2013). Frequent neurological assessments should be performed to evaluate for deviations from the patient's baseline. Patients on ECLS often require sedation and may need neuromuscular blockade. Therefore, the neurological assessment includes evaluation of pupillary reflexes, peripheral sensory/motor function, sedation monitoring, and peripheral nerve stimulation reactivity. Changes from the patient's baseline commonly indicate further diagnostic imaging such as EEG or CT.

Cardiovascular nursing assessment focus may vary among patients receiving VV or VA ECLS. As the ECLS serves as the perfusion source, assessing peripheral and central perfusion is necessary (Chung, Shiloh, & Carlese, 2014). Vital signs and hemodynamic parameters are continuously monitored; hemodynamic parameters include mean arterial pressure, cardiac output/index, central venous pressure, pulmonary artery pressure, systemic vascular resistance, and mixed venous oxygen saturation level (SvO_2). SvO_2 levels, which represent peripheral oxygen consumption, are used to adjust ECLS circuit flow rates and should remain more than 60% (Gay et al., n.d.). The nursing assessment includes cardiac rhythm monitoring and neurovascular extremity evaluation. Further nursing management includes monitoring the therapeutic impact of and for complications related to vasopressor and inotropic medications.

Most patients receiving ECLS require continuous mechanical ventilation. Thus, nursing assessments should include continuous pulse oximetry, endotracheal tube position, breath sounds, and the quantity and quality of pulmonary secretions. Ventilation goals focus on resting the lungs by limiting tidal volumes (less than 4 mL/kg predicted body weight [PBW]), plateau pressures (20–25 cmH_2O), and respiratory rate while maintaining elevated positive endexpiratory pressure (PEEP) levels (greater than or equal to 10 cm H_2O; Schmidt et al., 2014). Ventilator and ECLS flow settings are adjusted from the frequent monitoring of arterial and venous blood gases.

NURSING INTERVENTIONS, MANAGEMENT, AND IMPLICATIONS

Monitoring of the ECLS circuit is often a shared responsibility between the perfusion clinician and nurse. For example, monitoring of the inflow and outflow cannulas should be routinely assessed for bleeding and placement stability; bleeding or unstable cannula sites should be reported to the perfusion clinician and ICU team. The nurse should evaluate oxygenator function by monitoring blood gas values. The ECLS catheters should be evaluated for rhythmic shaking, known as *chattering*, which may indicate hypovolemia or improper cannula placement (Chung et al., 2014). The bedside nurse should be aware of the ECLS flow rates, oxygenator, and sweep settings for integration into the interpretation of laboratory values and assessment findings.

Regarding the genitourinary system, hourly urine output should be monitored—acute renal failure occurs in 70% to 85% of patients receiving ECLS, often necessitating dialysis. Moreover, the nurse should monitor for electrolyte abnormalities (Chen, Tsai, Fang, & Yang, 2014). The gastrointestinal system must be monitored for signs of ischemia or bleeding; stool should be assessed for color and consistency. Notably, patients receiving ECLS commonly receive gastric ulcer prophylaxis through proton pump antagonists or histamine antagonists (Zangrillo et al., 2013).

A patient receiving ECLS has vast hematologic and integumentary considerations. Anticoagulation is required during ECLS to prevent clot formation in the circuit related to blood–surface interactions; however, bleeding is the most common complication of ECLS (Bartlett, 2016). Serial hematologic laboratory testing, including activated clotting time, anti-factor Xa activity levels, activated partial thromboplastin time, complete blood counts, fibrinogen, and lactate dehydrogenase (Annich, 2015). Owing to anticoagulation and the invasive nature of the ECLS cannulas, monitoring for bleeding is imperative. Patients on ECLS receive many blood product transfusions to keep appropriate intravascular volume in addition to optimizing oxygen-carrying capacity (Sen et al., 2016). Patients receiving ECLS are at an increased risk of integumentary complications secondary to immobility—increasing the risk for pressure ulcer development. Ideally, the patient's body position should be changed every 2 hours with pressure points supported by a dry, wrinkle-free surface.

Summary

ECLS serves as an effective treatment modality for the patient suffering from severe pulmonary or cardiorespiratory failure. Care of the patient receiving ECLS is complex, requiring interdisciplinary cooperation and competent nursing care—with an emphasis on continuously analyzing the patient's clinical presentation and monitoring for complications. As the health care industry witnesses advances in vascular access, ECLS circuitry, anticoagulation therapy, and patient management, Bartlett (2016) envisions outcomes associated with ECLS therapy to improve, introducing health care to a population of ECLS patients he describes as "awake, extubated, spontaneously breathing (patients), without systemic anticoagulation, managed in step-down units, general care, or even at home" (p. 10). As ECLS therapy continues to evolve, nursing care remain as a primary determinant in ensuring positive patient outcomes.

Annich, G. (2015). Extracorporeal life support: The precarious balance of hemostasis. *Journal of Thrombosis and Haemostasis*. Retrieved from http://onlinelibrary.wiley.com/doi/10.1111/jth.12963/full

Aubron, C., Cheng, A. C., Pilcher, D., Leong, T., Magrin, G., Coper, D. J., . . . Pellegrino, V. (2013). Factors associated with outcomes of patients on extracorporeal membrane oxygenation support: A 5-year cohort study. *Critical Care, 17*(2), R73. doi:10.1186/cc12681

Bartlett, R. H. (2016). ECMO: The next ten years. *Egyptian Journal of Critical Care Medicine, 4*(1), 7–10. doi:10.1016/j.ejccm.2016.01.003

Chen, Y.-C., Tsai, F.-C., Fang, J.-T., & Yang, C.-W. (2014). Acute kidney injury in adults receiving extracorporeal membrane oxygenation. *Journal of the Formosan Medical Association, 113*(11), 778–785.

Chung, M., Shiloh, A. L., & Carlese, A. (2014). Monitoring of the adult patient on venoarterial extracorporeal membrane oxygenation. *ScientificWorld Journal, 2014*, 393258. doi:10.1155/2014/393258

Extracorporeal Life Support Organization. (2017). Retrieved from https://www.elso.org

Gaffney, A. M., Wildhirt, S. M., Griffin, M. J., Annich, G. M., & Radomski, M. W. (2010). Extracorporeal life support. *British Medical Journal, 341*, c5317. doi:10.1136/bmj .c5317

Gay, S. E., Ankney, N., Cochran, J. B., & Highland, K. B. (n.d.). Critical care challenges in the adult ECMO patient. *Dimensions of Critical Care Nursing, 24*(4), 15762–15764. Retrieved from http://www.ncbi.nlm.nih.gov/pubmed/16043975

Mehta, A., & Ibsen, L. M. (2013). Neurologic complications and neurodevelopmental outcome with extracorporeal life support. *World Journal of Critical Care Medicine, 2*(4), 40–47.

Schmidt, M., Pellegrino, V., Combes, A., Scheinkestel, C., Cooper, D. J., & Hodgson, C. (2014). Mechanical ventilation during extracorporeal membrane oxygenation. *Critical Care, 18*(1), 203.

Sen, A., Callisen, H. E., Alwardt, C. M., Larson, J. S., Lowell, A. A., Libricz, S. L., . . . Ramakrishna, H. (2016). Adult venovenous extracorporeal membrane oxygenation for severe respiratory failure: Current status and future perspectives. *Annals of Cardiac Anaesthesia, 19*(1), 97–111.

Williams, K. E. (2013). Extracorporeal membrane oxygenation for acute respiratory distress syndrome in adults. *AACN Advanced Critical Care, 24*(2), 149–158; quiz 159.

Zangrillo, A., Landoni, G., Biondi-Zoccai, G., Greco, M., Greco, T., Frati, G., . . . Pappalardo, F. (2013). A meta-analysis of complications and mortality of extracorporeal membrane oxygenation. *Critical Care and Resuscitation, 15*(3), 172–178. Retrieved from http://www.ncbi.nlm.nih.gov/pubmed/23944202

■ FLUID AND ELECTROLYTE IMBALANCES

Michael D. Gooch

Overview

Fluid and electrolyte balance is essential for homeostasis. Fluid balance ensures adequate cellular perfusion and function and is the key to maintaining electrolyte balance as well. Sodium (Na^+), potassium (K^+), calcium (Ca^{2+}), and magnesium (Mg^{2+}) play key roles in maintaining cell membrane stability, muscle contractions, cardiac and neuronal conduction, and bone health. This balance may be altered by numerous processes, including numerous medications, diseases, alterations in the pH, and nutrition. A thorough history, including medication review, physical examination, and analysis of laboratory data, is often needed to identify an imbalance, assess for complications, and formulate a plan of care. Nurses should be able to recognize the diagnostics needed to properly identify an imbalance, the associated clinical manifestations, and initial management of these derangements.

Background

Water makes up 50% to 60% of our total body weight, though this varies by age, gender, and muscle and fat composition (Hall, Matlock, Ward, Gray, & Clayden, 2016; Harring, Deal, & Kuo, 2014; Kamel & Halperin, 2017). Water is contained in various compartments and can be shifted around if needed by the body. The intracellular space accounts for two thirds of our total body water. The remainder is extracellular and includes intravascular (plasma) and interstitial spaces. Water balance is regulated by the hypothalamic– neurohypophyseal–renal axis; during acute illness this axis is often altered leading to imbalances in many hospitalized patients (Knepper, Kwon, & Nielsen, 2015). By releasing vasopressin or antidiuretic hormone (ADH), altering the thirst response, and altering renal water excretion, this axis works to maintain a serum osmolality of 280 to 295 mmol/kg, as with any lab the accepted values vary. Osmolality is a measure of the concentration of solutes in a solution (Hall et al., 2016; Harring et al., 2014; Kamel & Halperin, 2017). The higher the osmolality, the higher the concentration of solutes. Osmolality must be balanced between intracellular and extracellular compartments to maintain equilibrium and cell membrane integrity (Kamel & Halperin, 2017; Sterns, 2015). Sodium is the primary extracellular solute and directly influences osmolality, as well as how fluids shift among the body's compartments. Fluid movement is also influenced by plasma proteins, glucose, and other electrolytes.

Sodium is the most abundant extracellular cation, with an accepted normal range of 135 to 145 mEq/L. Hyponatremia is considered the most common electrolyte imbalance encountered in the hospitalized patient (Cho, Kim, Hong, Joo, & Kim, 2017). It is estimated that 15% of admitted adults have hyponatremia with an overall mortality rate of 3% to 29% (Harring et al.,

2014). The degree of hyponatremia is often assessed based on the serum and urine Na⁺ concentrations and osmolality. Isotonic hyponatremia (osmolality 280–295 mmol/kg) is characterized by a normal serum osmolality and may result from elevated serum lipids or proteins. Hypertonic hyponatremia (osmolality greater than 295 mmol/kg) may be caused by hyperglycemia or osmotic diuretics (Cho et al., 2017; Craig, Baker, & Rodd, 2015; Harring et al., 2014; Kamel & Halperin, 2017).

The most common problem is hypotonic hyponatremia (osmolality less than 280 mmol/kg). Hypotonic patients can be further categorized as hypovolemic, euvolemic, and hypervolemic. Hypovolemia occurs when there is a loss of both water and Na⁺ from the body, for example, excessive gastrointestinal (GI) or genitourinary (GU) losses. The Na⁺ loss usually exceeds the water loss, and these patients often appear dehydrated. Euvolemia occurs when excess free water is gained, most often related to ADH release or function, and there is no excess of serum Na⁺. This may include hypothyroidism; cortisol insufficiency; syndrome of inappropriate antidiuretic hormone (SIADH); exogenous free water intake; and use of certain drugs, including thiazide diuretics and 3,4-methylenedioxymethamphetamine (MDMA, ecstasy). As the free water is gained, the serum Na⁺ is lowered, but there is usually no loss of Na⁺. However, the patient does not appear dehydrated or volume overloaded. Hypervolemia occurs when there is an increased retention of both body water and Na⁺, often because of renal disease, heart failure, or cirrhosis. Water is retained more than Na⁺, leading to a decrease in the serum Na⁺. These patients usually appear volume overloaded (Cho et al., 2017; Craig et al., 2015; Harring et al., 2014; Kamel & Halperin, 2017; Sterns, 2015).

Hypernatremia is most often associated with a decrease in free water intake that leads to cellular dehydration and an increased osmolality. This can be seen in patients with a decreased thirst reflex and those without easy access to water, for example, those with limited mobility, extremes of age, and in comatose states. It is also associated with diabetes insipidus (DI); because of the lack of ADH, the kidneys cannot adequately regulate water balance. Excess water loss worsens hypernatremia, but unless the thirst reflex is altered or there is limited access to water, insufficient free water intake is the primary cause of hypernatremia (Cho et al., 2017; Craig et al., 2015; Harring et al., 2014; Kamel & Halperin, 2017).

Potassium is the most abundant intracellular cation with an accepted serum range of 3.5 to 5.0 mEq/L. Potassium plays a key role in maintaining the resting membrane potential of cardiac and muscle cells. Hypokalemia may be related to an increased loss from the GI or GU tract, cellular shifts from alkalosis and beta-2 stimulation, or inadequate dietary intake. Hypomagnesemia can also lead to hypokalemia. Hyperkalemia may result from medications that increase K⁺ levels, inadequate excretion as seen in renal failure, cellular shifts seen with acidosis and significant tissue trauma, or maybe a measurement error because of cell hemolysis from the lab draw, often referred to as *pseudohyperkalemia* (Combs & Buckley, 2015; Gooch, 2015; Hall et al., 2016; Kamel & Halperin, 2017; Medford-Davis & Rafique, 2014).

Calcium plays an essential role in neuromuscular function and bone health. A normal Ca^{2+} level is often considered to be 8.5 to 10.5 mg/dL or an ionized level of 4.6 to 5.3 mg/dL. About half of the serum Ca^{2+} is bound to proteins; the remainder is free or ionized. Almost all (99%) of the body's Ca^{2+} is stored in the bones. Hypocalcemia most often results from inadequate intake or GI absorption, a chronic kidney disease that results in vitamin D deficiency, hypoparathyroidism, or from massive blood transfusions. In the setting of hypoalbuminemia, hypocalcemia may be noted and is often considered a pseudohypocalcemia. Evaluating the ionized Ca^{2+} level can help determine whether a true imbalance exists. Hypercalcemia most often develops from hyperparathyroidism or in cases of higher levels; malignancy is a prime cause. It is estimated that 20% to 30% of cancer patients experience hypercalcemia (Chang, Radin, & McCurdy, 2014; Cho et al., 2017; Gooch, 2015; Hall et al., 2016; Love & Buckley, 2015).

Magnesium is the second most common intracellular cation and plays a similar role to Ca^{2+} in regard to the nervous system. When outside the normal range of 1.8 to 2.5 mg/dL, it may influence K^+ and Ca^{2+} levels. Hypomagnesemia is more common and often results from altered dietary intake or absorption or increased urinary excretion. Hypermagnesemia is rare and often associated with renal failure, but could be related to medications that increase the magnesium levels (Cho et al., 2017; Chang et al., 2014; Love & Buckley, 2015).

Clinical Aspects

ASSESSMENT

It is common for acutely ill patients to have one or more imbalance. The nurse should be observant for risk factors and signs or symptoms of these imbalances. Imbalances in electrolytes can result in symptoms or clinical manifestations that are not exclusive to a particular electrolyte. Often, to link the clinical manifestations associated with an electrolyte imbalance, laboratory data need to identify the imbalance and inform the treatment plan. The patient may have altered mental status, weakness, headache, or seizures. Management is guided by the lab values, clinical findings, and rapidity with which the symptoms started. Hypovolemia should be corrected as the patient's condition allows. In the stable hyponatremic patient, free water restrictions may be all that is required to stabilize the patient. In the unstable seizing patient, a bolus of hypertonic (3%) saline may be required. In most patients, increasing the serum Na^+ by 4 mEq/L is all that is needed to reduce cerebral edema and resolve the seizures. In patients with SIADH or hypervolemic hyponatremia, a vasopressin antagonist may be administered to block ADH receptors in the kidneys and limit the reabsorption of water (Cho et al., 2017; Craig et al., 2015; Gooch, 2015).

NURSING INTERVENTIONS, MANAGEMENT, AND IMPLICATIONS

Hypernatremia may be managed with isotonic intravenous (IV) fluids initially to restore perfusion. Loop diuretics may be used in volume overloaded patients to increase the excretion of water and Na^+. In the setting of DI, desmopressin (DDAVP) may be given. An important caveat to the management of Na^+ imbalances is that the level should not be rapidly changed. If the serum Na^+ is increased too quickly, osmotic demyelination or central pontine myelinolytic may occur. If the serum Na^+ is reduced too rapidly, cerebral edema often develops. A guideline to prevent complications is to correct the level by no more than 1 to 2 mEq/L/hr and no more than 10 mEq/day (Cho et al., 2017; Craig et al., 2015; Gooch, 2015; Sterns, 2015). The more chronic the condition, the slower the correction.

Any patient suspected of having a K^+ imbalance should have his or her EKG quickly assessed. Patients may experience muscle cramps or weakness, which could progress to respiratory failure. Flattened or inverted T waves, the appearance of U waves, and ST depression are often seen with hypokalemia. Hypokalemic management is also based on severity and may require oral or IV K^+ replacement. In the setting of hypomagnesemia, the Mg^{2+} imbalance will have to be corrected first (Cho et al., 2017; Combs & Buckley, 2015; Gooch, 2015; Medford-Davis & Rafique, 2014).

Of the electrolyte imbalances, hyperkalemia is the most lethal. If there is a concern for hyperkalemia, the EKG should quickly be assessed for the presence of peaked T waves, a prolonged PR interval, or a widened QRS. If these EKG changes are present, IV Ca^{2+} should be administered to stabilize the resting membrane potential of the cardiac cells and prevent life-threatening arrhythmias. Treatment should not be delayed while awaiting lab values. Hyperkalemia is managed in two ways. First, high-dose albuterol, insulin with glucose, or sodium bicarbonate may be given to shift the K^+ back in the cells temporarily. Subsequently, the excessive K^+ should be eliminated. This is most effectively accomplished through hemodialysis, but loop diuretics or cation exchange resins may also be used with caution (Cho et al., 2017; Combs & Buckley, 2015; Gooch, 2015; Medford-Davis & Rafique, 2014).

Hypocalcemia causes neuromuscular excitability, including muscle spasms, paresthesias, hyperactive deep tendon reflexes (DTRs), and eventually, seizures. The EKG should also be assessed for a prolonged QT interval and bradycardia. Symptomatic patients may be managed with oral or IV Ca^{2+} replacement. Patients with hypercalcemia may have lethargy, muscle weakness, hypoactive DTRs, and at higher levels a shortened QT and widened QRS may be noted on the EKG. Patients may develop atrioventricular blocks, which can progress to cardiac arrest in levels more than 15 mg/dL. Initially, IV fluids should be given to restore renal perfusion. Depending on the severity of the patient, hemodialysis may be used to remove the excess Ca^{2+}. In less severe cases, the patient may be given a loop diuretic, a bisphosphonate, a glucocorticoid, or calcitonin (Chang et al., 2014; Cho et al., 2017; Gooch, 2015; Love & Buckley, 2015).

Lastly, patients with low serum Mg^{2+} levels present similarly to those with hypokalemia and hypocalcemia and have weakness and muscle cramps. This can progress to neuromuscular and cardiac irritability. Treatment is focused on replacement with oral or IV Mg^{2+} depending on the patient's condition. Hypermagnesemia is similar to hypercalcemia, and patients experience blunted neuromuscular effects, including lethargy, paralysis, decreased DTRs, and eventually hypotension, cardiac and respiratory compromise. Calcium may be administered to antagonize the Mg^{2+} and reverse neuromuscular weakness. If needed, dialysis is effective at removing the excess electrolyte in severe cases (Chang et al., 2014; Cho et al., 2017; Love & Buckley, 2015).

Summary

Fluid and electrolyte balance is critical to maintaining all the body functions. Sodium and water have an important relationship and imbalances are common in patients with acute problems. Patients with Na^+ imbalances often present with neurological changes and the imbalance cannot be aggressively corrected. Potassium is crucial for cardiac and muscle function and an imbalance can be life-threatening, and often requires rapid identification and correction to prevent complications. Calcium and Mg^{2+} both play an important role in neuromuscular function and can affect cardiac function as well. Nurses should evaluate for these imbalances in the acutely ill patient, recalling that the patient may have more than one. Labs are often helpful, but history and physical examination findings are also important to identify the imbalance and manage the derangement.

Chang, W.-T., Radin, B., & McCurdy, M. T. (2014). Calcium, magnesium, and phosphate abnormalities in the emergency department. *Emergency Medicine Clinics of North America, 32*(2), 349–366.

Cho, K.-C., Kim, J.-J., Hong, C.-K., Joo, J.-Y., & Kim, Y. B. (2017). Perimesencephalic nonaneurysmal subarachnoid hemorrhage after clipping of an unruptured aneurysm. *World Neurosurgery, 102*, 694.e15–694.e19.

Combs, D. J., & Lu, Z. (2015). Sphingomyelinase D inhibits store-operated Ca2+ entry in T lymphocytes by suppressing ORAI current. *Journal of General Physiology, 146*(2), 161–172.

Craig, S. A., Baker, S. R., & Rodd, H. D. (2015). How do children view other children who have visible enamel defects? *International Journal of Paediatric Dentistry, 25*(6), 399–408.

Gooch, M. D. (2015). Identifying acid-base and electrolyte imbalances. *Nurse Practitioner, 40*(8), 37–42.

Hall, J. E., Matlock, J. V., Ward, J. W., Gray, K. V., & Clayden, J. (2016). Medium-ring nitrogen heterocycles through migratory ring expansion of metalated ureas. *Angewandte Chemie, 55*(37), 11153–11157.

Harring, T. R., Deal, N. S., & Kuo, D. C. (2014). Disorders of sodium and water balance. *Emergency Medicine Clinics of North America, 32*(2), 379–401.

Kamel, K. S., & Halperin, M. L. (2017). *Fluid, electrolytes, and acid–base physiology: A problem-based approach* (5th ed.). Philadelphia, PA: Elsevier.

Knepper, M. A., Kwon, T. H., & Nielsen, S. (2015). Molecular physiology of water balance. *New England Journal of Medicine, 372*(14), 1349–1358.

Love, J. W., & Buckley, R. G. (2015). Disorders of calcium, phosphate, and magnesium metabolism. In A. B. Wolfson (Ed.), *Harwood-Nuss' clinical practice of emergency medicine* (6th ed., pp. 1052–1057). Philadelphia, PA: Wolters Kluwer.

Medford-Davis, L., & Rafique, Z. (2014). Derangements of potassium. *Emergency Medicine Clinics of North America, 32*(2), 329–347.

Sterns, R. H. (2015). Disorders of plasma sodium. *New England Journal of Medicine, 372*(13), 1269.

■ FLUID RESUSCITATION

Laura Stark Bai

Overview

Intravenous fluid resuscitation is one of the most common treatments in acute medical care (Myburgh, 2015). It is used as a therapy in adults and children for a range of medical problems, including dehydration, sepsis, diabetic ketoacidosis (DKA) and hyperglycemic hyperosmolar state (HHS) trauma, burns, acute pancreatitis, and more. There are two types of fluids that are used for fluid resuscitation. Crystalloids are isotonic solutions composed of ions that are capable of passing through semipermeable membranes, such as a capillary wall. The examples include normal saline, Ringer's lactate, or dextrose 5% in water. Colloid solutions, conversely, consist of insoluble molecules, which enhance therapeutic expansion of intravascular spaces. An example of a colloid solution is albumin or fresh frozen plasma. Isotonic saline (0.9%), referred to as *normal saline*, is a crystalloid solution and the most commonly used intravenous fluid in the world (Myburgh, 2015).

Background

Fluid resuscitation is an important element in the treatment plan in many medical ailments. Crystalloid and colloid solutions are infused into the intravascular space to correct metabolic and electrolyte abnormalities, as well as manage hypotension and hypoperfusion through fluid expansion in the vascular space (Katz & Choukalas, 2013). Although fluid resuscitation is safe and effective, there are complications that must also be considered to maintain patient safety.

Sepsis is one of the more serious conditions that require proper fluid resuscitation, affecting an estimated 300 cases per 100,000 population (Mayr, Yende, & Angus, 2014). To correct sepsis-induced hypoperfusion, current guidelines recommend administration of crystalloid fluids for hypotension and elevated lactate at a dose of 30 mL/kg for adults and 20 mL/kg for children (Waltzman, 2015). Initiation of fluids should occur immediately on the recognition of sepsis, and total fluid administration should be complete in 3 hours as part of the treatment bundle (Rosini & Srivastava, 2013). This is important, as early fluid resuscitation has been linked to decreased mortality in patients with severe sepsis and septic shock (Lee et al., 2014).

Fluid resuscitation is a mainstay in the treatment of DKA and HHS to lower blood sugar levels, correct electrolyte levels, and ensure hemodynamic stability. Patients in DKA may be in deficit of 3 to 5 mL of fluid and need fluid resuscitation with an initial 1 L bolus of normal saline, followed by continuous infusion for maintenance therapy. When blood sugar levels stabilize below 250 mg/dL, then dextrose 5% is added to the infusion. Fluid replacement is also essential in HHS, as the fluid deficit is up to 10 L or more. The recommendation for fluid therapy is an initial 500 mL bolus of normal saline followed by 1 to 2 L over 2 hours. The total amount of fluid administered in the first 12 hours should be half of the estimated fluid loss. It is important that the correct rate of infusion is monitored, as too rapid a correction of hyperosmolality from fluid resuscitation can lead to cerebral edema.

Fluid loss and dehydration are one of the most serious issues as a result of a burn injury because of fluid shifts from the intravascular spaces. Therefore, fluid resuscitation is essential in the effective treatment of this patient population to maintain tissue oxygenation, correct hypovolemia, and improve survival. There are multiple formulas available to calculate the amount of fluid given in the first 24 to 48 hours based on the percentage of surface area burned and patient weight. Children, elderly patients, and patients with inhalation injury may require additional fluid requirements (Mitchell et al., 2013). Each formula has its recommendation on the type of fluid administered (Haberal, Abali, & Karakayali, 2010). It is important to be aware of an institution's policy for the treatment of burn patients.

Fluid therapy is a central part of the treatment of acute pancreatitis because of hypovolemia from vasodilation, capillary leakage, edema, and vomiting that may lead to decreased tissue damage if untreated. Prompt and aggressive fluid resuscitation is recommended to decrease morbidity and mortality. Specifically, 250 to 500 mL/hr should be administered to patients with pancreatitis, except patients with comorbidities putting them at risk for fluid overload. However, in practice, an estimated 3.5 to 4.5 L of fluids are typically administered in the first 24 hours. Fluid status should be reassessed every 6 to 8 hours by checking urinary output, heart rate, blood urea nitrogen (BUN) hematocrit, and central venous pressure (CVP; Bortolotti, Saulnier, Colling, Redheuil, & Preau, 2014).

Fluid resuscitation is also important in reducing morbidity and mortality in trauma and hemorrhagic shock, especially in the first 24 hours. However, new guidelines point toward lower target blood pressures in trauma patients for guiding fluid resuscitation. Current guidelines indicate less use of crystalloids and earlier use of plasma and platelets and allowance of permissive hypotension before bleeding control (Carrick, Leondard, Slone, Mains, & Bar-Or, 2016).

Care must be taken with fluid resuscitation as to avoid complications. With aggressive fluid administration, patients may be at risk for fluid overload, which may exhibit as orthopnea, dyspnea on exertion, shortness of breath, and extremity swelling. Fluid overload is reversible with the use of diuretics or dialysis to remove excess fluid.

Clinical Aspects

ASSESSMENT

Nursing assessment for patients in need of fluid resuscitation focus on assessment for signs and symptoms of fluid volume deficit. Physical examination includes assessment of skin turgor, mucous membranes, mental status, neck veins, and urine output to assess for hydration and volume status. Nurses should pay close attention to vital signs, particularly blood pressure and heart rate, as hypotension and tachycardia may indicate hypovolemia. Lab values that should be considered as part of the assessment include BUN, creatinine, specific gravity, and hematocrit. Important information to obtain the patient's history includes a full medical history, particularly for renal, cardiac, or liver disease, because of the risk of fluid overload. In addition, history of present illness, weight, and current medication list should also be gathered.

NURSING INTERVENTIONS, MANAGEMENT, AND IMPLICATIONS

Nursing problems that should be considered are fluid volume deficit, the risk for ineffective tissue perfusion, and risk for impaired skin integrity.

Interventions include careful and timely administration of prescribed crystalloid or colloid fluids. Monitoring of urine output, blood pressure, heart rate, specific gravity, electrolytes and renal function tests, and body weight are also paramount to treatment.

OUTCOMES

Nursing interventions for patients requiring fluid resuscitation focus on achieving goals for increasing fluid intake, eliminating signs of dehydration, maintaining blood pressure and urine output, proper electrolyte balance, and normal kidney function.

Summary

Fluid resuscitation is an important aspect of treatment for multiple medical conditions. Protocols for the amount and type of fluid and the time over which they should be administered vary based on the goals of therapy and patient weight. It is important for nurses to be aware of plans for fluid resuscitation and the rationale behind the therapy. Nurses must also closely monitor the patient status, vital signs, and laboratory values to evaluate the effectiveness of therapy. Deviations from the expected plan of care should be escalated to the medical care teams.

Bortolotti, P., Saulnier, F., Colling, D., Redheuil, A., & Preau, S. (2014). New tools for optimizing fluid resuscitation in acute pancreatitis. *World Journal of Gastroenterology, 20*(43), 16113–16122.

Carrick, M. M., Leonard, J., Slone, D. S., Mains, C. W., & Bar-Or, D. (2016). Hypotensive resuscitation among trauma patients. *BioMed Research International, 2016,* 8901938.

Haberal, M., Sakallioglu Abali, A. E., & Karakayali, H. (2010). Fluid management in major burn injuries. *Indian Journal of Plastic Surgery, 43*(Suppl.), S29–S36.

Katz, J., & Choukalas, C. (2013). Goal directed fluid resuscitation: A review of hemodynamic, metabolic, and monitoring based goals. *Current Anesthesiology Reports, 3*(2), 98–104.

Lee, S. J., Ramar, K., Park, J. G., Gajic, O., Li, G., & Kashyap, R. (2014). Increased fluid administration in the first three hours of sepsis resuscitation is associated with reduced mortality: A retrospective cohort study. *Chest, 146*(4), 908–915.

Mayr, F. B., Yende, S., & Angus, D. C. (2014). Epidemiology of severe sepsis. *Virulence, 5*(1), 4–11.

Mitchell, K. B., Khalil, E., Brennan, A., Shao, H., Rabbitts, A., Leahy, N. E., . . . Gallagher, J. J. (2013). New management strategy for fluid resuscitation: Quantifying volume in the first 48 hours after burn injury. *Journal of Burn Care & Research, 34*(1), 196–202.

Myburgh, J. A. (2015). Fluid resuscitation in acute medicine: What is the current situation? *Journal of Internal Medicine, 277*(1), 58–68.

Rosini, J. M., & Srivastava, N.; Surviving Sepsis Campaign. (2013). The 2012 guidelines for severe sepsis and septic shock: An update for emergency nursing. *Journal of Emergency Nursing, 39*(6), 652–656.

Waltzman, M. L. (2015). Pediatric shock. *Journal of Emergency Nursing, 41*(2), 113–118.

■ HEART TRANSPLANTATION

S. Brian Widmar

Overview

Heart transplantation is a surgical procedure for the treatment of end-stage heart failure or structural heart disease (McCalmont & Velleca, 2017). A total of 66,737 heart transplants have been performed since 1988, with 3,191 performed in 2016 alone (Organ Procurement and Transplantation Network, 2017). Important nursing considerations for care in the heart transplant recipient include assessment of normal alterations in anatomy and physiology, the administration and management of antirejection or immunosuppressant medications, monitoring for signs and symptoms of organ rejection and infection, and reduction of risk for opportunistic and hospital-acquired infections (Costanzo et al., 2010; Welbaum, 2015).

Background

Heart failure is a chronic, progressive clinical syndrome that develops from a structural or functional cardiac abnormality that reduces ventricular filling or ejection (McCalmont & Velleca, 2017). There are an estimated 6.5 million Americans living with heart failure, and of those, around 960,000 new heart failure cases are diagnosed annually (Writing Group et al., 2016). The causes of heart failure are numerous, including cardiomyopathy (secondary to ischemic heart disease, valvular disease, or hypertension), infections, metabolic disorders, electrolyte deficiencies, nutritional disorders, systemic diseases (e.g., connective tissue disorders, amyloidosis), and exposure to toxic substances (e.g., alcohol or illicit drug use, radiation therapy, chemotherapy, or chemical exposures; McCalmont & Velleca, 2017).

Across the trajectory of the heart failure syndrome, advanced, "end-stage" heart failure, or stage D heart failure, is classified as being refractory to optimized medical therapy and requires specialized interventions to improve symptoms and reduce risk of mortality (Hunt et al., 2001). Options for therapy in stage D heart failure include heart transplantation; chronic mechanical circulatory support; chronic inotropes; experimental surgery or drugs; and end-of-life care, or hospice (Hunt et al., 2001). Heart transplantation is indicated when heart failure symptoms persist and there is evidence of end-organ dysfunction despite optimized medical therapy, or when refractory angina cannot be relieved through surgical revascularization or optimized medical therapy (McCalmont & Velleca, 2017). Other indications for heart transplantation include refractory life-threatening arrhythmias or congenital heart disease with progressive heart failure that cannot be corrected through surgical repair (McCalmont & Velleca, 2017). Since 1988, around 2,000 to 3,000 heart transplants have been performed each year (Organ Procurement and Transplantation Network, 2017).

Research studies have shown an improvement in patient quality of life after transplantation (Grady, Jalowiec, & White-Williams, 1996). In addition to improvement in quality of life, heart transplantation has demonstrated an increase in life expectancy, and has shown to be cost-effective, adding an average of 8.5 years of life with less than $800,000 per quality-adjusted life year (QALY) relative to medical therapy (Writing Group et al., 2016). From 2008 to 2010, the 1-year survival rate for heart transplant recipients was 89.6%, and the 5-year survival rate was 77% (Colvin et al., 2017).

Major causes of posttransplant morbidity include renal dysfunction, hypertension, diabetes, osteoporosis, hyperlipidemia, and gout (Kittleson & Kobashigawa, 2014). Major causes of postoperative mortality in the heart transplant recipient include rejection, infection, cardiac allograft vasculopathy, and malignancy (Kittleson & Kobashigawa, 2014). The incidence of acute rejection in the first year after transplantation was 23% among recipients who underwent transplant between 2013 and 2014 (Colvin et al., 2017). The most common cause of death in the first postoperative year was infection, followed by cardio-vascular/cerebrovascular disease (Colvin et al., 2017). Malignancy was less frequently seen as a cause of death and was reported as the cause in 1.7% of deaths after 5 postoperative years (Colvin et al., 2017).

Clinical Aspects

Postoperatively, the heart transplant recipient has specific assessment findings related to the transplant surgery and will have a greater risk for rejection due to the postoperative immune response, and an increased risk for infection, due to the introduction of immunosuppression therapy. Immunosuppression drug therapy may increase postoperative morbidity due to drug-related side effects. Specific assessment findings and implications for care are discussed here.

Heart rate and blood pressure must be closely monitored. When excised from the donor, the transplanted heart is "denervated," meaning the sympathetic and parasympathetic nerve fibers are severed. This anatomical variant affects the resting and responsive heart rate. The normal resting heart rate in the heart transplant patient is generally higher than the normal range, usually 90 to 110 beats per minute (McCalmont & Velleca, 2017). Heart rates outside of this range should be reported. It is important to note that medications that act on the vagus nerve (atropine, digoxin) will be ineffective and should not be used (Moore-Gibbs & Bither, 2015).

The transplanted heart does not respond quickly to stress that requires an abrupt increase in heart rate to maintain adequate cardiac output (e.g., orthostatic hypotension, hypovolemia, etc.). Patients may become orthostatic if quickly transitioning from bed to chair and should be allowed to dangle before attempting transfer. Lastly, due to denervation, many heart transplant patients with myocardial ischemia or myocardial infarction will not feel the chest pain associated with angina, so clinical manifestations of ischemia or infarction, such as ST segment depression or elevation on electrocardiogram, patient complaints of shortness of breath, fatigue, and so on, should be closely monitored (McCalmont & Velleca, 2017).

Often, a heart transplant recipient may not exhibit signs and symptoms of rejection, and because of this, routine surveillance for rejection is standard practice in hospitals (McCalmont & Velleca, 2017). An endomyocardial biopsy (EMB) is the key diagnostic test used in grading the severity of rejection, and treatment is usually directed based upon results (Moore-Gibbs & Bither, 2015). However, in some heart transplant patients, signs and symptoms of rejection may be similar to the signs and symptoms of heart failure, especially if cardiac output is decreased. Pulse quality, the presence of edema, decreased urine output, and other signs and symptoms of heart failure (e.g., shortness of breath, hypotension, weight gain, activity intolerance, lethargy, and general malaise) should be closely monitored in the heart transplant recipient and should be reported. Hypertension is fairly common in heart transplant patients, most often due to immunosuppressant therapies (Moore-Gibbs & Bither, 2015).

Standard immunosuppressant therapy in the heart transplant recipient includes a three-drug approach, usually initiated at the time of transplantation. These drugs include a calcineurin inhibitor (tacrolimus or cyclosporine), an antimetabolite (mycophenolate mofetil), and corticosteroids (McCalmont & Velleca, 2017). Corticosteroids are often weaned to a low daily dose, or are weaned gradually to eventually be discontinued. Nurses should be familiar with their hospital's specific corticosteroid-tapering protocol, as these may vary across transplant programs (Moore-Gibbs & Bither, 2015).

Many patients will have renal dysfunction secondary to heart failure at the time of transplantation, and this can be exacerbated by hypovolemia and hypotension intraoperatively, as well as from nephrotoxic effects of immunosuppression therapy and antibiotic regimens postoperatively (McCalmont & Velleca, 2017). Oliguria or anuria should be promptly reported, as should electrolyte abnormalities, elevated blood urea nitrogen (BUN), and creatinine levels. Judicious use of volume administration or vasoactive medication therapy to maintain a mean arterial pressure between 60 and 80 mmHg may be necessary. Placement of a Foley catheter may be required to closely monitor urine output (McCalmont & Velleca, 2017).

Due to immunosuppressant therapy, heart transplant patients are at an increased risk for community-acquired infections, opportunistic infections, and nosocomial infections (McCalmont & Velleca, 2017). Corticosteroid therapy may reduce the patient's ability to produce pyrogens, and, as a result, the patient's body temperature may be lower than normal. Small increases in body temperature should be noted and reported. A temperature greater than 100.4°F may be used as a threshold for drawing blood cultures (McCalmont & Velleca, 2017).

Strict handwashing and proper technique is probably the most effective intervention for reducing hospital-acquired infections (McCalmont & Velleca, 2017). Wound care, dressing and device site care per hospital protocol, and the timely removal of any invasive lines or indwelling catheters as early as possible are vitally important to reducing risk of nosocomial infection (Moore-Gibbs & Bither, 2015). Perioperative antibiotics should be administered to reduce the incidence of surgical site infections. Additional antibiotic regimens will be used as prophylaxis against opportunistic infections such as cytomegalovirus, *Pneumocystis jiroveci*, or oral candidiasis (McCalmont & Velleca, 2017).

Summary

Heart transplantation is a surgical intervention indicated in patients with advanced, end-stage heart failure, which has been shown to increase life expectancy and improve heart failure symptoms and quality of life. However, due to physiologic alterations secondary to the operative procedure, and its required postoperative medication therapies, heart transplant recipients are at an increased risk for hemodynamic alterations, organ rejection, and increased potential for opportunistic and nosocomial infections. Nurses must be aware of the implications of these changes upon hemodynamic function and the suppressed immune response, and should closely monitor for signs and symptoms associated with organ rejection and infection, to ensure patient safety and adequately anticipate and provide appropriate interventions and care.

Colvin, M., Smith, J. M., Skeans, M. A., Edwards, L. B., Uccellini, K., Snyder, J. J., . . . Kasiske, B. L. (2017). OPTN/SRTR 2015 annual data report: Heart. *American Journal of Transplantation, 17*(S1), 286–356.

Costanzo, M. R., Dipchand, A., Starling, R., Anderson, A., Chan, M., Desai, S., . . . Lung Transplantation, G. (2010). The International Society of Heart and Lung Transplantation Guidelines for the care of heart transplant recipients. *Journal of Heart and Lung Transplantation, 29*(8), 914–956. doi:10.1016/j.healun.2010.05.034

Grady, K. L., Jalowiec, A., & White-Williams, C. (1996). Improvement in quality of life in patients with heart failure who undergo transplantation. *Journal of Heart and Lung Transplantation, 15*(8), 749–757.

Hunt, S. A., Baker, D. W., Chin, M. H., Cinquegrani, M. P., Feldman, A. M., & Francis, G. S. (2001). ACC/AHA guidelines for the evaluation and management of chronic heart failure in the adult: Executive summary. A report of the American College of Cardiology/American Heart Association Task Force on Practice Guidelines (Committee to revise the 1995 Guidelines for the Evaluation and Management of Heart Failure): Developed in collaboration with the International Society for Heart and Lung Transplantation; endorsed by the Heart Failure Society of America. *Circulation, 104*(24), 2996–3007.

Kittleson, M. M., & Kobashigawa, J. A. (2014). Long-term care of the heart transplant recipient. *Current Opinion in Organ Transplantation, 19*(5), 515–524. doi:10.1097/MOT.0000000000000117

McCalmont, V., & Velleca, A. (2017). Heart transplantation. In S. Cupples, S. Lerret, V. McCalmont, & L. Ohler (Eds.), *Core curriculum for transplant nurses* (pp. 307–412). Philadelphia, PA: Mosby.

Moore-Gibbs, A., & Bither, C. (2015). Cardiac transplantation: Considerations for the intensive care unit nurse. *Critical Care Nursing Clinics of North America, 27*(4), 565–575. doi:10.1016/j.cnc.2015.07.005

Organ Procurement and Transplantation Network. (2017). National data, from U.S. Department of Health and Human Services. Retrieved from https://optn.transplant .hrsa.gov

Welbaum, C. (2015). Caring for patients with solid organ transplants. *American Nurse Today, 10*(9). Retrieved from https://www.americannursetoday.com/ caring-patients-solid-organ-transplants

Writing Group, M., Mozaffarian, D., Benjamin, E. J., Go, A. S., Arnett, D. K., Blaha, M. J., . . . Stroke Statistics. (2016). Executive summary: Heart disease and stroke statistics—2016 update: A report from the American Heart Association. *Circulation, 133*(4), 447–454. doi:10.1161/CIR.0000000000000366

■ HEPATIC FAILURE

Leon Chen
Fidelindo Lim

Overview

The liver is an organ that is indispensable in maintaining the body's homeostasis. Therefore, hepatic failure (HF) is a critical condition that impacts multiple organ systems and is directly correlated with heightened estimates of mortality. Acute hepatic failure (AHF) is often described as "a severe liver injury, potentially reversible in nature with the onset of hepatic encephalopathy within eight weeks of the first symptoms in the absence of pre-existing liver disease" (Bernal & Wendon, 2013, p. 2525). Although the immediate effects of AHF can lead to neurological, respiratory, cardiovascular, renal, endocrinological, and coagulation dysfunctions, chronic liver disease is characterized by progressive hepatic injury that changes normal anatomy and physiology, and leads to complication that presents unique challenges (Singh, Gupta, Alkhouri, Carey, & Hanouneh, 2016).

Background

HF can be categorized as either acute or chronic. AHF is characterized by a rapid liver dysfunction and is notable for acute jaundice, encephalopathy, and coagulopathy in a patient with no previous diagnosis of liver disease. AHF can then be subdivided into categories based on the interval of symptom onset. Categories include hyperacute (symptoms onset less than 7 days), acute (8–28 days) and subacute (28 days to 28 weeks; Kim & Kim-Shluger, 2016). Drug-induced hepatitis from acetaminophen toxicity is the most common cause of AHF in the United States, followed by viral infections such as hepatitis A, B, C, and E virus. HF can also be caused by ischemic injuries in the setting of circulatory failure (Bernal & Wendon, 2013). With the failure of liver function, systemic complications ensue.

Hepatic encephalopathy (HE) is characterized by altered mental status in the setting of fulminant HF. The pathogenesis of this condition is poorly understood, but is likely multifactorial and leads to cerebral edema (Bernal & Wendon, 2013). The factors that contribute to cerebral edema include the breakdown of the blood–brain barrier, the release of neurotoxins, and osmotic alterations. Previously it was thought that the altered mental status was purely because of the build-up of serum ammonia under decreased hepatic clearance. However, the process is now believed to be more complex, although a serum ammonia level of over 200 mmol/L is highly predictive of cerebral edema (Kim & Kim-Shluger, 2016). Cerebral edema in AHF, if untreated, ultimately causes intracranial hypertension. The mortality of HF-associated intracranial hypertension is high and is the leading cause of death worldwide among liver failure patients (Romero-Gómez, Montagnese, & Jalan, 2013).

Respiratory failure because of altered mental status or metabolic derangement can occur in the setting of fulminant HF. In addition, because of the dysfunction in the immune system seen in HF, patients are at a higher risk for infection and up to one third of the patients develop acute respiratory disease syndrome and requires invasive respiratory support (Bernal & Wendon, 2013; Kim & Kim-Shluger, 2016).

Circulatory failure occurs because of the dysfunctional liver, clearance of vasoactive metabolites is decreased as a result there is vasoplegia and profound vasodilation. The result is a decrease in systemic vascular resistance and an alteration of cardiac output. The deceased vascular resistance increases cardiac output, and places increased demand on the heart. In some cases, this leads to high-output cardiac failure (Bernal & Wendon, 2013; Kim & Kim-Shluger, 2016). Often patients who have AHF are baseline hypovolemic because of poor oral intake and nausea/vomiting. In these cases, a decreased vascular resistance exacerbates an already low cardiac output state and leads to further cardiac circulatory compromise (Lee, 2012).

Renal failure can occur in up to 50% of patients with AHF. The cause of renal failure can be the toxic insult that caused the original HF or the alteration in volume status and circulatory failure. With the decrease in cardiac output, renal perfusion pressure decreases and the organ suffers from ischemic damage (Bernal & Wendon, 2013; Kim & Kim-Shluger, 2016). Maintaining euvolemia is crucial to sustaining renal function although renal-replacement therapy is often required to support the patient's kidney functions.

Profound hypoglycemia can be seen in AHF patients because of an impaired gluconeogenesis and glycogenolysis, both of which are essential in maintaining euglycemia through breaking down glycogen storage or formulating serum glucose (Lee, 2012).

The liver produces a cascade of coagulation factors, including factors II, VII, IX, and X along with factors C and S. With the disruption of the liver function, the production of coagulation factors is decreased and often these patients are prone to bleeding (Bernal & Wendon, 2013; Kim & Kim-Shluger, 2016).

Chronic hepatic failure (CHF) is the progressive fibrosis of liver tissue through chronic injury. Excessive alcohol consumption is implicated in the majority of the cases. However, autoimmune disease, such as Wilson's disease, can also lead to chronic liver disease. The anatomy of the liver is altered with scarring and stricture of the vasculature. This disruption leads to conditions such as portal hypertension (PH), esophageal varices, and spontaneous bacterial peritonitis (SBP; Bernal & Wendon, 2013; Kim & Kim-Shluger, 2016).

The progressive structural changes that cause PH include fibrosis, nodule formation, and vascular thrombosis inside the liver. All of these result in an increased vascular resistance in the portal venous system and pressure overload in vessels that drain into the system. PH is the main cause of complications such as esophageal varices and SBP (Mehta et al., 2014).

Fifty percent of patients with the chronic liver disease or cirrhosis develop esophageal varices. This distended esophageal vein is a resultant of increased portal venous pressure, and the severity of the varices is correlated with the severity of the underlying liver disease. Major esophageal variceal bleeding occurs in approximately 6% to 76%, and depending on the literature and mortality rates, approaches 20% (Kim & Kim-Shluger, 2016).

One of the most common complications of cirrhosis is ascites. This condition develops in 58% of patients within 10 years of diagnosis of cirrhosis, and these patients have a 1-year mortality of 15% and a 5-year mortality rate of 44% (Kim & Kim-Shluger, 2016). Ascites is the buildup of fluid because of an inadequate venous return at the portal system. This protein-rich fluid often becomes infected and causes SBP. SBP is diagnosed in 12% of all hospitalized patients with ascites and carries a mortality rate of 33% (Kim & Kim-Shluger, 2016). If left unrecognized and untreated, it is an extremely deadly complication of cirrhosis or chronic liver disease.

Clinical Aspects

The prevention, care, and cure of HF are complex and challenging. As in the management of any condition, better outcomes are achieved with collaborative, evidence-based, and patient-centered care. The American Association for the Study of Liver Diseases (AASLD) issued a data-supported position paper to inform the management of AHF and HE (Lee, Larson, & Stravitz, 2011; Vilstrup et al., 2014).

ASSESSMENT

Altered mental status, coagulopathy, and rapid clinical decline are the primary considerations in HF. The nurse should assess the patient for confusion, jaundice, petechiae, spider angiomas, melena, hematemesis, ascites, and peripheral edema. The key recommendations from the AASLD position paper include (Lee et al., 2011):

- Obtain details concerning all prescription and nonprescription drugs, herbs, and dietary supplements taken over the past year.
- To exclude Wilson disease, obtain ceruloplasmin, serum and urinary copper levels, slit lamp examination for Kayser–Fleischer rings, hepatic copper levels when liver biopsy is feasible, and total bilirubin/alkaline phosphatase ratio.
- Liver biopsy is recommended when autoimmune hepatitis is suspected.
- In patients who have a previous cancer history or massive hepatomegaly, consider underlying malignancy and obtain imaging and liver biopsy to confirm the diagnosis.
- Liver biopsy may be appropriate to attempt to identify a specific etiology if the etiological remains elusive after extensive initial evaluation.
- Periodic surveillance cultures are recommended to detect bacterial and fungal pathogens as early as possible.
- Monitor and trend serum ammonia, metabolic profile, complete blood count, and coagulation profile (activated partial thromboplastin time

[aPTT], partial thromboplastin time [PTT], and international normalized ratio [INR]).

HF inevitably affects every body system. The nurse needs to assess the patient's renal, respiratory, integumentary, and cardiac status while monitoring him or her.

NURSING INTERVENTIONS, MANAGEMENT, AND IMPLICATIONS

Taking into account the patient's overall scenario, relevant nursing diagnoses in HF include risk for injury related to delirium, substance intoxication, and delirium tremens; fatigue related to malnutrition; imbalanced nutrition: insufficient nutrients related to a loss of appetite, nausea, and vomiting; risk for deficient fluid volume; ineffective protection related to impaired blood coagulation and bleeding.

Nursing interventions in AHF are geared toward preventing and responding to life-threatening complications such as esophageal varices, bleeding, HE, hepatorenal syndrome, malnutrition, and SBP (Gluud, Vilstrup, & Morgan, 2016). Highlights from the 2014 AASLD guidelines in the management of HF (Lee et al., 2011) and HE include (Vilstrup et al., 2014):

■ For patients with known or suspected acetaminophen overdose in 4 hours of presentation, give activated charcoal just before starting N-acetylcysteine dosing.
■ Lactulose is the first choice for treatment and prevention of episodic overt HE.
■ Neomycin and metronidazole are choices for the treatment of HE.
■ Seizure activity should be treated with phenytoin and benzodiazepines with short half-lives. Prophylactic phenytoin is not recommended.
■ In the absence of intracranial pressure (ICP) monitoring, frequent (hourly) neurological evaluation is recommended to identify early evidence of intracranial hypertension.
■ Mannitol bolus (0.5–1.0 g/kg body weight) is recommended as first-line therapy for increase in ICP. The prophylactic administration of mannitol is not recommended.
■ Replacement therapy for thrombocytopenia and/or prolonged prothrombin time is recommended only in the setting of hemorrhage or previous invasive procedures.

Current research does not justify the routine use of parenteral nutrition, enteral nutrition, or oral nutritional supplements in patients with liver disease (Koretz, Avenell, & Lipmann, 2012). The comprehensive nursing care of the patient draws on current guidelines related to hemodynamic monitoring, fluid management, blood transfusion, and infection control.

OUTCOMES

Expected positive outcomes include excretion of excess fluid (reduced ascites and edema), the absence of respiratory distress, prompt resolution of bleeding episodes and HE, hepatic function test will return to normal or baseline, and the client will adhere to lifestyle modifications to improve and maintain hepatic health. The highest quality of life should be restored if possible.

Summary

Although AHF is a rare condition, expert nursing is essential in preventing life-threatening complications such coagulopathy and HE. The precise etiology of HF should be addressed to guide collaborative management, particularly for patients with HE. The nurse should be vigilant in protecting the patient's liver from further damage from medications and other comorbidities. As patients may deteriorate rapidly, arranging care in a center with expertise in managing patients with HF will secure the best possible outcomes for these patients.

Bernal, W., & Wendon, J. (2013). Acute liver failure. *New England Journal of Medicine, 369*(26), 2525–2534.

Kim, B., & Kim-Schluger, L. (2016). Liver failure: Acute and chronic. In J. M. Oropello, S. M. Pastores, & V. Kvetan (Eds.), *Lange critical care* (1st ed., pp. 469–480). New York, NY: McGraw-Hill.

Koretz, R. L., Avenell, A., & Lipman, T. O. (2012, May). Nutritional support for liver disease. *Cochrane Database of Systematic Reviews.* doi:10.1002/14651858.CD008344 .pub2

Lee, W. M. (2012). Acute liver failure. *Seminars in Respiratory and Critical Care Medicine, 33*(1), 36–45.

Lee, W. M., Larson, A. M., & Stravitz, R. T. (2011). AASLD position paper: The management of acute liver failure: Update 2011. Retrieved from https://www.aasld.org/sites/default/files/guideline_documents/alfenhanced.pdf

Mehta, G., Gustot, T., Mookerjee, R. P., Garcia-Pagan, J. C., Fallon, M. B., Shah, V. H., . . . Jalan, R. (2014). Inflammation and portal hypertension—The undiscovered country. *Journal of Hepatology, 61*(1), 155–163.

Romero-Gómez, M., Montagnese, S., & Jalan, R. (2015). Hepatic encephalopathy in patients with acute decompensation of cirrhosis and acute-on-chronic liver failure. *Journal of Hepatology, 62*(2), 437–447.

Singh, T., Gupta, N., Alkhouri, N., Carey, W. D., & Hanouneh, I. (2016). In reply: Acute liver failure. *Cleveland Clinic Journal of Medicine, 83*(8), 557.

Vilstrup, H., Amodio, P., Bajaj, J., Ferenci, P., Mullen, K. D., Weissenborn, K., & Wong, P. (2014). Hepatic encephalopathy in chronic liver disease: 2014 Practice Guideline by the American Association for the Study of Liver Diseases and the European Association for the Study of the Liver. *Hepatology, 60*(2), 715–735.

■ HEPATITIS

Ramona A. Sowers
Linda Carson

Overview

Hepatitis is a term used for a variety of viral, bacterial, and noninfectious causes of inflammation of the liver. It is believed to have been first described by Hippocrates. Some persons have no symptoms, whereas others may develop fever, headache, malaise, anorexia, nausea, vomiting, diarrhea, abdominal pain, clay-colored stools, pruritus, dark-colored urine, and jaundice of the skin, sclera, and mucous membranes. Known causes of hepatitis include heavy alcohol and/or drug use; toxins such as carbon tetrachloride; medications, prescribed or over-the-counter such as acetaminophen; herbal and dietary supplements; and medical conditions, including genetic disorders, poor hygiene, environmental conditions, and viruses. According to the World Health Organization (WHO), hepatitis is a major public health problem globally, with more than 1,000,000 deaths annually from viral hepatitis. The Centers for Disease Control and Prevention (CDC) also notes that the most common forms of hepatitis in the United States are viral.

Background

There are several types of hepatitis that are related to viral infections. The first of these types of hepatitis is hepatitis A (HAV), which is highly contagious. The usual transmission is oral–fecal, either person to person or by consumption of contaminated food or water. Microscopic amounts have been found on objects that infected persons have come in contact with. HAV infection has an incubation period that averages 28 days and is generally a self-limited illness that does not progress to a chronic condition. A decrease in the number of outbreaks can be accredited to extensive education regarding handwashing and food preparation as well as the global use of HAV immunization. Lifelong immunity occurs following an infection or after receiving the HAV vaccine. (CDC, 2017).

Hepatitis B (HBV) was previously known as *serum hepatitis*. Transmission occurs when blood, serum, or other bodily fluids from an infected person enter the body of someone who is uninfected. This may be through sexual contact, sharing needles and syringes, mother to baby during birth, or poor infection control in health facilities. Symptoms may occur any time between 2 weeks and 6 months postexposure. The illness may be acute or short term but can become chronic with 15% to 25% of infected patients developing cirrhosis, liver cancer, and liver failure. Treatment is supportive. HBV vaccine is effective in preventing the disease (CDC, 2017).

Hepatitis C (HCV) is a serious blood-borne illness previously called *non-A, non-B hepatitis*. Infection occurs through exposure to infected blood and blood products, solid organ transplantation before 1992, shared needles or other equipment used to inject drugs, and unprotected sex with multiple sexual partners who are infected. Mayo Clinic experts estimate that one third of the global population is infected, most undetected for decades as they are not clinically ill. In the United States, approximately 2% of the population is infected (Krebbeks & Cunningham, 2013). The federal government has recommended screening for HCV in persons born between 1945 and 1965. HCV is the most common cause of liver transplantation (Glund & Glund, 2009). Diagnosis is often made during routine medical testing. HCV can now be "successfully cured" with the recent treatment options of antiviral medications such as Harvoni (ledipasvir/sofosbuvir). To date, there is no vaccine available to provide immunity against HCV (CDC, 2017).

Hepatitis D, "delta hepatitis," is uncommon in the United States. It is caused by the hepatitis D virus (HDV) and only occurs in individuals also infected with the hepatitis B virus. HDV is an incomplete virus that needs HBV to replicate. It can be acute, short term, or long-term chronic. It is transmitted percutaneously or through mucosal contact with infected blood. The incubation period is 65 to 104 days. Treatment is supportive and currently there is no vaccine to provide immunity (CDC, 2017).

Hepatitis E virus (HEV) infection is self-limiting and does not result in chronic illness. It is rare in the United States but common in many parts of the world such as Asia and Africa. Transmission is through ingestion of fecal matter, even microscopic amounts, usually associated with a contaminated water supply in countries with poor sanitation. Incubation period is 16 to 65 days. There is no vaccine. As with HAV, good hygiene and handwashing as well as avoiding any contact with the HEV virus is the best method of prevention (CDC, 2017).

Clinical Aspects

Viral hepatitis has two components: the active phase, which is seen in all five forms of the virus, and the chronic phase of the disease, seen only in hepatitis B, C, and D. The five viruses known to cause the various forms of viral hepatitis cause many of the same symptoms in the infected patient during the acute phase. Symptoms are dependent on the cause and severity of liver involvement. The most commonly reported signs and symptoms include complaints of anorexia, low-grade fever, significant abdominal pain, generalized fatigue and malaise, nausea and vomiting, jaundice (having a yellow hue to the mucous membranes and skin), dark-colored urine and clay-colored stools, and unexplained arthralgia or joint pain.

Many patients in the chronic phases of hepatitis B and C remain asymptomatic. It can take decades following exposure for the patient to become symptomatic.

ASSESSMENT

A focused health history will determine the patient's risk factors for hepatitis: age (more than 75% of patients with HCV were born between 1945 and 1965);

medications, prescribed (sulfonamides, phenothiazides) and over-the-counter (acetaminophen); travel; alcohol use; exposure to toxins; sexual history; any known exposure (health care worker with needlestick); long-term dialysis; blood transfusion or solid organ transplant before 1992; use of clotting factor concentrates before 1987; use of injected illegal drugs; and HIV. Diagnostic studies, including complete blood count (CBC), urinalysis, and liver function studies (LFTs), will provide insight into the liver status. An acute viral hepatitis panel is used to help detect and/or diagnose acute liver infection and inflammation that is due to one of the three most common hepatitis viruses: HAV, HBV, or HCV (CDC, 2017).

■ Hepatitis A antibody, immunoglobulin M (IgM)—These antibodies typically develop 2 to 3 weeks after first being infected and persist for about 2 to 6 months. Hepatitis A IgM antibodies develop early in the course of infection, so a positive hepatitis A IgM test is usually considered diagnostic for acute hepatitis A in a person with signs and symptoms.
■ Hepatitis B core antibody, IgM—This is an antibody produced against the hepatitis B core antigen. It is the first antibody produced in response to a hepatitis B infection and, when detected, may indicate an acute infection. It may also be present in people with chronic hepatitis B when flares of disease activity occur.
■ Hepatitis B surface antigen (HBsAg)—This is a protein present on the surface of the hepatitis B virus. It is the earliest indicator of an acute infection but may also be present in the blood of those chronically infected.
■ Hepatitis C antibody—This test detects antibodies produced in response to an HCV infection. It cannot distinguish between an active or previous infection. If positive, it is typically followed up with other tests to determine whether the infection is a current one.

Additional studies may include the following:

■ HAV antibody, total and HBV core antibody, total—These tests detect both IgM and immunoglobulin G (IgG) antibodies and may be used as part of the panel to determine whether someone has had a previous infection.
■ HBV surface antibody—The test for this antibody may sometimes be included in a panel to help determine whether an infection has resolved or a person has developed the antibody after receiving the hepatitis B vaccine and achieved immunity for protection against HBV (National Library of Medicine, 2014).

NURSING INTERVENTIONS, MANAGEMENT, AND IMPLICATIONS

The goals of the nursing intervention and management during the acute phase are to decrease demand on the liver, minimize complications, and prevent transmission of the infecting virus by providing education about the disease process, treatment, and prognosis. Appropriate hand hygiene and personal protective equipment is used to prevent the transmission of all hepatitis viruses. Monitoring of the patient should include vital signs, pain assessment, cardiac status via EKG and telemetry, and urinary output. Auscultation of the heart and lungs will help provide an accurate assessment of the patient's current cardiopulmonary status.

During the chronic phase of viral hepatitis, nursing interventions will be no different than those for any other patient requiring medical care: vital signs, height, weight, and pain assessment are required.

OUTCOMES

The patient's vital signs will return to baseline, urinary output will be greater or equal to 30 mL/hr, indicating normalizing renal function, and all peripheral pulses will be palpable, indicating return of adequate circulatory perfusion. SaO_2 saturation on room air will return to greater than 90% or there will be reduction in the required supplemental oxygen required by the patient. The patient's mental status will return to baseline, indicating that cerebral perfusion has occurred. The patient and his or her family members will be able to answers questions regarding the prevention and transmission of viral hepatitis, during both the acute phase and the chronic phase.

Summary

Hepatitis can be caused by viral, bacterial, and noninfectious conditions that precipitate inflammation of the liver. Symptom severity is dependent on the amount of liver involvement. Today's challenge is to identify at-risk patients for vaccination, testing, and treatment utilizing current medical guidelines (Krebbeks & Cunningham, 2013). Vaccination is effective in preventing HAV and HBV. Advances in antiviral therapy can halt and even reverse the progression of liver disease and decrease mortality in patients infected with HBV and HCV (Zhou et al., 2016).

Centers for Disease Control and Prevention. (2017, May 16). Viral hepatitis. Retrieved from https://www.cdc.gov/hepatitis

Krebbeks, V., & Cunningham, V. (2013). A DNP nurse-managed hepatitis C clinic, improving quality of life for those in a rural area. *Online Journal of Rural Nursing, 13*(1). Retrieved from http://rnojournal.binghamton.edu/index.php/RNO/article/view/104

National Library of Medicine. (2014, November 20). Hepatitis viral panel. Retrieved from http://www.nlm.nih.gov/medlineplus

Zhou, K., Fitzpatrick, T., Walsh, N., Kim, J. Y., Chou, R., Lackey, M., . . . Tucker J. D. (2016). Interventions to optimize the care continuum for chronic viral hepatitis: A systematic review and meta-analysis. *Lancet, 16*(12), 1409–1422.

∎ HYPERGLYCEMIA AND HYPOGLYCEMIA

Laura Stark Bai

Overview

Hyperglycemia and hypoglycemia are two terms that refer to abnormalities in blood sugar levels. Hyperglycemia occurs when blood sugar is higher than the normal range for a patient and hypoglycemia is when blood sugar is lower than the normal range. Both conditions are not diseases in themselves but are associated with a greater disease process that requires prompt medical attention. They are each associated with different symptoms and occur for different reasons. Most often, hyperglycemia and hypoglycemia are complications of diabetes mellitus, which affects approximately 9.3% of Americans.

Background

Hyperglycemia is a deviation of one's blood sugar level above the normal range. For healthy individuals, normal blood sugar is approximately 70 to 99 mg/dL when fasting. Postprandial blood sugar, which is taken 2 hours after a meal consumption, should be less than 140 mg/dL. Blood sugar that is tested and results in a number higher than this is indicative of hyperglycemia. Both adults and children can develop hyperglycemia. It is difficult to assess the incidence of hyperglycemia because of its wide range of causes. However, glucose levels can vary from 40% to 90% based on the testing threshold used to define hyperglycemia (Viana, Moraes, Fabbrin, Santos, & Gerchman, 2014). Hyperglycemia has multiple causes, including stress, medications (i.e., steroids), excess consumption of carbohydrates, inactivity, illness, infection, and surgery. Most often, it is caused by two serious, and potentially fatal, complications of diabetes mellitus (DM).

Diabetic ketoacidosis (DKA) is an acute condition that is associated with blood sugar levels of about 250 to 600 mg/dL, severe metabolic acidosis, hyperosmolality, and ketonemia. It most commonly affects patients with type 1 DM but is often seen in patients with type 2 DM. Mortality rates range from about 1% to 5%, based on the patient's age and comorbidities (Nyenwe & Kitabchi, 2016). Hyperglycemic hyperosmolar state (HHS) is similar to DKA with its presence of hyperglycemia and hyperosmolality. However, HHS is associated with blood glucose levels more than 600 mg/dL, severe dehydration without ketosis, and is most often seen in elderly patients with type 2 DM (Pasquel & Umpierrz, 2014). Although the incidence of HHS is not known, it accounts for fewer than 1% of hospitalizations for patients who have DM. The mortality rate is estimated to be 10% to 20% (Pasquel & Umpierrz, 2014).

Both DKA and HHS are most often precipitated by lack of/or inadequate levels of insulin in the blood or infectious processes. They can both also be attributed to other bodily stressors, such as myocardial infarction, stroke, or pancreatitis. Symptoms include polyuria, polydipsia, polyphagia, nausea, vomiting, weakness, abdominal pain, dehydration, confusion, and lethargy and/or coma. Treatment focuses on correction of hyperglycemia and electrolyte imbalances, as well as rehydration. In extreme circumstances, patients may require a critical level of care if intubation or hourly blood sugar checks are indicated. DKA is considered resolved when blood sugar is below 200 mg/dL plus two of the following three criteria: anion gap less than 12 mEq/L, serum bicarbonate more than 15 mEq/L, or venous pH more than 7.3 (Van Ness-Otunnu & Hack, 2013). HHS is resolved when serum osmolality returns to normal range and vital signs and mentation return to baseline (Van Ness-Otunnu & Hack, 2013).

Hypoglycemia occurs when an individual's blood sugar drops below the normal range to 69 mg/dL or less. Symptoms include diaphoresis, hunger, weakness, lightheadedness, shaking, anxiety, seizures, nausea, and vomiting. In some cases, patients may even experience stroke-like symptoms, such as blurry vision, confusion, or slurred speech. The most common causes of hypoglycemia are DM, particularly when patients decrease their food consumption, increase activity levels, or overdose on insulin administration. Other causes include overproduction of insulin after a meal, excess alcohol consumptions, anorexia, pregnancy, dumping syndrome, and medical conditions that affect the heart, liver, or kidneys. Treatment for hypoglycemia is based on the precipitating cause of the decrease in blood sugar levels. Typically, a 15-g dose of a carbohydrate, such as orange juice, increases blood sugar levels. Commercially prepared glucose products are also available and can be used for hypoglycemia. However, if a person is not alert enough to orally consume glucose, dextrose can be administered parenterally.

The key to prevention of hyperglycemia and hypoglycemia is proper health maintenance. Patients who are at risk for these conditions should be careful to maintain consistency in their diets and exercise routines. Avoiding carbohydrates and sugars in excessive quantities will help to avoid hyperglycemia. Frequent monitoring of blood sugar levels with adherence to a proper medication regimen as prescribed by a physician is also crucial.

Clinical Aspects

ASSESSMENT

When assessing patients with suspected hyperglycemia or hypoglycemia, assessment and maintenance of airway, breathing, and circulation are of vital importance, as coma and death are symptoms of both. Subsequently, a finger stick for blood sugar level is crucial to identify hyperglycemia or hypoglycemia quickly. Furthermore, serum electrolytes, serum osmolality, urinalysis, complete blood count, pH, arterial blood gas, and an electrocardiogram are needed to help identify the cause of the syndrome and guide nursing interventions and treatment. In addition, if the patient is conscious or if a third party is available, a thorough history of present illness, past medical history, surgical history, and a list of medications should be obtained to gather precipitating information that can inform a cause. Further assessment should evaluate the adequacy of circulation, activity level, elimination, knowledge deficits, pain, fluid and nutrition status, and respiratory status.

NURSING INTERVENTIONS, MANAGEMENT, AND IMPLICATIONS

When it comes to hypoglycemia and hypoglycemia, nurses play a very important role. Some patients may have a knowledge deficit that requires education by a nurse on how to properly manage blood sugar. Patients are also at risk for multiple issues secondary to hyperglycemia and hypoglycemia, such as infection, skin integrity, the risk for falls, the risk for altered sensory perception, fluid volume deficit, fluid and electrolyte imbalance, ineffective therapeutic regimen, and altered or imbalanced nutrition.

Although medical treatment is different, the nursing interventions for hyperglycemia and hypoglycemia are largely focused on health maintenance and self-monitoring. Nursing interventions include monitoring of blood sugar levels, diet management, and education, monitoring for signs and symptoms of hyperglycemia or hypoglycemia and electrolyte imbalance, and administration of blood glucose lowering or elevating agents as indicated.

Treatment for hyperglycemia focuses lowering blood sugar, correcting electrolyte imbalances, and rehydration. In critical cases, patients may require endotracheal intubation and strict nursing management to monitor glucose and electrolyte levels. Treatment for hypoglycemia is usually a 15-g dose of a carbohydrate, such as orange juice, to increase blood sugar levels. However, if a person is not alert enough to orally consume glucose, it can be administered intramuscularly or intravenously. Long-term management of both hyperglycemia and hypoglycemia involves proper medication administration, diet, and activity management, which should be discussed with a primary care physician and possibly a registered dietician. Hemoglobin A1c (HbA1c) should be monitored as well to track blood sugar trends over a 2- to 3-month period to determine compliance with/or effectiveness of treatment for people at risk for hyperglycemia.

OUTCOMES

With rapid recognition and treatment initiation, morbidity and mortality associated with hyperglycemia and hypoglycemia can be reduced. A thorough history and physical in conjunction with the appropriate assessment and laboratory testing must be completed to rule out all possible precipitating causes of hyperglycemia and hypoglycemia (Van Ness-Otunnu & Hack, 2013). By following the recommended guidelines for the management of each syndrome, a positive prognosis can be expected.

Summary

Hyperglycemia and hypoglycemia are two syndromes associated with deviation from normal blood sugar levels. Although multiple factors can cause each, they are both most often caused by the complications of DM. Either condition can ultimately be fatal, however, with proper nursing and medical management, resolution is very achievable. Prevention is key through close management of medications, diet, and activity level.

Nyenwe, E. A., & Kitabchi, A. E. (2016). The evolution of diabetic ketoacidosis: An update of its etiology, pathogenesis, and management. *Metabolism: Clinical and Experimental, 65*(4), 507–521.

Pasquel, F. J., & Umpierrez, G. E. (2014). Hyperosmolar hyperglycemic state: A historic review of the clinical presentation, diagnosis, and treatment. *Diabetes Care, 37*(11), 3124–3131.

Van Ness-Otunnu, R., & Hack, J. B. (2013). Hyperglycemic crisis. *Journal of Emergency Medicine, 45*(5), 797–805.

Viana, M. V., Moraes, R. B., Fabbrin, A. R., Santos, M. F., & Gerchman, F. (2014). Assessment and treatment of hyperglycemia in critically ill patients. *Revista Brasileira de terapia Intensiva, 26*(1), 71–76.

■ HYPERTENSIVE CRISIS AND HYPERTENSION

Kathleen Bradbury-Golas

Overview

A hypertensive crisis is a sudden and severe rise in blood pressure (BP). There are two types of hypertensive crises—both require immediate medical attention (American Heart Association, 2016). Hypertensive urgency occurs when the BP reading is equal to or greater than 180/110 mmHg, and remains there for two or more readings within a 10-minute span without indication of end-organ damage. The hypertensive patient may be asymptomatic or exhibit symptoms of headache, shortness of breath, or epistaxis. A hypertensive emergency (previously referred to as *malignant hypertension*) occurs with a persistent systolic BP (SBP) reading of 180 mmHg or a diastolic BP (DBP) reading of 120 mmHg. Symptoms include altered level of consciousness, confusion, stupor, chest pain, and possible stroke symptoms. In general, hypertension, defined as a BP reading higher than 140/90 mmHg on two or more occasions, can be attributed to many causes such as pain, anxiety, tobacco smoking, obesity, illicit drug use, excessive alcohol or salt use, and age.

If the BP is not maintained at a normal reading (less than 140/90), whether it is slightly elevated over a long period or severely elevated for a short period of time, the sequelae can result in myocardial infarction, heart failure, cardiomyopathy, aortic dissection, intracranial infarction/hemorrhage, retinal hemorrhage/infarct, and renal damage/failure (Stafford, Will, & Brooks-Gumbert, 2012). Emergency nursing care for adults with hypertensive crises is focused on early recognition, prompt evaluation, and emergency pharmacotherapy initiation for BP reduction in order to avoid permanent end-organ damage.

Background

In 2009, the American Heart Association (2016) estimated that 77.9 million Americans older than 20 years had some degree of hypertension. According to the Centers for Disease Control and Prevention (CDC), hypertension affects approximately 32% of the American population, averaging one in every three American adults (CDC, 2015). Having hypertension costs the United States more than $48 billion yearly and increases the risk of heart disease and stroke, the leading causes of death in the United States (CDC, 2015). Hypertension is more prevalent in adults older than 55 years (gender equal at this age), African Americans, those individuals who are overweight or obese due to lack of physical activity and high sodium intake, and those who have the genetic predisposition for the disease (National Institutes of Health, 2015). Because only 50% of patients known to have hypertension maintain adequate control of their BP, the resulting end-organ damage can occur markedly with time.

Most patients who suffer from hypertensive crises are known hypertensive patients, with poor or inadequate control (Marik, 2015). However, hypertensive crises can also occur from preeclampsia/eclampsia, pheochromocytoma (adrenal tumor), primary aldosteronism, hyperthyroidism, Cushing syndrome (excess glucocorticoid), or central nervous system disorders (head trauma or brain tumors).

Hypertension and prehypertension in children and adolescents have been increasing due to the strong association of high BP and increased weight and obesity within this population. The National Institutes of Health guidelines (2005) continue to define hypertension in children and adolescents as SBP and/or DBP, that is, on repeated measurement, at or above the 95th percentile. BP between the 90th and 95th percentile in childhood has been designated "high normal." However, secondary hypertension (disorders such as pheochromocytoma, Turner syndrome, coarctation of the aorta, or diabetes) is more common in children than in adults (National Institutes of Health, 2005; Rodriquez-Cruz & Pantnana, 2015). Therefore, all pediatric/adolescent patients with elevated BPs should be assessed for an underlying disorder causing the hypertension.

Clinical Aspects

ASSESSMENT

Completing an accurate history and assessment is a critical component of nursing care. Obtaining a full history of other comorbid conditions, such as hyperlipidemia, diabetes mellitus, coronary artery disease, renal disease, and sleep apnea is crucial when assessing a patient with a hypertensive crisis. In addition, current medications and obtaining recall of previous BP readings will assist in determining medication compliance.

All patients should be questioned regarding their use of over-the-counter medications and other drugs, including cocaine, methamphetamines, phencyclidine, and alcohol. In addition, patients who take monoamine oxidase inhibitors (MAOIs) are at increased risk for serious medication interactions, as combined use of MAOIs and other antidepressants can lead to a hypertensive reaction (Stafford et al., 2012). Prolonged use of nonsteroidal anti-inflammatories, decongestants, oral contraceptives, and various herbal products (i.e., bitter orange and ephedra) can also lead to a hypertensive crisis.

The physical assessment should focus on changes in the following body systems: cardiac (BP in both arms, heart rate, abnormal heart sounds [S3, S4, gallop], and volume status), vascular (carotid, aortic or renal bruits, edema), respiratory (adventitious breath sounds [crackles], oxygen saturation), and neurological (focal changes as commonly seen in cerebral vascular accidents, seizures; Batchelor, Gillman, Goodin, & Schwytzer, 2015). The nurse will need to be knowledgeable of various diagnostic indicators to assist in determining the degree of organ damage that has occurred. These include 12-lead electrocardiogram (myocardial infarction, ischemic changes, ventricular hypertrophy); urinalysis for blood, protein, glucose, and microalbumin; renal function tests (blood urea nitrogen and creatinine); and radiographs (chest x-ray for left ventricular/cardiac enlargement; Emergency Nurses Association, 2013). CT scans and echocardiography may also be indicated depending on presenting symptomatology.

NURSING INTERVENTIONS, MANAGEMENT, AND IMPLICATIONS

Distinguishing between the two hypertensive crises is essential to ensuring that proper treatment is initiated. During triage, it is essential for the nurse to differentiate hypertensive emergency from urgency to allow for quick initiation of treatment. Patients presenting with a hypertensive emergency should immediately receive a rapid-acting, titratable intravenous antihypertensive agent within a critical/emergency care area for BP reduction (Marik, 2015). During this time, the BP should be monitored continuously, which may require the insertion and use of an arterial line. Urine output is also monitored hourly to ensure adequate renal perfusion. The patient is assessed as per protocol and by physiologic response to determine response to therapy and extent of end-organ damage (Emergency Nurses Association, 2013).

Patients with hypertensive urgency, without other serious symptoms, should have their BP reduced slowly with an oral antihypertensive agent within a 24- to 48-hour period. Rapid-onset oral antihypertensive agents, such as clonidine, labetalol, or captopril, are often used for gradual, short-term reduction of BP while being observed in either an observational unit or emergency department, though treatment rarely requires hospitalization. Once stabilized, the patient will be changed to a long-term antihypertensive agent, stabilized, and then monitored in the outpatient primary care setting.

OUTCOMES

The initial goal of therapy for a hypertensive emergency is to reduce the mean arterial pressure by 25% over the first 24 to 48 hours. In contrast, there is no evidence to suggest a benefit from rapidly reducing the BP in patients with hypertensive urgency. Actually, too rapid a reduction in this state could yield organ damage from hypoperfusion.

Classifications of medications often used for rapid reduction of BP include nitrates (i.e., nitroprusside and nitroglycerin), beta-adrenergic blockers (i.e., labetolol and atenolol), calcium channel blockers (i.e., nicardipine, dilitazem, verapamil), and angiotensin-converting enzyme inhibitors (i.e., enalapril; Bisognano, 2015). Hydrazine is the preferred agent for pregnant patients. The nurse should have a thorough knowledge of the action, administration techniques, side effects, and adverse reaction for all medications that he or she administers. Associated end-organ effects may require specific treatment for specific disorders.

Long-term prognosis and outcomes depend upon patient compliance with medications and the extent of secondary end-organ damage. Once the patient's BP is reduced to a therapeutic level, the nurse should provide education on lifestyle modifications, medication adherence, and health care compliance.

Summary

Hypertension remains the "silent" killer of vascular disease here in the United States. In the essential form, hypertension has no symptoms, yet it continues to damage multiple organ sites throughout the body when not treated. Hypertensive crisis results for many different reasons, which include but are not limited to poor BP control, noncompliance with antihypertensive medications, and secondary physiologic disorders. Early recognition, differentiation in triage, and subsequent nursing care and pharmacotherapy are essential elements in reducing the short- and long-term complications that can occur in hypertensive crisis.

American Heart Association (2016). Hypertensive crisis: When you should call 9-1-1 for high blood pressure. Retrieved from https://www.heart.org/ HEARTORG/Conditions/ HighBloodPressure/ AboutHighBloodPressure/ Hypertensive-Crisis_UCM_301782_Article.jsp#.WDMfh03fN1s

Batchelor, N., Gillman, P., Goodin, J., & Schwytzer, D. (2015). *Medical surgical nursing* (4th ed.). Silver Spring, MD: American Nurses Association.

Bisognano, J. (2015). Malignant hypertension. *Medscape.* Retrieved from http:// emedicine.medscape.com/article/241640-overview#a5

Centers for Disease Control and Prevention. (2015). High blood pressure facts. Retrieved from http://www.cdc.gov/bloodpressure/facts.htm

Emergency Nurses Association. (2013). *Sheehy's manual of emergency care* (7th ed.). St. Louis, MO: Mosby

Marik, P. (2015). *Hypertensive crises, Part III. Evidence-based critical care* (pp. 429–443). Cham, Switzerland: Springer International Publishing. doi:10.1007/978-3 -319-11020-2_28

National Institutes of Health. (2005). Diagnosis, evaluation, and treatment of high blood pressure in children and adolescents. Retrieved from https://www.nhlbi.nih.gov/files/ docs/resources/heart/hbp_ped.pdf

National Institutes of Health. (2015). Exploring high blood pressure. Retrieved from http://www.nhlbi.nih.gov/health/health-topics/topics/hbp/atrisk

Rodriquez-Cruz, E., & Pantnana, S. (2015). Pediatric hypertension. Retrieved from http://emedicine.medscape.com/article/889877-overview

Stafford, E., Will, K., & Brooks-Gumbert, A. (2012). Management of hypertensive urgency and emergency. *Clinician Reviews, 22*(10), 20. Retrieved from http:// www.mdedge.com/ clinicianreviews/ article/ 79156/ nephrology/management -hypertensive-urgency-and-emergency

■ HYPOTHERMIA

Marian Nowak

Overview

Hypothermia is defined as a core body temperature of 95°F (35°C). Hypothermia occurs when the heat loss to the environment cannot be compensated by the heat produced by the body (*Free Medical Dictionary*, 2016). It is a potentially life-threatening condition. Exposure to extreme cold is a leading cause of preventable weather-related mortality. Variables that increase the risk for hypothermia-related death include advanced age, mental illness, male gender, and drug intoxication.

Nursing care for adults with hypothermia is focused on the early recognition of the deleterious effects of the exposure to low temperatures and the gradual rewarming to mitigate the body's defense of peripheral vasoconstriction. Accurate nursing assessment and response can optimize the effectiveness of an individual's ability to recover from this potential life-threatening condition (Lewis, Dirksen, Heitkemper, & Bucher, 2014).

Background

Extreme cold weather resulting in hypothermia is associated with excess morbidity and mortality. Moreover, it may result in death because it can exacerbate preexisting chronic conditions (including cardiovascular and respiratory diseases). A total of 13,419 deaths occurred from hypothermia during the period of 2003 to 2014; an unadjusted annual rate ranged from 0.3 to 0.5 per 100,000 persons. Data concerning hypothermia- related deaths for the United States overall were obtained from the Centers for Disease Control and Prevention's (CDC's) multiple cause-of-death files and "hypothermia" defined as any death with an underlying or contributing cause of death from exposure to excessive natural cold. Males accounted for 9,050 (67%) decedents (CDC, 2015). Mortality rates were highest among persons of advanced age. Several studies suggest that alcohol usage or drug poisoning contributes to a 10% increase in the cause of death in hypothermic patients. During 2006 to 2010, 10,649 deaths of U.S. residents were attributed to weather-related causes. This includes exposure to excessive natural heat, heat stroke, and sun stroke, which contributed to 3,332 (31%) of these deaths, and exposure to extreme environmental temperatures, a significant reduction in a person's core body temperature, or both was cited for 6,660 (63%) of deaths (Berko, Deborah, Saha, & Ingram, 2014).

Among deaths attributed to natural cold during 2006 to 2010, the death rate for infants was 1 death per million, which was higher than the rate for children aged 5 to 14 years but lower than the rate for persons aged 25 and over. Cold-related death rates were lowest for children aged 5 to 14 years of age (0.2 deaths per million) and increased progressively with age, as was the case for heat-related mortality, with rates increasing from 1.3 to 7.8 deaths per million among persons aged 15 to 74. The cold-related death rates for persons aged 75 and over are substantially higher than the rates for younger persons: 15.5 deaths per million among persons aged 75 to 84 and 39.6 deaths per million among persons aged 85 and older (Berko et al., 2014).

Persons with conditions that impair thermoregulatory function and those taking various medications are more susceptible to the effects of cold. Subpopulations at risk for cold-related mortality include older adults, infants, males, Black persons, and persons with preexisting chronic medical conditions. Alcoholics, persons using recreational drugs, homeless persons, and those with inadequate winter clothing or home heating are at increased risk of cold-related mortality. Other persons at risk include those who live in places with rapid temperature changes, large shifts in nighttime temperatures, or are at high elevations (Berko et al., 2014). Most body heat is lost in the form of radiant heat. *Radiant heat* refers to the heat given off by the body in the form of waves through the air (Lewis et al., 2014).

The greatest loss is from the head, lungs, and thorax. Severe environmental conditions, such as freezing temperatures, prolonged exposure to cold weather, cold winds, inadequate clothing, and exhaustion, predispose clients to hypothermia. Wet clothing increases evaporation heat loss up to five times and emersion in cold water increases evaporation up to 25 times (Iowa Great Lakes Water Safety Council, 2016).

Peripheral vasoconstriction is the body's first defense mechanism to attempt to compensate for heat loss. As cold temperature persists, shivering occurs in an attempt to produce heat. To prevent body cooling and hypothermia of seriously ill or injured casualties during transportation, casualty coverings must provide adequate thermal insulation against cold, wind, and moisture. Studies indicate that variables that affect the development of hypothermia include the time of exposure as determined by temperature and wind speed (Jussila, Rissanen, Parkkola, & Anttonen, 2014).

Clinical Aspects

ASSESSMENT

Assessment findings vary with the severity of the condition. Hypothermia may mimic cerebral or metabolic disturbances. Presenting symptoms may include ataxia, confusion, and withdrawal (Lewis et al., 2014)

Patients With Mild Hypothermia

Assessment findings also vary with the severity of the condition. Patients with mild hypothermia (93.2°F–96.8°F) often display shivering, lethargy, confusion, irrational behavior, and minor heart rate changes. Moderate hypothermia (86°F–93.2°F) patients exhibit rigidity, bradycardia, decreased respirations, respiratory acidosis, and hypovolemia. The blood pressure in patients with mild hypothermia is typically obtained by Doppler. In addition to decreases in peripheral arterial blood pressure, decreased renal flow leads to impaired water absorption and results in dehydration. Consequently, hematocrit increases and intravascular volume decreases. Due to increased viscosity of the blood, patients become prone to risk for myocardial infarction, stroke, pulmonary embolism, and renal failure (Samaras, Chevalley, Samaras, 2010).

Severe hypothermia, at or below 86°F, is potentially life-threatening. Symptoms include pale, cyanotic skin, fixed and dilated pupils, bradycardia, slow respiratory rate, ventricular fibrillation, or asystole. Warming is the treatment for all stages (Samaras et al., 2010).

NURSING INTERVENTIONS, MANAGEMENT, AND IMPLICATIONS

Nursing care of adults with hypothermia should initially focus on removing the patient from the cause (e.g., remove wet clothing if resent), maintaining arterial blood gases (ABGs), correcting dehydration, treating dysrhythmias, and rewarming the patient. High-flow oxygen should be provided via nonrebreather mask.

Passive or spontaneous rewarming methods include moving the patient to a warm dry place, removing wet clothing, using radiant lights, and placing warm blankets on the patient. Active surface rewarming method includes fluid or warm air-filled warming blankets or warm water emersion (98.6°F–104°F). Monitor the patient for vasodilation, which results in hypotension during the rewarming process. In severe hypothermia, alternative methods include applying heat directly to the core by using warm IV fluids (98.6°F), humidified oxygen (111.2°F), and peritoneal lavage with warm fluids (up to 113°F) while closely monitoring the patient for arrhythmias. Warming of the central trunk first to limit rewarming shock using extracorporeal circulation with rapid infuser or hemodialysis may also be done (Hoskin, Melinyshyn, Romet, & Goode, 1986; Kumar et al., 2015).

OUTCOMES

The expected outcomes of evidence-based nursing care are centered on preventing the progression of hypothermic complications and progression. The hospital use of minimally invasive rewarming for nonarrested, otherwise healthy, patients with primary hypothermia and stable vital signs has the potential to decrease morbidity and mortality. Ongoing monitoring is needed for ABG's temperature, level of consciousness, vital signs, oxygen saturation, heart rate and rhythm, electrolytes, and glucose. Active surveillance for changes in physical assessment is key in prevention progression of injury (Paal et al., 2015). Patients with moderate to severe hypothermia should have the core rewarmed before the extremities. As rewarming takes place, patients are at risk for after a further drop in core temperature. Monitoring of vital signs and gentle progression of rewarming are imperative. Gentle rewarming will avoid rewarming shock that can produce hypotension and dysrhythmias (Paal et al., 2015).

Summary

Exposure to cold is a leading cause of weather-related mortality and is responsible for approximately twice the number of deaths annually as due to exposure to heat in the United States (CDC, 2015). Prompt recognition of the signs and symptoms of hypothermia is necessary for reducing mortality. Recognition of hypothermia and intervention of symptoms include the application of evidence-based nursing rewarming guidelines. Following rewarming therapy guidelines and observing for potential systemic complications can assist the practitioner in avoiding complications.

Patients should be rewarmed by using external warming (e.g., blankets or forced heated air) for mild hypothermia and internal warming methods (e.g., body cavity lavage) for severe hypothermia. In the event of cardiac arrest, cardiopulmonary resuscitation should be performed during rewarming in accordance with published standard guidelines.

Berko J., Ingram, D., Saha, S., & Parker, J. D. (2014). Deaths attributed to heat, cold, and other weather events in the United States, 2006–2010. *National Health Statistics Report, 76*, 1–15.

Centers for Disease Control and Prevention. (2015). Hypothermia-related deaths, 2003–2013. *MMWR Weekly, 64*(6), 141–143.

Hoskin, R. W., Melinyshyn, M. J., Romet, T. T., & Goode, R. C. (1986). Bath rewarming from immersion hypothermia. *Journal of Applied Physiology, 61*, 1518–1522.

Iowa Great Lakes Water Safety Council. (2016). Cold water immersion. Retrieved from http://www.watersafety council.org/coldwaterimmersion/index.html

Jussila K., Rissanen S., Parkkola K., & Anttonen H. (2014). Evaluating cold, wind, and moisture protection of different coverings for prehospital maritime transportation—A thermal manikin and human study. *Prehospital and Disaster Medicine, 29*(6), 1–9.

Kumar, P., McDonald, G. K., Chitkara, R., Steinman, A. M., Gardiner, P. F., and Giesbrecht, G. G. (2015). Comparison of distal limb warming with fluid therapy and warm water immersion for mild hypothermia rewarming. *Wilderness and Environmental Medicine, 26*, 406–411. doi:10.1016/j.wem.2015.02.005

Lewis, S., Dirksen, S, Heitkemper, M., & Bucher, L. (2014). *Medical surgical nursing* (9th ed.). St. Louis, MO: Elsevier Mosby.

Paal, P., Gordon, L., Strapazzon, G., Brodmann Maeder, M., Putzer, G., Walpoth, B., . . . Brugger H. (2015). Accidental hypothermia—An update. The content of this review is endorsed by the International Commission for Mountain Emergency Medicine (ICAR MEDCOM). *Scandinavian Journal of Trauma, Resuscitation and Emergency Medicine, 24*(1), 111. doi:10.1186/s13049-016-0303-7

Radiant. (2016). In *The Free medical dictionary*. Retrieved from http://medical-dictionary.thefreedictionary.com/radiant+heat

Samaras, N., Chevalley, T., & Samaras, D. (2010). Older patients in the emergency department: A review. *Annals of Emergency Medicine, 56*, 261.

■ INTEGUMENTARY EMERGENCIES

Susanna Rudy

Overview

Serious, life-threatening skin disorders are rare. Presentation to the emergency department (ED) with a dermatological complaint can be frustrating for both patient and provider, particularly if there is no clear cause for the annoyance of symptoms such as rash and itching. Although most rashes are benign and self-limiting, there are serious dermatological emergencies that pose a lethal threat to health and mortality if they are not immediately differentiated or diagnosed on presentation. A delay in the identification, specialty consultation, and supportive intensive care treatment can result in a permanently debilitating or fatal outcome for the patient. A systematic approach to identification and management of some of the most common and acutely deadly rashes are reviewed.

Background

On an average, the prevalence of dermatological complaints requiring medical treatment ranges between 19% and 27%, with the majority of these cutaneous conditions being benign (Baibergenova & Shear, 2011). The epidemiology of outpatient presentation accounts for approximately 5% to 8% of these conditions. Only 3.3% present urgently to the ED and of that 94 % are discharged home after evaluation and treatment. Approximately 4% require hospital admission. Skin infections, in the form of cellulitis, account for approximately 33% of the admissions (R. A. Schwartz, McDonough, & Lee, 2013).

Of all of the types of skin rashes, there are approximately 10 that present as a predictor for potential life-threatening sequelae of pain, prolonged illness, multisystem organ failure, and, in some cases, death. The following all present with characteristic symptoms and rash that require expedient diagnoses and management: erythema multiforme major (EM), Stevens–Johnson syndrome (SJS), toxic epidermal necrolysis (TEN), drug hypersensitivity syndrome (DHS) otherwise known as *drug rash with eosinophilia and systemic symptoms* (DRESS) syndrome, staphylococcal scalded skin syndrome (SSSS), staphylococcal/streptococcal toxic shock syndrome (TSS), *Neisseria* meningitis (meningococcemia), necrotizing fasciitis, pemphigus vulgaris (PV), vibrio, and Rocky Mountain spotted fever (RMSF). For purposes of discussion, the blistering cutaneous disorders of SJS, TENS, SJS/TENS, and DRESS are reviewed in brief.

SJS, TEN, and an overlap of SJS/TEN are severe mucocutaneous diseases thought to be extensive examples of erythema multiform (EM). They are rare and involve the loss of the epidermal layers of the skin resulting in fluid losses, potential for shock, respiratory failure, sepsis, gastrointestinal (GI) hemorrhage, and multiorgan system failure (Papadakis & McPhee, 2017; Stone & Humphries,

2011). The overall combined incidence in the worldwide population of all three is approximately two to seven per million/annually and a 1,000-fold increase in patients with HIV (R. A. Schwartz et al., 2013). TEN, SJS, and SJS/TEN are often listed together as they are all variants of the same histopathologic disease continuum differing only by severity and body surface affected. All variants are thought to be caused by an immune-mediated hypersensitivity response from specific drugs; reactions occur in 80% to 95% of cases (Pereira et al., 2007). Reactions can be delayed toward an initial exposure or rapid reexposure. This disease occurs in all age groups.

Research supports a genetic predisposition of certain individuals to hypersensitivity reactions to certain metabolite complexes formed with the breakdown of certain medications. Specific implication applies to certain antibiotics classes and drugs such as sulfa, nonsteroidal anti-inflammatory drugs (NSAIDs), anticonvulsants, and antigout medications. Other triggers of cutaneous disorders can be exposure to bacterial and viral infections, malignancy, certain vaccinations, contrast medium, and graft versus host disease (R. B. Schwartz, Sattin, & Hunt, 2013). When exposed to the triggers, certain individuals develop an immune-mediated cytotoxic reaction that results in apoptosis (cell death) of the keratinocytes in the epidermis and tissue necrosis. The diseases are hallmarked by skin peeling, separating the epidermal layer of the skin from the dermis. They are all systemic diseases that involve the integumentary, pulmonary, ophthalmic, and genitourinary systems; internal involvement results from the massive release of proinflammatory cytokines that result in epithelial sloughing (Papadakis & McPhee, 2017).

The spectral diseases are separated only by a percentage of body surface area and epidermal detachment that occurs. Features of TEN occur with or without purpura (spots). TEN with spots includes widespread purpuric macules and progression of flaccid blistering bullae, skin erosions, and painful epidermal denudation of the skin or sloughing involving the epithelium layers of the eyes, lungs, GI tract, and genitals (Papadakis & McPhee, 2017). Skin can easily be separated with gentle lateral pressure known as *Nikolsky's sign.* The course progression can occur over a period of 1 day to 3 weeks after exposure to the trigger. Total body surface area affected in TEN is more than 30% and can be as life-threatening as a severe burn (Pereira et al., 2007). The rash is central and can involve at least two mucosal sites. The active phase of blistering and skin loss occurs in 2 weeks (R. A. Schwartz et al., 2013). The cutaneous sequelae are prominent with the most concerning involving ocular complications that can result in blindness (R. B. Schwartz et al., 2013). Patients with TEN with spots are very ill with acute skin failure and mortality rate is between 10% and 70%; primary causes of death result from septicemia and multisystem organ failure (Cohen, 2016).

SJS shares most of the same features and morphology as TEN but is differentiated from TEN in that it has less than 10% body surface area (BSA) involvement. The overlap of SJS/TEN has an affected BSA of 10% to 30% (Cohen, 2016; R. A. Schwartz et al., 2013).

DRESS syndrome is also in the same class of drug eruption (DE) life-threatening cutaneous diseases as TEN and SJS; the pathogenesis is consistent among them

(Camous, Calbo, Picard, & Musette, 2012). Difficult to diagnose because of the similarities to other cutaneous diseases, as well as a delay in symptomology, DRESS is predominantly a drug-induced hypersensitivity reaction caused by the same trigger medications seen with the other spectral diseases mentioned with antiepileptic's and allopurinol being the most common. There is a strong genetic link associated with how certain populations metabolize the trigger medications that form complexes that trigger antibody formation (Camous et al., 2012). DRESS is caused by a T cell mediated response to the foreign complexes lending to the overwhelming proinflammatory response. Reactivation of the herpes virus in combination with exposure to suspected trigger drugs is specific to DRESS (Camous et al., 2012). Symptoms of DRESS appear in 2 to 6 weeks after exposure to the medications. The syndrome is characterized by a viral prodrome, high fevers, lymphadenopathy, organ involvement, hematologic abnormalities, hallmarked facial edema, skin eruptions of a morbilliform rash of more than 50% BSA. Resolution is gradual with the removal of the offending agent; typically, 6 to 9 weeks with the possibility of persistence for months with intermittent periods of remission and exacerbation (Camous et al., 2012; Papadakis & McPhee, 2017).

Clinical Aspects

ASSESSMENT

A good patient history and timely physical assessment are important to prompt treatment and management of the spectrum of life-threatening cutaneous disorders. A previous history of exposure to one of the trigger medications, a previous history or genetic predisposition to these diseases, the physical symptoms, the appearance of the affected skin, percentage involved, and time of onset can all help differentiate a diagnosis. A skin biopsy for histology and frozen section are a definitive diagnostic tools used to confirm a diagnosis.

NURSING INTERVENTIONS, MANAGEMENT, AND IMPLICATIONS

Patients with cutaneous-related problems require aggressive medical management and close monitoring. Nursing need to manage patient pain issues, fluid loss, monitoring of hemodynamics, and accurate intake and output. Patients in the early phases of blister formation affecting the mucosal areas have difficulty with eating, swallowing, and may be at risk for dehydration and poor nutrition, decreased protein intake that leads to poor wound healing. Patients also have pain and require adequate pain management. Attention to pain scores and follow-up assessments are of primary importance. Owing to the potential for skin loss, exposed skin need to be managed with dressing changes and creams; overall acuity of patients with these cutaneous diseases is higher and require more nursing time. Deterioration in respiratory, GI, and hemodynamics should be anticipated and monitored closely. Close monitoring of patient's neurological status, hemodynamics, intake and output, nutritional intake, and pain should be ongoing. Early consultation with nutrition and ophthalmology for baseline assessment should be a priority (Papadakis & McPhee, 2017; R. A. Schwartz et al., 2013).

Primary management of these dermatological emergencies involves removal of the trigger drug if the patient is still on it. It will also be noted in the patient's chart. Aggressive management includes fluid resuscitation, nutritional supplementation, and extensive wound management (Papadakis & McPhee, 2017; Stone & Humphries, 2011). Specialty care in intensive care or the burn unit is necessary to manage large cutaneous injuries, the large amounts of fluid loss, and the anticipated worsening progression of the diseases to involve the eyes, lungs, GI, and skin. The expediency of an offending drug removal and admission to intensive care improve overall prognosis. Ocular sequelae associated with these conditions can lead to blindness. Eyes should be managed with eye drops and ointments to prevent the abrasions and dry eye associated with these skin conditions. Opthalmology consult is mandatory (Papadakis & Humphries, 2017; Pereira et al., 2007; Stone & Humphries, 2011).

Pan culturing is appropriate on admission, but the administration of empiric antibiotics should be avoided because of an increased risk of resistance and no evidence of improved outcomes to support the use of empiric broad spectrum antibiotics (Pereira et al., 2007). Skin debridement may be necessary for TEN patients, and large denuded areas should be covered with allograft skin. Consideration of adjuvant treatments with intravenous immunoglobulin (IVIG), cyclosporine, plasmapheresis, tumor necrosis factor (TNF)-alpha inhibitors is a matter of clinical judgment. There is promising evidence to support the benefit of high-dosed, pulsed steroid dosing arresting disease in a shorter interval of time than without (Pereira et al., 2007). The patient should be educated on the triggers and causative mechanisms, and how to avoid them and similar classes of medications. Human leukocyte antigen (HLA) tissue typing can determine predisposition to developing life-threatening cutaneous disorders in certain patient populations and should be considered before starting therapy.

OUTCOMES

Identification and management of integumentary emergencies can be very challenging but is imperative to promote positive patient outcomes. Differentiating TEN, SJS, SSSS, and other potentially life-threatening disorders must be identified and managed appropriately. Utilizing the assessment skills and interventions discussed in this entry will assist the nurse to successfully promote positive outcomes.

Summary

Using a systematic approach to evaluating, identifying, and differentiating a presenting dermatological complaint can improve the outcome of life-threatening cutaneous rashes if identified early. The pathogenesis of apoptosis in these cutaneous diseases is rapid in onset and, once triggered, is irreversible. Timing is critical. Discontinuation of the offending medication and aggressive resuscitative management in a burn unit are essential and the overall primary predictors of overall prognosis or mortality.

Baibergenova, A., & Shear, N. H. (2011). Skin conditions that bring patients to emergency departments. *Archives of Dermatology, 147*(1), 118–120.

Camous, X., Calbo, S., Picard, D., & Musette, P. (2012). Drug reaction with eosinophilia and systemic symptoms: An update on pathogenesis. *Current Opinion in Immunology, 24*(6), 730–735.

Cohen, V. (2016). Toxic epidermal necrolysis. *Medscape.* Retrieved from http://emedicine.medscape.com/article/229698-overview

Papadakis, M. A., & McPhee, S. J. (2017). *Current medical diagnosis & treatment* (56th ed.). New York, NY: McGraw-Hill.

Pereira, F. A., Mudgil, A. V., & Rosmarin, D. M. (2007). Toxic epidermal necrolysis. *Journal of the American Academy of Dermatology, 56*(2), 181–200.

Schwartz, R. A., McDonough, P., & Lee, B. W. (2013). Toxic epidermal necrolysis. Part 1. Introduction, history, classification, clinical features, systemic manifestations, etiology, and immunopathogenesis. *Journal of American Academy of Dermatology, 69(4),* 173.e1–173.e13. doi:10.1016/j.jaad.2013.05.003

Schwartz, R. B., Sattin, R. W., & Hunt, R. C. (2013). Medical response to bombings: The application of lessons learned to a tragedy. *Disaster Medicine and Public Health Preparedness, 7*(2), 114–115.

Stone, K., & Humphries, R. (2011). *Current diagnosis & treatment: Emergency medicine* (7th ed.). New York, NY: McGraw-Hill.

■ INTRA-AORTIC BALLOON PUMP

Grant Pignatiello

Overview

With more than 70,000 annual insertions, the intra-aortic balloon pump (IABP) is the most commonly used circulatory assistive device (Parissis et al., 2016; Parissis, Soo, & Al-Alao, 2011). Positioned in the ascending aorta, the IABP uses pulsations coordinated with the patient's innate cardiac cycle to assist patients with left ventricular dysfunction by augmenting diastolic pressure, reducing systemic vascular resistance (SVR), and enhancing coronary and cerebral perfusion. Although empirical data support the benefit provided through use of the IABP, its use is not free of risk; therefore, nurses caring for patients receiving circulatory support from an IABP must possess a thorough breadth of knowledge related to cardiovascular physiology and hemodynamics, IABP functional mechanisms, and factors concerned with maintenance of patient safety and therapeutic discontinuation (Lewis, Ward, & Courtney, 2009).

Background

The first successful application of an IABP was reported in 1967 within a 45-year-old female suffering from severe cardiogenic shock after an acute myocardial infarction; subsequent testing and evaluation through the latter portion of the 20th century and mechanical/engineering developments through the early 21st century have refined the IABP as a reliable therapeutic modality for circulatory support (Parissis et al., 2016). The IABP is most commonly inserted through the femoral artery; however, it can also be inserted through the subclavian artery (Parissis et al., 2016; Raman, Loor, London, & Jolly, 2010). Ideally, the balloon, which contains a volume of 40 mL and a length ranging from 22 to 27.5 cm, should be placed such that the tip is just distal to the left subclavian branch of the aortic arch and the proximal end superior to the renal arteries.

The functionality of the IABP is contingent upon its coordination with the cardiac cycle; following counterpulsation principles, the balloon is inflated during diastole (the T-P interval of an electrocardiogram tracing) with helium gas and deflated during systole (QRS-T interval of an electrocardiogram tracing). This possesses numerous consequences for the systolic and diastolic phases of the cardiac cycle. Systolic consequences associated with IABP counterpulsation include (a) a decrease in systolic and end-diastolic blood pressure from systolic unloading by the IABP and subsequent afterload reduction and (b) decrease in left ventricular wall tension, and increased left ventricular ejection fraction and cardiac output due to afterload reduction. Diastolic consequences related to IABP counterpulsation include (a) decreased left ventricular diastolic volume secondary to enhanced ventricular unloading, (b) enhanced coronary artery perfusion due to retrograde displacement of blood pushed back through the aortic arch during diastole, (c) enhanced myocardial oxygen supply related to an increase in diastolic pressure time index and a decrease in tension time index, and (d) increased peripheral blood flow related to the increased arterial pressure from the balloon inflation resulting in an increased arterial–venous gradient (Parissis et al., 2016).

Because of the IABP's ability to reduce systemic afterload, enhance coronary perfusion, and augment diastolic pressure, it is an ideal supportive modality for clinical situations in which the patient's volume status is optimized and the patient is experiencing acute ventricular failure refractory to maximum inotropic support. Parissis et al. (2016) identify several objective clinical parameters that would indicate IABP use in the setting of acute ventricular failure: (a) cardiac index less than 1.8 L/min, (b) systolic arterial pressure less than 90 mmHg, (c) left or right atrial pressure greater than 20 mmHg, (d) urine output less than 20 mL/hr, (e) SVR greater than 2,100 dynes, and (f) metabolic acidosis. Moreover, IABPs are used after 5% to 10% of cardiac surgeries for patients who are unable to wean from cardiopulmonary bypass and may also be indicated for myoconservation during periods of unstable angina, following acute myocardial infarctions with or without tachyarrhythmia, acute ischemic mitral incompetence, ischemic rupture of the ventricular septum, severe cardiogenic shock, and during percutaneous coronary intervention (Parissis et al., 2011, 2016).

Use of IABP is associated with decreased risk of mortality; a meta-analysis conducted by Fan et al. (2016) of 33 clinical trials containing 18,889 patients found that patients who received IABP therapy who were suffering from acute myocardial infarction were more likely to be alive 6 months later when compared to those who did not receive an IABP (odds ratio [OR]: 0.66, 95% confidence interval [CI]: 0.48–0.91, p = .010). Nevertheless, despite the IABP's effectiveness in improving patient outcomes, Krishna and Zacharowski (2009) identify several absolute and relative contraindications. Absolute contraindications to IABP placement include aortic regurgitation, aortic dissection, end-stage heart disease with no anticipated recovery, and aortic stents; whereas, the relative contraindications include uncontrolled sepsis, abdominal aortic aneurysm, tachyarrhythmia, severe peripheral vascular disease, and arterial reconstruction surgery. Moreover, use of IABP is associated with risks that must be considered for those providing nursing care to the patient.

Clinical Aspects

ASSESSMENT

Nursing care of the patient receiving IABP therapy requires skilled physical assessment and a thorough understanding of human physiology to evaluate the patient's clinical progression and for signs and symptoms of complications (Lewis et al., 2009). To maintain a global perspective on the patient's physiological status, intricate patient monitoring is necessary. Commonly, patients possess central venous catheters and intra-arterial catheters; patients may also have pulmonary artery catheters. Through this, clinicians can receive relevant clinical information in addition to vital signs on demand, such as arterial blood pressure, central venous pressure, pulmonary artery pressures, cardiac output/index, and pulmonary wedge pressures. Moreover, supportive imaging, such as radiography and echocardiography, can provide additional data indicative of cardiac function. Furthermore, assessment of the IABP's effectiveness is evaluated by monitoring diastolic augmentation and the timing of the balloon's inflation/deflation with the patient's cardiac cycle. Moreover, as the patient's hemodynamic and cardiovascular function widely impacts other physiological processes, other indicators of cardiac function include pulmonary status (oxygenation, arterial oxygen saturation, etc.), lactate levels, renal function, and metabolic measures (Lewis et al., 2009).

In addition, IABP therapy is associated with an increased risk of specific complications. The most common complication is IABP-induced thrombocytopenia and access site bleeding (Lewis et al., 2009; Parissis et al., 2011). The IABP can cause destruction of platelets, contributing to thrombocytopenia and site bleeding. Access site bleeding should be managed by either the addition of a suture to the site or through gentle compression—excessive pressure should be avoided as it narrows the arterial lumen and may contribute to distal limb ischemia (Lewis et al., 2009). Therefore, nursing care involves regular evaluation of the insertion site for signs of bleeding and/or hematoma formation. Also, the IAPB can cause red blood cell destruction; it is not uncommon for recipients of IABPs to require intermittent blood transfusions.

Hypoperfusion of limbs and/or organ systems is another common complication of IABP therapy. Distal limb ischemia is a risk most prevalent in patients with existing peripheral vascular disease and often occurs shortly after placement of the IABP. Nursing care involves regular monitoring of extremity in neurovascular status, such as extremity temperature, color, movement, and sensation; moreover, distal pulses (dorsalis pedis and posterior tibial) should be regularly evaluated. In addition, vascular assessments should include all extremities—although unlikely, there is possibility of balloon migration and subsequent obstruction of additional vessels. Similarly, urine output should be regularly monitored—a sudden decline in urine output may indicate occlusion of the renal arteries emerging from the distal aorta. Lactate values can be monitored as an indicator of tissue perfusion (Lewis et al., 2009).

OUTCOMES

As the combination of ventilation and pharmacologic support in combination with the IABP contributes to restoration of cardiac function, IABP support should be reduced and ideally discontinued. An indication of readiness for lessening IABP support is the gradual tolerance of weaning pharmacological inotropic agents. Lessening of IABP support can be through either frequency or volume weaning. Frequency weaning involves reducing the number of assisted beats provided by the IABP; for example, full assistance by the IABP indicates a 1:1 frequency—every heartbeat is supported by IABP augmentation. Eventually, as the patient's condition improves, IABP support can be diminished to frequencies of 1:2, 1:3, and 1:4. Whereas, volume weaning involves the gradual reduction of the volume within the balloon—decreasing augmentation provided by the IABP and increasing cardiovascular workload (Lewis et al., 2009). Once the IABP is discontinued, the nurse must continue to regularly assess the access site for signs of bleeding and/or hematoma formation and distal extremity neurovascular status.

Summary

IABPs provide effective circulatory support to patients suffering acute ventricular failure by augmenting diastolic pressure, reducing afterload, and enhancing coronary artery perfusion. These patients, often critically ill, require nursing care that incorporates a proficient understanding of pathophysiology and human hemodynamics. Furthermore, nursing care requires the nurse to perform thorough physical assessments and apply such data to the patient's clinical context to anticipate and recognize signs/symptoms of complications or progress associated with IABP therapy. As mechanical circulatory devices continue to develop, the nursing discipline can anticipate the provision of more complex circulatory modalities that not only augment the diastolic phase of the cardiac cycle, but the systolic phase as well (Parissis et al., 2016).

Fan, Z.-G., Gao, X.-F., Chen, L.-W., Li, X.-B., Shao, M.-X., Ji, Q., . . . Tian, N.-L. (2016). The outcomes of intra-aortic balloon pump usage in patients with acute myocardial infarction: A comprehensive meta-analysis of 33 clinical trials and 18,889 patients. *Patient Preference and Adherence, 10,* 297–312. doi:10.2147/PPA.S101945

Krishna, M., & Zacharowski, K. (2009). Principles of intra-aortic balloon pump counterpulsation. *Continuing Education in Anaesthesia, Critical Care and Pain, 9*(1), 24–28. doi:10.1093/bjaceaccp/mkn051

Lewis, P. A., Ward, D. A., & Courtney, M. D. (2009). The intra-aortic balloon pump in heart failure management: Implications for nursing practice. *Australian Critical Care, 22*(3), 125–131. doi:10.1016/j.aucc.2009.06.005

Parissis, H., Graham, V., Lampridis, S., Lau, M., Hooks, G., & Mhandu, P. C. (2016). IABP: History-evolution-pathophysiology-indications: What we need to know. *Journal of Cardiothoracic Surgery, 11*(1), 122. doi:10.1186/s13019-016-0513-0

Parissis, H., Soo, A., & Al-Alao, B. (2011). Intra-aortic balloon pump: Literature review of risk factors related to complications of the intra-aortic balloon pump. *Journal of Cardiothoracic Surgery, 6,* 147. doi:10.1186/1749-8090-6-147

Raman, J., Loor, G., London, M., & Jolly, N. (2010). Subclavian artery access for ambulatory balloon pump insertion. *Annals of Thoracic Surgery, 90*(3), 1032–1034. doi:10.1016/j.athoracsur.2009.11.082

■ MENTAL AND BEHAVIORAL HEALTH EMERGENCIES

Lia V. Ludan

Overview

Nurses in emergency departments and critical care settings are likely to encounter individuals experiencing mental and behavioral health emergencies. Mental and behavioral health emergencies encompass a variety of psychiatric disorders that include substance abuse, depression with suicidal ideations, acute delirium, generalized or situational anxiety, and psychosis. In recent years, there has been an increase of patients presenting to the acute care and outpatient settings for care in states of a mental or behavioral health crisis. The nursing care for patients suffering from mental or behavioral health emergencies must be focused on the safety of the patient and the health care staff and should include a detailed history and physical examination, nursing care coordination, and community resources to optimize the health of the patients with a mental or behavioral health emergency.

Background

Mental health illness can affect one's mood, thinking, or feelings (National Alliance on Mental Illness, 2016). There are multiple factors that can increase one's risk for developing a behavioral health illness, such as substance abuse, chronic illness, stressful lifestyle, genetics, traumatic life events, biochemical processes, and basic brain structure. Approximately, 48 million Americans aged 18 years and older have experienced a mental or behavioral health event in a given year (National Alliance on Mental Illness, 2016). About 10 million Americans suffer an event that is serious enough to disrupt their life's activities. Hispanic and African Americans use behavioral health resources at half the rate of Caucasian Americans, and Asian Americans use mental health services at one third the rate of Caucasian Americans (National Alliance on Mental Illness, 2016).

Individuals who have mental illness have a life expectancy decreased by 10 years. When behavioral health issues are present, it increases early mortality from other disease processes such as cardiovascular problems, diabetes, and HIV/AIDS. This can be caused by the individual's general neglect of their health, decrease in physical activity, increase in substance abuse, unhealthy eating habits, and side effects from medications. Other risk factors are low income, lower levels of education, and homelessness.

Mental illness affects youths as well as adults. One in every five youth (aged 13–18 years) undergoes a mental health event sometime during his or her life (National Alliance on Mental Illness, 2016). Half of all chronic behavioral health illness starts as early as 14 years of age, and three quarters of these issues present by the age of 24 years. An estimated 70% of youths in the justice system have at least one behavioral health issue (National Alliance on Mental Illness, 2016). About 20% of individuals have more than one behavioral health issue. Many children do not receive the services needed for their mental health illness. Researchers have calculated that approximately 50% of youths receive services for mental illness (National Alliance on Mental Illness, 2016). Of children who have died from suicidal attempts, 90% had a previous mental illness.

The elderly population is also at risk for mental illness. With the risk of cognitive decline and dementia, the elderly become more vulnerable (Yasamy, Dua, Harper, & Saxena, 2012). Loss of friends and partners can produce a feeling of loneliness, which can develop into depression. Certain chronic diseases can cause a decrease in mobility and independence, which can result in social isolation. The elderly are at risk for neglect or abuse (World Health Organization, 2012), which poses a negative influence on their psychological well-being.

When an individual suffers a serious mental illness, the individual may put his or her life on hold, meaning a loss of earnings. Each year, the American economy loses $193 billion in wages because of serious behavioral events (National Alliance on Mental Illness, 2016). According to the National Institute of Mental Health (Insel, 2015), mental disorders cost $2.5 trillion globally in 2010. The cost is projected to be $6 trillion by 2030 (National Institute of Mental Health, 2016).

According to the American College of Emergency Physicians (ACEP; 2014), psychiatric inpatient beds have decreased to less than 50,000 nationwide. This drastic decrease has forced patients to seek treatment at outpatient facilities, community resources, and other outpatient medical management groups. The outpatient facilities have been under strain because of lack of staff and budget cuts. This forces an increasing number of individuals to seek treatment at acute care settings, such as emergency rooms, for acute mental or behavioral health symptoms that require immediate nursing and medical care (ACEP, 2014).

Clinical Aspects

ASSESSMENT

One of the vital aspects of effective nursing care of a mental and behavioral health patient is obtaining a complete history and physical assessment and laboratory data. The assessment of the patient allows the nurse to identify the patient's problem and establish a relationship with the patient (Karas, 2002). The first step in the assessment process is to assess the behavior of the patient—that is, whether the patient is violent, withdrawn, overactive (manic state), or flat. If the patient is violent and can put the staff or himself or herself at risk of harm, trained security should be notified. If the patient cannot be calmed, then physical or chemical restraints may be indicated. The preferred routes of medication are: oral, intramuscular (IM), then intravenous (IV). Most clinicians start with butyrophenone, such as haloperidol, with or without a benzodiazepine such as lorazepam (ACEP, 2014). The nurse should be aware that antipsychotics are linked to prolonged QT syndrome, extrapyramidal side effects, and anticholinergic effects (ACEP, 2014). Most patients may be responsive to supportive measures alone (Karas, 2002). Placing a patient in a quiet environment, reducing noise, and ensuring a sensation of safety may promote a positive encounter. Once safety has been established, then the professional can determine whether the patient is medically or behavioral stable, and ascertain whether the patient needs oxygen, fluids, cardiac monitoring, or medications (Karas, 2002).

The first step is obtaining the client's demographics, such as age, gender, current living situation, ethnicity, and religion. Subsequently, one should determine the nature of the patient's chief complaint; this should be given in the patient's own words. This can be very different from what is reported from the ambulance personnel, family, or other witnesses. Then the nurse, should obtain the history of present illness. Questions that can be asked include: "What time was the onset of the event? What factors precipitated the event? What was the duration of the event?" (Karas, 2002). Questions regarding allergies, medications are taken daily, psychiatric history, substance abuse, and medical history should be answered. Then the nurse performs the physical examination, including taking the patient's vital signs, blood pressure, heart rate, oxygen saturation, respirations, and temperature. Performing a head-to-toe examination, inspecting the head for trauma and an ocular examination can be very helpful. Pinpoint or dilated pupils can represent the use of narcotics or other substances. Inspection of the neck and chest can be very helpful as well (Karas, 2002). Auscultation of breath sounds can reveal an indication of congestive heart failure or pneumonia. In the elderly, these disease processes can cause delirium. Adverse heart sounds can be caused by atrial fibrillation, metabolic derangements, or drug toxicities. An abdominal examination can display signs of infection, ascites, or hepatomegaly, which can cause the patient to have a change in their mental state. The nurse should inspect the skin for rashes, needle marks, diaphoresis, petechiae, or purpura (Karas, 2002).

The psychiatric examination starts with the appearance of the patient; the nurse also assesses how the patient is dressed and groomed. Subsequently, the nurse observes motor function for abnormal movement, assessing muscle tone, posture, and gait. During assessment, the nurse should note whether the patient's speech is low, fast (manic), or slow (depression) when answering questions (Zun, 2016). He or she should then inquire about suicidal ideation or violent thoughts by asking whether the patient wants to hurt himself or herself or others. The nurse should then assess the patient's insight and judgment (Zun, 2016), and whether the patient understands that there is a problem and what needs to be done to correct it. The abnormal thought process can be a key indicator for schizophrenia and psychotic disorders. The nurse should obtain a urine drug screen, alcohol testing, bedside blood glucose levels, and urine pregnancy test for all women of child bearing age (Zun, 2016). If the physical examination reveals any adverse finding, the nurse should anticipate further diagnostic testing such as medical imaging, cardiogram, and laboratory studies. Subequently, the patient should have a psychiatric screening from a trained professional, such as a behavioral health counselor or a psychiatrist (Zun, 2016).

NURSING INTERVENTIONS, MANAGEMENT, AND IMPLICATIONS

A common nursing issue that occurs when a patient with a mental or behavioral health emergency seeks care in an ED is the delayed transfer of patients to definitive psychiatric inpatient care. Often, the prolonged boarding times in ED for patients with a mental or behavioral health emergency occur because of lack of insurance, need to transfer to an outside facility, and the lack of inpatient facility throughout the nation (ACEP, 2014). Another known issue is stigma from health care providers toward patients in states psychiatric emergency. Nurses should recognize their personal biases toward mental illness and take appropriate courses of action to prevent stigmatization of these patients (Trossman, 2011). Lastly, the majority of ED and critical care nurses lack continuing education on how to address patients with mental or behavioral health emergencies. However, nurses in these care settings should seek educational offerings to enhance the safety, manage stigma, and initiate plans of nursing care to support the needs of patients with mental or behavioral health emergencies (Trossman, 2011).

OUTCOMES

The primary outcome of nursing care for patients experiencing a mental or behavioral health emergency is safety, psychological recovery, and optimization of other acute or chronic physical conditions. This is ensured by continued assessment and close observation of the patient while in the acute care and inpatient setting. Subsequently, the nurse assesses the patient's disposition, and determines whether the patient should be discharged or become an inpatient. If the patient can be discharged from the acute care setting, the nurse should provide follow-up and community resources to the patient. He or she should ensure the patient's understanding of the follow-up instructions and how to access the community resources. Another important aspect is to educate the patient about how and when to seek care if a behavioral crisis is happening. If the patient is to be admitted the nurse must ensure that proper arrangements have been made for the transfer and set a plan for the patient's current behavioral health issue. Having an established plan helps when inpatient beds are not readily available. For the patient to have a positive outcome, care must be developed and implemented on a multidisciplinary level with evidence-based treatment plans.

Summary

Mental illness is a disease process that can be difficult to treat because it involves the consideration of many factors. When caring for a patient with mental health, nurses must keep in mind that risk factors, safety issues, and detailed assessment skills are vital in providing care to this population type. Having a complete understanding of the complex dynamics of the disease process ensure that the nurse and the patient are providing and receiving high-quality, evidence-based nursing care.

American College of Emergency Physicians. (2014). Care of the psychiatric patient in the emergency department: A review of the literature. Retrieved from https://www.acep .org/uploadedFiles/ACEP/Clinical_and_Practice_Management/Resources/Mental_ Health_and_Substance_Abuse/Psychiatric%20Patient%20Care%20in%20the%20 ED%202014.pdf

Insel, T. (2015). Post by former NIMH director Thomas Insel: Mental health awareness month: By the numbers. Retrieved from https://www.nimh.nih.gov/about/directors/ thomas-insel/blog/2015/mental-health-aware ness-month-by-the-numbers.shtml

Karas, S. (2002). Behavioral emergencies: Differentiating medical from psychiatric disease. *Emergency Medicine Practice, 4*(3), 1–20. Retrieved from http://www .ebmedicine.net/topics.php?paction=showTopic&topic_id=61

National Alliance on Mental Illness. (2016). Mental health by the numbers. Retrieved from https://www.nami.org/Learn-More/Mental-Health-By-the-Numbers

Trossman, S. (2011, April). Overcoming stigma. Retrieved from http://www.the americannurse.org/2011/04/12/overcoming-stigma

Yasamy, M. T., Dua, T., Harper, M., & Saxena, S. (2012). *Mental health of older adults, addressing a growing concern* (pp. 4–9). Retrieved from http://www.who.int/mental_ health/world-mental-health-day/WHO_paper_wmhd_2013.pdf

Zun, L. (2016). Care of psychiatric patients: The challenge to emergency physicians. *Western Journal of Emergency Medicine, 17*(2), 173–176.

■ NEUROTRAUMA

Anita Sundaresh

Overview

Neurotrauma is prevalent in adults as well as the pediatric population. It can be categorized by mechanisms of injury, clinical severity, radiological appearance, or anatomic distribution. The effects of the trauma can last from hours to days. Seat belts and helmets often protect individuals from a neurologic injury, which is the main focus of public health efforts. Migraines and strokes, common neurological disorders that affect individuals worldwide, will be discussed.

Background

Migraine is derived from the Greek word *hemicrania* (Silberstein, 2004). It is a disorder that is associated with significant neurological, gastrointestinal, as well as autonomic changes. It can be associated with episodes of headache that are pulsating in quality, unilateral or bilateral, and can be exacerbated by physical activity (Kurth & Diener, 2012). Some of the contributing factors of migraine include nonsteroidal anti-inflammatory drugs, combination analgesics, dopamine antagonists, corticosteroids, opioids, and migraine-specific medications. Migraine is a common disorder that affects about 11% of the world's total population. Females are at higher risk than males; of females, 17.6% are affected with migraines, whereas 5.7% of males are affected. Migraines are prevalent in 3% of the pediatric population aged between 2 and 7 years, increasing to 8% to 23% in children aged 11 years and older (Semenov, 2015). One's quality of life is deeply affected by migraines as they can be very debilitating. "Migraines yearly cost to employers is about US $13 billion and yearly medical costs exceed $1 million" (Silberstein, 2004, p. 381).

The World Health Organization (1978) has defined *stroke* as "a clinical syndrome, of presumed vascular origin, typified by rapidly developing signs of focal or global disturbance of cerebral functions lasting more than 24 hours or leading to death" (as cited in Intercollegiate Stroke Working Party, 2012, p. 27). Eight-five percent of strokes are due to cerebral infarction, 10% are attributed to primary hemorrhage, and 5% are caused by subarachnoid hemorrhage (SAH). Transient ischemic attack (TIA) occurs when symptoms last fewer than 24 hours. It is due to an inadequate cerebral or ocular blood supply that can result in thrombus or an embolism (Hankey & Warlow, 1994). SAH can occur with a sudden onset of headache or vomiting, and can also present with loss of consciousness. It occurs as result of a hemorrhage from a cerebral blood vessel, aneurysm, or vascular malformation.

Causes of stroke include cardioembolic, atherosclerotic, dissections, vasculitis, hypertension, and atrial fibrillation. Some of the nonmodifiable risk factors include age, gender, race, ethnicity, and genetics. Some of the modifiable risk factors include hypertension, diabetes mellitus, atrial fibrillation, and dyslipid-emia, and individuals afflicted with these risk factors. Stroke is a leading cause of morbidity and results in significant financial burdens, which have been estimated at $34 billion per year for health care services, medications, and decreased days of work (Boehme, Esenwa, & Elkind, 2017).

Clinical Aspects

ASSESSMENT

The most common symptom that patients experience with a migraine is a headache. "It results from activation of meningeal and blood vessel nocicep-tors combines with a change in central pain modulation" (Silberstein, 2004, p. 382). Nurses need to be aware of the clinical features associated with migraines, such as the positive phenomena of migraines, which are seeing stars, spark photopsia, and complex geometric patterns (Diener & Kurth, 2012). Some of the symptoms associated with migraine headache include nausea, vomiting, photophobia, and phonophobia. Migraine stroke is suspected when aura symptoms of migraine attacks last for more than 24 hours (Diener & Kurth, 2012).

The diagnostic criteria for migraine without aura include at least five attacks, a headache that lasts for 4 to 72 hours, and a headache that results in at least two of the following characteristics: unilateral location, pulsating quality, mod-erate or severe intensity, and aggravation by or avoidance of routine physical activity. The following can also occur: nausea/vomiting or photophobia and phenophobia. The diagnostic criteria with aura, known as the *classic migraine*, include at least two attacks and a typical aura, hemoplegic aura, and basilar type aura. Some of the symptoms of atypical aura include visual, sensory, or speech symptoms, homogeneous or bilateral visual symptoms. "Visual phenom-ena, which are usually benign, occurred in 1.22% of women and in 1.08% of men in a general population sample" (Silberstein, 2004, p. 384).

A nursing-related problem that can occur is when nurses are not able to iden-tify aura that trigger migraines. Therefore, nurses should encourage patients to keep a headache diary to identify triggers that the patient experiences. The nurse should also provide patients with dietary and lifestyle approaches that can pre-vent headaches. Lifestyle approaches can include limiting caffeine intake, daily exercise, stress management, a low-tyramine diet, and regular sleep patterns. The diary must include time and date of all headaches and activities that lead to migraine headaches. Nurses should anticipate medications that are used to pro-vide relief of migraines, such as the triptans that include sumatriptan, rizatriptan, and eletriptan. Sumatriptan can provide short-acting relief, and naratriptan can be used to provide long-lasting relief. Nurses should also encourage follow-up appointments with a neurologist to discuss symptom relief, treatment, and management of migraines. Cognitive behavioral therapy and biofeedback help patients to develop management skills and ways to prevent headaches (Parker & Waltman, 2012).

Nurses should facilitate rapid diagnosis and initiation of treatment as they work together with physicians and nurse practitioners. A thorough history and neurological examination are key to identifying patients who may have suffered a stroke. Sudden numbness or weakness of face, arm, or leg, especially on one side of the body, sudden confusion, trouble speaking, severe headache, difficulty seeing, and dizziness are signs and symptoms that should warn nurses that the patient is having a stroke (Goldstein & Simel, 2005). Nurses should address the need to prevent hypertension as treating the disease reduces the risk of stroke. "The Systolic Hypertension in the Elderly Program (SHEP) study shows that treatment of isolated systolic hypertension in the elderly decreases the risk of stroke by 36%" (Gorelick et al., 1999, p.1113). Nurses must also educate stroke patients that stroke can lead to myocardial infarction (MI). The importance of adhering to oral anticoagulant agents can reduce the possibility of stroke in patients with MI. The use of anticoagulants, antiplatelet agents, and lipid-lowering agents can prevent stroke after a patient has suffered an MI. "The incidence of ischemic stroke is approximately one to two percent per year after MI. This risk is greatest in the first month after MI (31%)" (Gorelick et al., 1999, p. 1114).

Another risk factor for stroke is atrial fibrillation, which increases the risk of stroke approximately six times. It is important for health care professionals to consider the risk of stroke against the risk of hemorrhage in patients with stroke. Diabetes mellitus is another risk factor for stroke. Nurses can help patients understand the importance of taking diabetes medication or insulin therapy to control blood sugar levels. "The likelihood of stroke increased with the following acute neurological deficits: facial droop, arm drift, or a speech disturbance" (Goldstein & Simel, 2005, p. 2401) It is important for nurses to anticipate the need for neuroimaging studies to examine the extent of an injury for a patient with neurological deficits. A change is mental status needs to be reported by nurses for early intervention and treatment of care (Goldstein & Simel, 2005).

NURSING INTERVENTIONS, MANAGEMENT, AND IMPLICATIONS

It is important for nurses to be aware of effective strategies that are needed to prevent migraine and stroke in patients. Some of the risk factors for stroke include hypertension, atrial fibrillation, arterial obstruction, and hyperlipidemia. Nurses must clarify with health care professionals the parameters needed to initiate blood pressure therapy for patients with hypertension, as well as parameters to resume blood pressure therapy. "Goals for target BP level or reduction from pretreatment baseline are uncertain and should be individualized, but it is reasonable to achieve a systolic pressure <140 mmHg and a diastolic pressure <90 mmHg" (Kernan et al., 2014, p. 2170). It is also important for nurses to know the risk factors for recurrent stroke, including sleep apnea and aortic arch atherosclerosis. Therefore, it is necessary to rely on updated guidelines to manage stroke. Nurses should also be aware of patients who are diabetic as well as prediabetic to enhance the role of lifestyle modification in patient's daily lives.

This will help reduce vascular problems among patients. Nurses should also help patients understand the benefit of weight loss in preventing cardiovascular risk factors that can lead to stroke. Evidence-based guidelines must be incorporated into practice to prevent stroke among patients (Kernan et al., 2014).

OUTCOMES

Nurses should facilitate rapid assessment and initiation of treatment as they work together with physicians and nurse practitioners to provide positive outcomes for patients. Education on identification of signs and symptoms of neurotrauma events is foundational in preventing initial and/or recurring events. It is also important for the nurse to provide counseling and education to the patient and family regarding medications, medication interactions, consequences of noncompliance with medications, and therapy to prevent complications and negative outcomes of the event.

Summary

Nurses must also be educated on many aspects of migraines. Migraines are worsened by physical activity and associated with cooccurring symptoms such as nausea, vomiting, and photophobia. Preventative therapy can help patients and reduce the severity of their migraine attacks (Marmura, Silberstein, & Schwedt, 2015). There is consistent evidence that individuals with migraine are approximately two times more likely to develop an ischemic stroke and vigilant nursing care should include stroke-prevention strategies to mitigate cardiovascular morbidity (Kurth & Diener, 2012, p. 3421).

Boehme, A. K., Esenwa, C., & Elkind, S. V. (2017). Stroke risk factors, genetics, and prevention. *Circulation, 120*, 472–495.

Goldstein, L. B., & Simel, D. L. (2005). Is this patient having a stroke? *Journal of the American Medical Association, 293*(19), 2391–2402. doi:10.1001/jama.293.19.2391

Gorelick, P. B., Sacco, R. L., Smith, D. B., Alberts M., Mustone-Alexander, L., Rader, D., . . . Rhew, D. C. (1999). Prevention of a first stroke: A review of guidelines and a multidisciplinary consensus statement from the National Stroke Association. *Journal of the American Medical Association, 281*(12), 1112–1120. doi:10.1001/jama.281.12.1112

Hankey, G. J., & Warlow, C. P. (1994). Transient ischemic attacks of the brain and eye. In R. J. Davenport (Ed.), *Major problems in neurology*. Philadelphia, PA: Saunders.

Intercollegiate Stroke Working Party. (2012). *National clinical guideline for stroke* (4th ed.). London, UK: Royal College of Physicians.

Kernan, W. N., Ovbiagele, B., Black, H. R., Bravata, D. M., Chimowitz, M. I., Ezekowitz, M. D., & Johnston, S. C. C. (2014). Guidelines for the prevention of stroke in patients with stroke and transient ischemic attack. *Stroke, 45*(7), 2160–2236.

Kurth, T., & Diener, H. (2006). Current views of the risk of stroke for migraine with and migraine without aura. *Current Pain and Headache Reports, 10*(3), 214–220. doi:1007/S11916-006-0048-5

Kurth, T., & Diener, H. C. (2012). Migraine and stroke. *Stroke, 43*(12), 3421–3426.

Marmura, M. J., Silberstein, S. D., & Schwedt, T. J. (2015). The acute treatment of migraine in adults: The American Headache Society Evidence Assessment of Migraine Pharmacotherapies. *Headache: The Journal of Head and Face Pain, 55*(1), 3–20.

Parker, C., & Waltman, N. (2012). Reducing the frequency and severity of migraine headaches in the workplace: Implementing evidence-based interventions. *Workplace Health & Safety, 60*(1), 12–18. doi:10.3928/21650799-20111227-02

Silberstein, S. D. (2004). Migraine pathophysiology and its clinical implications. *Cephalgia: An International Journal of Headache, 24*(Suppl. 2), 2–7.

■ OBSTETRICAL AND GYNECOLOGICAL EMERGENCY CARE

Vicki Bacidore

Overview

Patients with OB/GYN problems are frequently seen and receive treatment in emergency departments (EDs). Obstetrical emergencies not only affect the health and well-being of the mother, but also the unborn child. Gynecological emergencies affect the female reproductive system, can be life-threatening, and may have an effect on sexual function and fertility. The role of the emergency nurse is to rule out life-threatening complications associated with abnormal uterine bleeding and to obtain emergent, urgent, or routine gynecologic consultation as needed. The management of OB/GYN emergencies requires excellent assessment skills and rapid interventions.

Background

An increasing number of women, despite having a primary care provider, utilize the ED for OB/GYN-related complaints for a variety of different reasons such as access barriers, physician referrals, convenience, tradition, and the feeling that their condition warrants emergency care (Burns & Sacchetti, 2016). The most frequent OB/GYN emergencies are abnormal vaginal bleeding, miscarriage, ectopic pregnancy, acute or chronic pelvic pain, and previously undiagnosed cancer of the female genital tract and trauma (ENA, 2013).

Abnormal uterine bleeding, formerly referred to as *dysfunctional uterine bleeding*, reflects a disruption in the normal cyclic pattern of ovulatory hormonal stimulation to the endometrial lining. The most common cause of abnormal uterine bleeding during the reproductive years is abnormal pregnancy and threatened abortion, incomplete abortion, and ectopic pregnancy (Behera, 2016).

Pelvic pain is a common chief complaint and can be due to a variety of etiologies. The uterus, cervix, and adnexa all share the same visceral innervation as the lower ileum, sigmoid colon and rectum, making it difficult to distinguish pain originating from reproductive or gastrointestinal organs. Pelvic pain can be classified as acute, chronic, or cyclical (ENA, 2010) and can be of sufficient severity to cause functional disability or lead to medical care. Nearly 4% of women are thought to have ongoing chronic pelvic pain (Davila, 2016).

Pelvic inflammatory disease (PID) is an infectious and inflammatory disorder of the upper female genital tract, including the uterus, fallopian tubes, and adjacent pelvic structures. Infection and inflammation may spread to the abdomen and surrounding hepatic structures. Typically affected is a menstruating woman aged younger than 25 years with multiple sex partners, who does not use contraception, and lives in an area with a high prevalence of sexually transmitted infections (STIs). The two most common organisms causing PID are *Neisseria gonorrheoeae* and *Chlamydia trachomatis* (Moore, 2017). A diagnosis of PID is typically based on the history and physical exam and, if untreated, can have significant long-term complications such as infertility, chronic pelvic pain, and ectopic pregnancy (ENA, 2010).

Spontaneous miscarriage is the death or expulsion of the fetus or products of conception before the age of viability and accounts for approximately 5% to 15% of all pregnancies (Gaufberg, 2017). Early pregnancy loss is primarily due to embryonic chromosomal defects and should be considered a possibility in any woman presenting to the ED with vaginal bleeding. Miscarriage after the first trimester is more likely due to advanced age, prior miscarriage, severe hypertension, endocrine dysfunction, abnormal embryologic development, or trauma (ENA, 2013).

Approximately 2% of all pregnancies in the United States are ectopic, meaning the embryo implants at a site other than the endometrium of the uterus, typically in the fallopian tube. This usually appears in the sixth week of gestation and, unless recognized, the fallopian tube will rupture, causing death of the fetus and threatening the life of the mother. The classic clinical presentation triad of ectopic pregnancy is abdominal pain, amenorrhea, and vaginal bleeding. Other signs include sudden onset of severe, unilateral pelvic pain, nausea, vomiting, dizziness, or weakness. Abdominal rigidity, involuntary guarding, evidence of shock all suggest a surgical emergency (Sepilian, 2016).

Pregnancy-induced hypertension (PIH) is described as hypertension related to pregnancy and is synonymous with preeclampsia–eclampsia, which typically occurs after the 20th week of pregnancy. Preeclampsia is the second leading cause of maternal mortality and is a multisystem condition characterized by hypertension, proteinuria, and edema. Eclampsia is a worsening of preeclampsia, is characterized by seizure activity, and has a high risk of cerebral hemorrhage, morbidity, and mortality (ENA, 2013).

Placenta previa occurs when the placenta implants in the lower uterine segment or over the cervical os, rather than its normal implantation in the upper uterine wall. As the fetus grows within the uterus, implantation may be disrupted as this area gradually thins in preparation for labor, causing painless bleeding through the cervix. *Placental abruption* is defined as the premature separation of the placenta from the uterus after the 20th week of gestation. Patients typically present with hemorrhage, uterine contractions, and fetal distress. Placental abruption is associated with high fetal and maternal morbidity and mortality and is the most common cause of fetal demise following maternal trauma (ENA, 2013).

Births in the ED are rare, but are considered high-risk deliveries. When a pregnant patient presents to the ED in labor, imminent delivery is primarily determined by crowning of the fetus and the mother's urge to push (ENA, 2013). A rapid decision is made whether or not to deliver in the ED, or, if time permits, transfer to a sterile, more desirable environment such as the labor and delivery unit. Emergency nurses must be prepared for potential delivery complications and to manage neonatal resuscitation as necessary. In the United States, there are approximately 4 million births annually, with a birth rate of 12.5 per 1,000 population (Centers for Disease Control and Prevention [CDC], 2014). The majority of these pregnancies and births are considered low risk and occur without complications. However, an increasing number of obstetrical patients do present to the ED with complications.

The Emergency Nurses Association's (ENA) position statement on obstetrical patients in the ED outlines safe care in this practice setting (ENA, 2011).

Clinical Aspects

ASSESSMENT

Obtaining a thorough history is crucial to the assessment process and to all patients. Vital components of the history include chief complaint; symptom onset; pain assessment (onset, provocation, palliation, quality, radiation, severity, and timing); history of trauma; presence of vaginal discharge or bleeding; obstetrical and sexual history, including last normal menstrual period; medical/surgical history; family and social history; medications; and allergies. All females of childbearing age should be evaluated for possible pregnancy. Patients with obstetrical or gynecological emergencies can experience significant blood loss and hypovolemia. Assessment priorities should always be airway, breathing, and circulation. Focused assessment must include the patient's general appearance and vital signs, assessment of the skin, respiratory, cardiovascular, abdominal, and genitourinary systems. A complete pelvic examination should be performed. For pregnant patients, gestational age and fetal viability are determined, including the possibility of impending delivery (ENA, 2007).

Diagnostics may include laboratory studies such as a complete blood count with differential, coagulation profile, serum chemistries, urinalysis, pregnancy test, type and crossmatch with Rh factor, the Kleihauer–Betke test to assess and measure the presence of fetomaternal hemorrhage, and screening for sexually transmitted infections (STIs). Imaging studies may include pelvic or transvaginal sonography with Doppler and CT. Electronic fetal monitoring for uterine contractions and fetal heart rate may also be required (ENA, 2007).

NURSING INTERVENTIONS, MANAGEMENT, AND IMPLICATIONS

Differential diagnoses and collaborative nursing-related problems include acute pain, fluid volume deficit, ineffective tissue perfusion, fear and anxiety, risk for infection, knowledge deficit, and anticipatory grieving. Emergency nurses need to continuously assess patients for pain, bleeding amount, and mental status. Patients have the potential to decompensate quickly due to blood loss.

Nursing interventions include (a) maintaining airway, breathing, and circulation; (b) providing supplemental oxygen as indicated; (c) establishing intravenous access for the administration of fluids and medications as needed; (d) preparing for and assisting with medical procedures; (e) administering pharmacological therapy as ordered; (f) assisting with admission and/or transfer if necessary; (g) providing patient and family education, and (h) ensuring follow-up care.

OUTCOMES

The OB/GYN patient in the ED must have continuous evaluation and ongoing monitoring of pain relief, normalization of maternal and/or fetal respiratory, circulation and perfusion status, a demonstrated increase in psychological functioning, and adequate knowledge of health status. Preservation of maternal and fetal life are the primary concerns for positive outcomes.

Summary

The patient with OB/GYN problems can offer challenging opportunities for the ED nurse. Utilizing the nursing process in order to assess and prioritize care for these women is essential to assess and manage potential threats to life. Emergency nursing knowledge of how to care for common OB/GYN emergencies promotes optimal outcomes for these women and their children.

Behera, M. A. (2016). Abnormal (dysfunctional) uterine bleeding. *Medscape*. Retrieved from http://emedicine.medscape.com/article/257007-overview

Burns, J. & Sacchetti, A. (2016). Enrollment with a primary care provider does not preclude ED visits for patients with woman's health related problems. *American Journal of Emergency Medicine, 34*(2) 266–268.

Centers for Disease Control and Prevention. (2014). Births and natality. Retrieved from https://www.cdc.gov/nchs/fastats/births.htm

Davila, G. W. (2016). Gynecologic pain. *Medscape*. Retrieved from http://emedicine.medscape.com/article/270450-overview

Emergency Nurses Association. (2007). *Emergency nursing core curriculum* (6th ed.). Philadelphia, PA: Elsevier Saunders.

Emergency Nurses Association. (2010). *Sheehy's emergency nursing: Principles and practice* (6th ed.). St. Louis, MO: Elsevier Mosby.

Emergency Nurses Association. (2011). Position statement: The obstetrical patient in the emergency department. Retrieved from https://www.ena.org/SiteCollectionDocuments/Position%20Statements/OBPatientED.pdf

Emergency Nurses Association. (2013). *Sheehy's manual of emergency care* (7th ed.). St. Louis, MO: Elsevier Mosby.

Gaufberg, S. V. (2017). Early pregnancy loss in emergency medicine. Medscape. Retrieved from http://emedicine.medscape.com/article/795085-overview

Moore Shepherd, S. (2017). Pelvic inflammatory disease. *Medscape*. Retrieved from http://emedicine.medscape.com/article/256448-overview

Sepilian, V. P. (2016). Ectopic pregnancy. *Medscape*. Retrieved from http://emedicine.medscape.com/article/2041923-overview

■ OPHTHALMIC EMERGENCIES

Shannon M. Litten

Overview

Ophthalmic emergencies in the general population account for 2% of emergency department (ED) visits in the United States annually (Cheung et al., 2014; Sharma & Brunette, 2014). Worldwide, this number reaches 55 million and results in poor unilateral vision in 23 million people (Gardiner, 2016a). A recent review of 1,400 EDs found the vast majority of ED visits (27%) result from ocular trauma, including 73% corneal abrasions, 6% blunt eye trauma, and 5% corneal foreign body (Walker & Adhikari, 2016). In the United States, eye injuries account for 3% to 5% of all occupational injuries (Sharma & Brunette, 2014). The second most common ocular condition seen in the ED is conjunctivitis (15%), followed by glaucoma or retinal problems (6%) (Walker & Adhikari, 2016). Nurses are frequently the first health caregiver to encounter these presentations and must be prepared to obtain correct information for prompt evaluation, treatment, and consult (Sharma & Brunette, 2014).

Background

An ophthalmic emergency consists of any eye condition that requires immediate medical attention to avert vision loss or impairment (Parekh, 2016). The most common eye emergencies can be categorized into trauma, infection, and neurovascular conditions (Parekh, 2016). Top diagnoses requiring an emergent ophthalmology consult include penetrating injury, chemical injury, acute glaucoma, sudden vision loss, and orbital cellulitis (Field, Tillotson, & Whittingham, 2015).

An estimated 2.5 million traumatic eye emergencies are seen annually, including blunt or penetrating trauma and chemical burns, which threaten visual loss in up to 60,000 cases (Gardiner, 2016a; Parekh, 2016). Ocular emergencies are more prevalent in middle-aged, White men and affect as many as 80% when the emergency results from trauma (Cheung et al., 2014; Parekh, 2016; Saccomano & Ferrara, 2014). Recent literature also identifies the elderly population at higher risk for ocular emergencies, particularly when related to falls (Cheung et al., 2014). In a study conducted by Cheung et al. (2014), the most common causes of traumatic injury occurred from motor vehicle crashes (MVC), falls, and assault (17.4%, 14.4%, and 11.1%, respectively). Blunt traumatic eye injuries include trauma to the eye (ocular trauma), the orbit (periocular trauma), or both and can lead to fractures, hemorrhage, or damage to the globe (Gardiner, 2016a; Parekh, 2016). The leading traumatic injuries from MVCs or falls are open globe and orbital fractures of which open globe carries the poorest outcomes; 66.7% lead to legal blindness (Cheung et al., 2014). However, orbital fractures are much more common than open globe injuries (45.3% vs. 6.1%) and result in 1.5% of legal blindness (Cheung et al., 2014).

Chemical injury from alkaline (lye, ammonia, fertilizers, pesticides) or acids (car batteries, bleach, and some refrigerants) can be just as detrimental to vision (Parekh, 2016; Patel, 2016; Sharma & Brunette, 2014). Alkaline destroys cell structure and leads to tissue destruction that continues until the agent is removed. Acids are less destructive due to coagulation necrosis, which precipitates tissue proteins, limiting depth of injury. Both can lead to corneal scarring (Parekh, 2016; Patel, 2016; Sharma & Brunette, 2014).

In children, corneal abrasions are the most common nonpenetrating eye injury (Saccomano & Ferrara, 2014). Although corneal abrasions affects all age groups, newborns and infants are frequently injured with an untrimmed fingernail, younger children with a toy, and adolescents during sports (Saccomano & Ferrara, 2014; Walker & Adhikari, 2016). Contact lens wearers are frequently affected from tangential impacts or foreign body debris. Other causes of corneal abrasion include dust, chemicals, sand, animal paws, and makeup brushes (Saccomano & Ferrara, 2014; Walker & Adhikari, 2016). If not treated immediately, opportunistic bacteria, virus, or fungi can infect the eye risking the development of inflammatory iritis (Walker & Adhikari, 2016).

Other causes of ocular emergency rates in Cheung et al.'s (2014) study were: infectious, 14.3%; preexisting conditions, 14%; unknown, 11.5%; and other traumatic causes, 7.5%. Ophthalmic emergencies in females were mostly a result of infectious agents or neurologic etiologies (Cheung et al., 2014). There are many causes of infectious eye conditions with varying degrees of severity. Conjunctivitis was the second most common infectious condition, affecting 15% of all eye emergencies seen in the ED and typically characterized by itchy, red eyes and discharge without visual acuity changes (Saccomano & Ferrara, 2014; Walker & Adhikari, 2016).

Although frequently viral and self-limiting, it is important to consider serious bacterial or corneal herpetic involvement that could result in vision loss without aggressive treatment (Walker & Adhikari, 2016). Common bacterial pathogens are *Staphylococcus aureus*, *Pseudomonas aeruginosa*, and *Acanthamoeba* (Parekh, 2016). Herpes zoster (HZV) and herpes simplex virus (HSV) are common viral infections. In the United States, HSV is the most common cause of corneal blindness. Fungal infections (*Fusarium* and *Candida*) are often transmitted via plants or soil and seen with agricultural workers or persons living in warm climates (Parekh, 2016). In addition to conjunctivitis, ophthalmic infections can lead to many eye conditions, such as periorbital cellulitis (infection of the eyelids), orbital cellulitis (infection of the orbital soft tissues), anterior uveitis or iritis (inflammation in anterior eye structures), keratitis (inflammation of the cornea), hordeolum (stye), endophthalmitis (inflammation in the vitreous chamber), and corneal ulcers (Parekh, 2016; Walker & Adhikari, 2016).

Neurovascular causes of ophthalmic emergencies often result from preexisting conditions such as hypertension and diabetes mellitus (Parekh, 2016). Examples include acute angle closure glaucoma, retinal detachment, and central retinal artery occlusion (CRAO) with the peak incidence between ages 50 and 70 years (Arroyo, 2016; Parekh, 2016; Sharma & Brunette, 2014; Walker & Adhikari, 2016). Acute angle closure glaucoma is precipitated by pupillary dilatation, such as from dimly lit rooms, emotional upset, or various anticholinergic or sympathomimetic medications (Sharma & Brunette, 2014). If left untreated it can lead to increased intraocular pressure, optic neuropathy, and visual loss (Walker & Adhikari, 2016). Retinal detachment can be traumatic or nontraumatic (Arroyo, 2016). Nontraumatic retinal detachment usually occurs over weeks to months with a common complaint of floaters in the visual field (Arroyo, 2016). In addition to inflammation and trauma, risk factors include myopia (nearsightedness), previous eye surgery, and family history (Arroyo, 2016; Parekh, 2016). Central retinal artery occlusion is a rare condition characterized by painless, acute visual loss that results from vascular occlusion and leads to an ischemic stroke of the retina, requiring immediate intervention (Sharma & Brunette, 2014).

Clinical Aspects

ASSESSMENT

The goal of treatment in eye emergencies is to prevent loss of function, vision, infection, and to relieve symptoms (Saccomano & Ferrara, 2014). The initial patient encounter with an ocular emergency is frequently with the nurse, who leads the triage process; the patient assessment, relevant history, and physical exam findings inform the next steps required (Field et al., 2015). Fear of blindness is terrifying to patients, therefore prompt and accurate triage is of the utmost importance (Patel, 2016). Triage includes history of the presenting complaint, past and present illnesses, current medications, allergies, previous ophthalmological history, and family history of eye problems (Field et al., 2015; Saccomano & Ferrara, 2014). Asking open-ended questions helps obtain the most accurate subjective information (Field et al., 2015). Ocular history must include vision changes; glasses or contact lens use; history of eye trauma, duration of symptoms, sudden or gradual onset; foreign body sensation; use of protective eyewear; details of any chemical injury, including immediate actions taken; excessive eye rubbing or scratching; and use of eye makeup (Saccomano & Ferrara, 2014). Visual acuity assessed by use of a Snellen chart helps inform the degree of severity as decreased visual acuity suggests severe eye emergency such as trauma, glaucoma, or iritis (Parekh, 2016; Saccomano & Ferrara, 2014). Assessing visual acuity will not be priority if the patient is seriously ill or there has been a chemical injury, in which case irrigation overrides assessment of visual acuity (Field et al., 2015; Parekh, 2016). After completing a visual acuity, the eye exam must assess for corneal transparency (smooth, clear, shiny), inflammation or redness, discharge, foreign body, rash or lesions, and extraocular movements (Parekh, 2016; Saccomano & Ferrara, 2014).

NURSING INTERVENTIONS, MANAGEMENT, AND IMPLICATIONS

At this point, the nurse will decide on the most appropriate care pathway and urgency required, such as consulting the emergency provider on duty (physician, nurse practitioner, or physician's assistant). For example, nurses can quickly and easily identify a full-thickness injury to the outer membranes of the eye, as seen in globe rupture, on visual exam alone (Patel, 2016). Another example of a complaint that is not readily obvious by traumatic etiology but can be identified by the nurse as potentially serious is acute angle closure glaucoma. These patients frequently complain of sudden-onset severe ocular pain, headache, nausea and vomiting, and vision changes such as halos or lights. Conversely, sudden painless loss of vision could indicate central retinal artery occlusion (CRAO). A painful rash around the eye that does not cross the dermatome accompanied with pain, fever, and red eye could indicate the possibility of herpes zoster ophthalmicus and the need for urgent evaluation (Patel, 2016).

Interventions that nurses can implement immediately are part of the nursing process and are directly related to positive patient outcomes. Immediate irrigation of the patient's eyes with an isotonic solution, such as normal saline or lactated Ringer's can stop the process of the chemical reaction (Field et al., 2015; Patel, 2016; Parekh, 2016). For patients with suspected globe injuries, a nursing priority is to avoid further evaluation and treatment methods that can place pressure on the globe (eyeball; Gardiner, 2016b). When indicated, pain control is essential for the well-being of the patient and should be part of nurse advocacy.

After the initial interventions have been implemented and the treatment plan determined, the nurse provides patient teaching that includes further prevention strategies, treatment plan, instructions for proper eye medication use, indications of infection, expectations, and follow-up required (Saccomano & Ferrara, 2014).

OUTCOMES

Optimal patient outcomes are best achieved with rapid recognition and early intervention (Gardiner, 2016a). One study of 11,000 eyes found 61% visual improvement when treatment was implemented early (Gardiner, 2016a). Nurses are at the forefront of early recognition for potentially vision-threatening etiologies, making their assessment skills and knowledge of eye emergencies an important part of their nursing practice.

Summary

Ophthalmic emergencies can present in many different ways, including traumatic, infectious, or neurovascular. Having a broad knowledge of these types of emergencies and their most common causes and presentations can direct care and promote positive patient outcomes (Cheung et al., 2014; Saccomano & Ferrara, 2014; Sharma & Brunette, 2014). Clinical preparation for recognition of specific signs or symptoms promotes prompt detection, triage, and treatment required, such as immediate eye irrigation for chemical injuries, pain control, or emergent ophthalmology consultation. These critical steps offer the best chance for sustaining vision and providing the best possible outcomes.

Arroyo, J. G. (2016). Retinal detachment. Retrieved from http://uptodate.com

Cheung, C. A., Rogers-Martel, M., Golas, L., Chepurny, A., Martel, J. B., Martel, J. R. (2014). Hospital-based ocular emergencies: Epidemiology, treatment, and visual outcomes. *American Journal of Emergency Medicine, 32*, 221–224.

Field, D., Tillotson, J., & Whittingham, E., (2015). *Eye emergencies: The practitioner's guide* (2nd ed.). Cumbria, UK: M&K Publishing. Retrieved from http://web.b.ebscohost.com.proxy.library.vanderbilt.edu/ehost/ebookviewer/ebook/bmxlYmtfXzk4NTkyMF9fQU41?sid=71bac6bb-ccd2-44fd-be50-3e9a0382ac04@sessionmgr101&vid=0&format=EB&rid=1

Gardiner, M. F. (2016a). Approach to eye injuries in the emergency department. Retrieved from http://uptodate.com

Gardiner, M. F. (2016b). Overview of eye injuries in the emergency department. Retrieved from http://uptodate.com

Patel, P. S. (2016). Top 10 eye emergencies. Retrieved from https://www.aao.org/young-ophthalmologists/yo-info/article/top-10-eye-emergencies

Parekh, S. J. S. (2016, May). Ophthalmic emergencies. Lecture presented at the 8th Annual Emergency Medicine Symposium, Wayne, NJ.

Saccomano, S. J., & Ferrara, L. R. (2014). Managing corneal abrasions in primary care. *Nurse Practitioner, 39*(9), 1–6. doi:10.1097/01.NPR.0000452977.99676.cf

Sharma, R., & Brunette, D. D. (2014). Ophthalmology. In R. M. Walls (Ed.), *Rosen's emergency medicine: Concepts and clinical practice* (8th ed., pp. 909–930). Philadelphia, PA: Elsevier/Saunders.

Walker, R. A., & Adhikari, S. (2016). Eye emergencies. In J. E. Tintinalli (Ed.), *Tintinalli's emergency medicine: A comprehensive study guide* (8th ed., pp. 1543–1579). Columbus, OH: McGraw-Hill.

■ ORTHOPEDIC EMERGENCIES IN ADULTS

Cindy D. Kumar

Overview

Musculoskeletal injuries with hemodynamic or neurovascular compromise require emergent intervention. Orthopedic emergencies are musculoskeletal injuries that pose an imminent threat to a person's life or limb (Azmy, 2016; Williams, 2009). In orthopedic emergencies, care by the nurse should be centered around observation and assessment for blood loss; altered tissue perfusion, motor, and sensory functions to tissue distal to injury; and prevention of systemic complications secondary to a musculoskeletal injury.

Background

In the United States, approximately 77% of injury-related health care visits are for musculoskeletal complaints (Weinstein & Yelin, 2016). The leading cause of orthopedic injuries for 18- to 44-year-olds is trauma (Weinstein & Yelin, 2016), whereas falls account for the most orthopedic injuries in adults older than 44 years (Bratcher, 2014, p. 195; Weinstein & Yelin, 2016). Falls are the number one cause of injury-related deaths in those older than 72 (Bratcher, 2014).

Once discharged from the hospital, more than 50% of those older than 65 years with musculoskeletal injuries require further medical care or treatment in rehabilitation facilities (Yelin, 2016), contributing to health care cost. Orthopedic injuries are the leading cause of lost work days in people aged 18 to 64 years, thereby creating additional health care cost burden.

Any orthopedic injury has potential for serious complications; however, there are specific injuries that necessitate prompt identification and intervention. These emergencies are open-book pelvic fractures, long-bone fractures, open fractures, compartment syndrome, and amputations. Some would argue cauda equina, joint dislocations, and septic joints also as orthopedic emergencies. There are specific reasons for the heightened concern of each injury. Open-book pelvic fractures are associated with a higher mortality rate due to their higher incidence of hemodynamic instability. Femur fractures increase the risk for fat or thromboembolism. Open fractures have an increased risk for infection and often occur in the presence of concurrent injuries. Compartment syndrome can lead to neurovascular injury and loss of tissue. Amputations are associated with blood loss. Cauda equina is concerning for possible permanent loss of sensory and/or motor function. Diagnosis of these injuries is made by radiologic imaging such as plain film radiographs or computed tomography. In some cases, magnetic resonance imaging is preferred or recommended (Azmy, 2016).

There is also lack of consensus over which injuries truly qualify as emergencies. Even the most benign complaints can have the potential to become emergent (Ewen, personal communication, January 8, 2017). What is known is that one third of patients presenting to the emergency department have orthopedic injuries (Bratcher, 2014, p. 195). The most common injuries are fractures, sprains, and strains, and the extremities are the most commonly injured part of the body. Injury may involve the bone, soft tissue structures, and joint spaces. Types of injuries include "fractures, dislocations, amputations, sprains, strains, penetrating injuries, ligament tears, tendon lacerations, and neurovascular compromise" (Bratcher, 2014, p. 195). The mechanism of injury is an important aspect in the identification and management of orthopedic injuries. Mechanisms include, but are not limited to, falls, motor vehicle collisions, assaults, sports injuries, crush injuries, or blast injuries (Bratcher, 2014). "A musculoskeletal injury that potentially will lead to complications, future impairment, or loss of life or limb if not treated with appropriate expeditious care" is an orthopedic emergency (Crum, 2016).

There are many risk factors that can either contribute to the mechanism of injury or precipitate an orthopedic emergency after the fact. Examples of risk factors include weakness from a previous injury, preexisting disabilities, concurrent acute illness (i.e., infection, arthritis flare), disruption of equilibrium from infection or intoxication, and peripheral neuropathy. Some medications can predispose a patient to increased risk for injury (i.e., diuretics, sedatives, narcotics, steroids) by affecting balance, bone density, or cognition. Bone disorders, such as osteoporosis, Paget's disease, and osteogenesis imperfecta, place a patient at greater risk before, during, and after an injury. (Cerepani & Ramponi, 2016)

In the aging population, there are additional factors that increase the risk of orthopedic emergencies (Fleischman & Ma, 2016). With age, there is a loss of bone and mass; bones become more brittle. There is also a loss of vertebral body height, and age-related muscle atrophy leads to decreased strength (Cerepani & Ramponi, 2016), all of which can affect gait and can cause fatigue more easily. Degenerative changes also decrease mobility. Due to decreased strength, an elderly person may lie injured for a long period of time before help arrives. This can increase the risk for hypo/hyperthermia, dehydration and electrolyte imbalances, and rhabdomyolysis. Special consideration must be given to the pediatric population, however, that is beyond the scope of this chapter.

Clinical Aspects

ASSESSMENT

Obtaining history of present illness and past medical history is essential to nursing care of orthopedic emergencies. Mechanism of injury, determination of fall risk, previous functional status of the individual, age, and comorbidities will affect nursing care and patient outcomes. Current medications, alcohol use, and illicit drug use must be addressed. Strong assessment skills are needed for monitoring of complications in these emergencies. Skills include but are not limited to inspection, palpation, and hemodynamic monitoring. Assessment of the six Ps: pain, pallor, pressure, pulses, paresthesia, and paralysis, must be incorporated into the nursing assessment before and after any intervention or diagnostic study.

Working knowledge of anatomy and physiology is needed to support understanding of processes involved with orthopedic emergencies (Bratcher, 2014).

Blood loss is the leading cause of preventable deaths in trauma (Bratcher, 2014, p. 196). Large volumes of blood loss can occur with pelvic or long-bone fractures, which can lead to hypotensive shock if left unmanaged. Pelvic fractures have an estimated blood loss potential of 2 L, whereas a femur fracture has a potential for blood loss of 1.5 L (Azmy, 2016). Blood loss may be obvious or internal. When arterial blood flow is compromised, tissue becomes ischemic. Ischemia leads to increased pain and decreased pulses. Assessment findings may include pallor, cool skin, cyanotic tissue, and prolonged capillary refill time. The nurse should anticipate the need for hemoglobin and hematocrit values.

The nurse needs to assess for concurrent injuries. For example, calcaneal fractures often have associated spinal injury/fracture (Dean, Hatch, & Pauly, 2016). Femur fractures may also have an associated posterior hip dislocation (Bratcher, 2014, p. 195). Clavicle fractures may have an associated pulmonary contusion, pneumothorax, or brachial plexus injury (Clugston, Hatch, & Taffe, 2016). The nurse should anticipate preparing the patient for additional studies, such as additional radiographic imaging, complete blood count, chemistry panel, and, in the presence of a crush injury or a patient who has been injured and stays down for a significant amount of time, a creatinine kinase and renal function should be evaluated for the presence of rhabdomyolysis or acute kidney injury.

NURSING INTERVENTIONS, MANAGEMENT, AND IMPLICATIONS

Priority nursing assessment should focus on hemodynamic and neurovascular status and the monitoring of related complications. In addition to assessment, nursing management needs to focus on the whole patient. Patient preparation for diagnostic studies and interventions, such as surgery or reductions, is the responsibility of the nurse. Documentation should include vital signs, neurovascular status, pain level, assessment findings, and responses to interventions. In the assessment, the nurse needs to include the patient's ability to understand teaching regarding splint/cast care, and signs and symptoms of complications such as infection or compartment syndrome.

Timely identification of the following potential systemic complications is crucial: nerve injury, hyperkalemia, rhabdomyolysis, and acute kidney injury. Hyperkalemia, in the presence of an orthopedic emergency, should be assessed for when there has been a resuscitative period, lengthy extraction, or a delay in transport (Bratcher, 2014). Potassium levels peak around the 12-hour mark and may be associated with tissue destruction (Bratcher, 2014, p. 198). Nerve injury can result from compression of bone from displacement or joint dislocation. Alterations in sensation and motor function can occur. The nurse should always check neurovascular status before and after any intervention. Concerning signs are paresthesia or numbness, cold skin, cyanosed tissue, and decreased or absent pulse. Crush injuries, in particular, raise concerns for severe muscle and tissue damage. Myoglobin is released into the bloodstream and when present in large amounts, can lead to kidney injury. Signs the nurse must assess for are increased muscle pain, change in sensation to affected limb, muscle weakness, and dark- or tea-colored urine (Bratcher, 2014).

OUTCOMES

Evidence-based nursing management of orthopedic emergencies is focused on restoring and/or preserving function. Close monitoring and keen observation for changes in physical assessment can reduce or prevent complications such as hypovolemic shock, compartment syndrome, venous thromboembolism or fat embolism, infection, and acute kidney injury. Expected outcomes of nursing care should concentrate on decreasing blood loss, increasing limb perfusion, minimizing tissue damage, and avoiding systemic effects (Williams, 2009).

Summary

The role of the nurse and evidence-based nursing care are key to management of orthopedic emergencies. Patient outcomes in the presence of orthopedic emergencies are dependent on ongoing assessment of hemodynamics, neurovascular status, and prompt identification of potential complications. Orthopedic emergencies truly are a matter of life or limb.

Azmy, D. A. (2016, December 30). Orthopedic emergencies. Retrieved from http://www .slideshare.net/AhmedAzmy/orthopaedic-emergencies?next_slideshow=1

Bratcher, C. M. (2014). Chapter 14: Musculoskeletal trauma. In B. B. Jacobs (Ed.), *Trauma nursing core course: Provider manual* (pp. 193–203). Des Plaines, IL: Emergency Nurses Association.

Cerepani, M. J., & Ramponi, D. R. (2007). Orthopedic emergencies. In K. S. Hoyt & J. Selfridge-Thomas (Eds.), *Emergency nursing core curriculum* (6th ed., pp. 585–603). Philadelphia, PA: Elsevier.

Clugston, J. R., Hatch, R. L., & Taffe, J. (2016). Clavicle fractures. *UpToDate*. Retrieved from https://www.upto date.com/contents/clavicle-fractures?source=search_result&s earch=CLAVICLE+FRACTURE&selectedTitle=1% 7E51

Crum, D. J. (2016). Orthopedic emergencies. Retrieved from http://c.ymcdn.com/sites/ www.txosteo.org/ resource/ resmgr/ imported/ Orthopedic%20Emergencies%20 -%20Joshua%20Crum.pdf

Dean, C., Hatch, R. L., & Pauly, K. R. (2016, August 9). Calcaneal fractures. *UpToDate*. Retrieved from https://www.uptodate.com/contents/calcaneus-fractures?source =search_result&search=calcaneal+fracture&selected Title=1%7E18

Fleischman, R. J., & Ma, O. (2016). Trauma in the elderly. In D. M. Cline, O. Ma, G. D. Meckler, J. Stapczynski, J. E. Tintinalli, & D. M. Yealy (Eds.), *Tintinalli's emergency medicine: A comprehensive study guide* (8th ed., pp. 1688–1691). Dallas, TX: American College of Emergency Physicians. Retrieved from http://access emergencymedicine.mhmedical.com/content.aspx?bookid=1658&Sectionid=109445304

Weinstein, S. L., & Yelin, E. H. (2016, December 15). The burden of musculoskeletal diseases in the United States. Retrieved from http://www.boneandjointburden.org

Williams, D. S. (2009). Orthopedic emergencies. Retrieved from https://fhs.mcmaster .ca/surgery/documents/OrthopaedicEmergenciesof23Sep2009byDrDaleWilliams.pdf

Yelin, E. H. (2016, December 16). The burden of musculoskeletal diseases in the United States. Retrieved from http://www.boneandjointburden.org

■ PEDIATRIC EMERGENCIES

Rachel Tkaczyk

Overview

In 2010, the Centers for Disease Control and Prevention (CDC) database reported a total of 129.8 million emergency department visits in the United States. Of those visits, 25.5 million visits consisted of patients younger than 15 years, and an additional 20.7 million visits were patients between 15 and 24 years (Centers for Disease Control and Prevention, 2012). When it comes to the emergency room setting, there is not one universal definition as to what constitutes a "pediatric emergency." Subsequently, levels of care and the associated acuity in the emergency setting often differ among various institutions. Despite varying definitions and management techniques, the approach to identifying, assessing, and treating a pediatric emergent situation must be systematic. In order to achieve successful outcomes, the medical staff must be equipped with the knowledge to appropriately recognize and treat all pediatric emergency scenarios.

Background

Pediatric patients, who accounted for 17.4% of the emergency room visits in 2010 in the United States, present unique challenges that can ultimately hinder an emergency department's ability to provide the best possible care (Macias, 2013). Obtaining a complete history and performing a thorough assessment in the pediatric population can be accompanied by many unique challenges. Particularly in the emergency setting, the time constraint alone can elicit a sense of urgency that affects the overall quality of the patient intake and triage. This section explores several challenges that may be encountered during the evaluation and treatment of pediatric emergencies.

One identified difficulty when attempting to obtain an accurate history is the lack of an established rapport with the patients and their family. This can contribute to an incomplete, and often, inadequate extraction of critical information. Oftentimes, obtaining history is not given enough time and a therapeutic relationship is not established. This is problematic as the health history typically provides 85% of the information that is needed in order for the medical team to make a diagnosis (Reuter-Rice & Bolick, 2012). As stated previously, another barrier is the element, and possibly lack thereof, of time. In the trauma scenario, resuscitation will take precedence over the acquisition of a health history. However, it is important to realize that this does not negate the significant of the health history. Rather it is necessary to recognize the limitation and employ strategies to overcome (Reuter-Rice & Bolick, 2012).

There are several key elements of the pediatric emergent intake. While obtaining a history is clearly significant, another key element is the pediatric assessment and physical examination (Halden et al., 2014). Both components are usedin order to answer the critical questions. Is there an immediate life threat? In terms of severity, where does the patient fall? Will the patient need admission? What evidence supports the providers' differential diagnoses? In summary, the goal of assessing the pediatric patient in the emergent setting is to determine the severity of the situation and whether or not treatment is indicated. Oftentimes, this requires the initial assessment but also reassessment. When it comes to the overall treatment of a seriously ill or injured child, the goal is to provide a systematic approach that is consistent across all institutions. The recommended model for all pediatric life-support courses consists of the general assessment, secondary assessment, and tertiary assessment (American Heart Association, 2015).

For example, in the case of a pediatric patient who presents with concern for sepsis, there are four physical exam signs that are recommended for early detection of pediatric septic shock, before hypotension occurs. They include alteration in mental status, decreased capillary refill, cold extremities, and peripheral pulse quality (Halden et al., 2014). These changes can be subtle, particularly to the provider who does not have an established baseline for a patient as a primary care provider may have had (Reuter-Rice & Bolick, 2012). Research has shown that several barriers to this practice of frequent reassessment exist and include a lack of time, increased workload, and at times a lack of nursing knowledge specific to the situation (Pretorius, Searle, & Marshall, 2014). This again reinforces the need to provide a systematic and standardized approach to assessment of the pediatric patient. With those skills, the medical team will be equipped with the tools to recognize signs of impending respiratory distress, failure, and shock. Without the ability to assess and intervene quickly, pediatric patients are at greater risk and can progress to cardiopulmonary failure that can lead to arrest (AHA, 2015).

Clinical Aspects

ASSESSMENT

In order to the meet the need for high-quality care in this population, several health care systems have integrated quality improvement methods to improve access, safety, and ultimately better the care delivered to this patient population (Macias, 2013). As discussed, one of the barriers to obtaining a thorough history from the beginning of the medical course is the lack of a developed therapeutic relationship with the patient and family. The American Academy of Pediatrics and the American College of Emergency Physicians continually recognizes the patient and family as significant decision-makers in the patient's overall care. Patient- and family-centered care is a method in health care that recognizes the essential role of the patient and family. The goal is to focus on and implement collaboration among the patient, family, and medical professionals (American Academy of Pediatrics, 2006).

NURSING INTERVENTIONS, MANAGEMENT, AND IMPLICATIONS

The American Academy of Pediatrics (AAP) and American College of Emergency Physicians have issued several recommendations to better improve the patient and medical team therapeutic relationship, which comes with its own emergency room-specific challenges. They continue to reinforce the necessity to validate a family and patient's concerns. The family member should be given the option to be present for all aspects of their child's care while in the emergency room. It is also essential that information be provided to the family during all interventions, despite their decision to be present or not (AAP, 2006).

OUTCOMES

In addition to information gathering, one of the key elements to improved outcomes in the pediatric emergency setting is early recognition and intervention. As stated previously, the sense of urgency and time constraint, increased work load, and inadequate knowledge can contribute to poor outcomes. Objective observation was recently studied in order to assess strengths and weaknesses during a pediatric resuscitation. The overall goal was to assess how well the medical providers in a pediatric emergency room adhered to cardiopulmonary resuscitation (CPR) guidelines during a resuscitation. During this study, 33 children received CPR under video recording. The results demonstrated appropriate compression rate, duration of pauses, and compression depth. It did show that there tended to be hyperventilation as well as the inability to coordinate the compression–ventilation ratio during the resuscitation. The overall recommendations included various training modalities for CPR among staff and evaluation of its effectiveness (Donoghue, 2015). This particular study is only one example of how a pediatric institution implemented a quality initiative to assess potential limitations and areas that required additional education. It demonstrates an overall approach to identify barriers to care, assess any shortcomings, and ultimately provide education to correct and improve certain practices.

Summary

The pediatric population is unique in many aspects when compared to the adult population, particularly in the emergency care setting. There are several challenges that the medical team faces, beginning from the moment the patient enters into their care and extends throughout treatment. Several strategies can be utilized in order to overcome those challenges and provide optimal care. It is of paramount importance that the medical team identifies any barriers to obtaining a thorough history and performing an in-depth assessment. Continued focus on ever-evolving education is also essential. With a consistent and systematic approach to pediatric emergency care, outcomes continue to improve.

American Academy of Pediatrics. (2006). Patient and family centered care and the role of the emergency physician providing care to a child in the emergency department. *Pediatrics, 118*(5), 2242–2244.

American Heart Association. (2015). *Pediatric advanced life support.* Elk Grove, IL: American Academy of Pediatrics.

Centers for Disease Control and Prevention. (2012). Reasons for emergency room use among U.S. children: National Health Interview Survey. Retrieved from https://www .cdc.gov/nchs/products/databriefs/db160.htm

Donoghue, A., Hsieh, T. C., Myers, S., Mak, A., Sutton, R., & Nadkarmi, V. (2015). Videographic assessment of cardiopulmonary resuscitation quality in the pediatric emergency department. *Resuscitation, 91,* 19–25. doi.10.1016/ j.resuscitation.2015.03.007

Halden, F.., Scoot, H. F., Donoghue, A. J., Gaieski, D. F., Marchese, R. F., & Mistry, R. D. (2014). Effectiveness of physical exam signs for early detection of critical illness in pediatric systemic inflammatory response syndrome. *BMC Emergency Medicine, 14*(24). doi:10.1186/1471-227X-14-24

Macias, C. (2013). Quality improvement in pediatric emergency medicine. *Academic Pediatrics, 13*(6), S61–S68.

Pretorius, A., Searle, J., & Marshall, B. (2014). Barriers and enablers to emergency department nurses' management of patients' pain. *Pain Management Nursing, 16*(3), 372–379. doi:10.1016/j.pmn.2014.08.015

Reuter-Rice, K. & Bolick, B. (2012). *Pediatric acute care: A guide for interprofessional practice* (1st ed.). Burlington, Ontario, Canada: Jones & Bartlett.

■ PSYCHIATRIC DISORDERS: SUICIDE, HOMICIDE, PSYCHOSIS

George Byron Peraza-Smith
Yolanda Bone

Overview

A psychiatric disorder is a syndrome characterized by a clinically significant disturbance in a person's cognition, emotional regulation, and/or behavior that reflects a dysfunction in the psychological, biological, or developmental processes underlying mental functioning (American Psychiatric Association (APA), 2009). Psychiatric disorders are accompanied with significant distress in social, occupational, or other important life activities. Suicide, homicide, and psychosis are common psychiatric disorders requiring emergency services. The Centers for Disease Control and Prevention (CDC, 2011) reported that there were an estimated 4.5 million emergency department visits nationwide with patients having a primary psychiatric disorder, accounting for 3.5% of all emergency department visits. Nursing care for psychiatric disorder emergencies is focused primarily on conducting a risk assessment, stabilizing clinical significant disturbances, and maintaining patient/staff safety.

Background

Over the past 40 years, psychiatric services for patients with psychiatric disorders have become increasingly deinstitutionalized (American College of Emergency Physicians, 2014). Services have shifted away from inpatient facilities to community-based care. Today, there are approximately 28 adult psychiatric beds per 100,000 populations with a projected need of 39 adult psychiatric beds per 100,000 populations to provide adequate services (Fuller Torrey, 2016). The resources to adequately treat psychiatric disorders in the patient with psychiatric disorders have not kept pace with the growing demand for services. This has forced patients to seek other avenues for treatment, including outpatient facilities, outpatient medical management groups, and community resources. Incarceration has become a default placement for the treatment and housing for persons with psychiatric disorders.

The insufficient numbers of psychiatric beds, inadequate funding for community-based programs, and insufficient access to treatment has caused many individuals with psychiatric disorders to utilize the emergency department for crisis management. Estimates are that the U.S. emergency departments collectively experience over 136 million patients annually (CDC, 2016) with an estimated 3% to 5% of those encounters being primarily for a psychiatric disorder (CDC, 2013, 2011). Psychiatric emergencies for suicide, homicide, and psychosis that could have been better managed and treated in the community are now overburdening emergency departments.

Suicide is the tenth leading cause of death in the United States with nearly 42,000 deaths by suicide in 2014 (CDC, 2015b). The American Foundation for

Suicide Prevention (2017) categorizes suicide risk in three factors: (a) health factors (mental health condition, substance abuse disorder, chronic medical condition or pain); (b) environmental factors (overwhelming stressful life event, prolonged stressful situation, access to lethal means, exposure to another person's suicide or violence); and (c) historical factors (previous suicide attempt, family history of suicide). A visit to an emergency department may be the suicidal patient's last effort or hope for intervention. Emergency department nurses should use a comprehensive approach to suicide prevention. The nurse should ensure the patients safety, reinforce coping skills and provide the family/significant others emotional support.

Homicides by persons with mental health conditions have entered our national consciousness due to several highly publicized public shootings and murders covered in the media. Homicides in the United States accounted for 15,809 deaths in 2014 with five deaths per 100,000 populations (CDC, 2015a). Youth homicide in the United States is even more grave as the second leading cause of death among those aged 15 to 24 years and accounts for more deaths in this age group than cancer, heart disease, birth defects, influenza, diabetes and HIV combined (CDC, 2014). The emergency department nurse may be both the target of violence, as well as responsible for assessing the homicidal risk by an individual and implementing safety protocols to prevent homicides.

In a survey of more than 1,700 emergency physicians, three quarters reported seeing a patient at least once a shift requiring hospitalization for psychiatric treatment (American College of Emergency Physicians, 2016). Patients with psychosis who present to the emergency department exhibit varying clinical presentations including functional or toxic/metabolic psychosis, the behavioral side effects of medications, complications of substance abuse, and coexisting medical and psychiatric illnesses. Delirium and dementia are the most frequent nonmedication-related causes of psychosis seen in the emergency department. Caring for patients with psychosis confers special challenges because the history of these patients is often poor or unobtainable. In addition, patients with psychosis lack insight into their illness and may present with bizarre affect, agitation, and violent behavior. The emergency department nurse should ensure the safety of the patient with psychosis, manage the anxiety, identify potential causes for the psychosis, and provide the family/significant others with emotional support.

Clinical Aspects

Although it is the goal of all members of the health care team to provide improved outcome-oriented care to persons, nursing is unique in its holistic approach. Nursing views individuals, especially during crises, as a person with multiple variables influencing and driving the crisis. It is the goal of nursing to care for the patient while implementing safety measures for all involved.

ASSESSMENT

During psychiatric emergencies, such as risk of suicide and homicide and/or the psychotic patient, the person affected, family members, and care team members are at risk for injury. Assessments to evaluate risk are essential to identify problems and minimize risk to all. Nursing should use tools that assess at-risk individuals for appearance and atmosphere, behavior, communication, potential for danger, and environment (Wright & McGlen, 2012).

When assessing for appearance and atmosphere, the nurse should be observing the patient and ask himself or herself:

■ How does the patient look?
■ Are there signs of injury?
■ Are there signs of alcohol or drugs?
■ Is the patient making or averting eye contact?

With respect to behavior, how is the patient behaving? For example, is the patient guarded, engaging, fearful, angry, sad or exhibiting bizarre behavior? In addition, how does the patient communicate? Is the at-risk individual communicating at all? Does the person speaking coherently or are thoughts disorganized? Is the person responding to "voices"? Other observatory/mental questions nursing should consider are potential physical barriers such as equipment, furniture, doorways, and so on. These "barriers" have the potential to cause a dangerous environment for the at-risk individual leading to harm to self and/or others. Finally, nurses should assess the patient's environment. Where does the patient think he or she is? Does the emergency room/critical care environment affect the communication/response of the at-risk person? For the suicidal, homicidal, and/or psychotic patient, nurses need to be conscious of the patient and staff; consequently, assessment measures do not end at the initial encounter. Rather, the assessment of the patient continues until the safety and stability of the patient are ensured.

NURSING INTERVENTIONS, MANAGEMENT, AND IMPLICATIONS

Psychiatric emergencies can cause anxiety for patients and staff alike. It is essential that emergency department nurses be aware of his or her own biases, concerns, and areas of weakness, to provide care that will ensure best outcomes. Complexities associated with at-risk patients present additional challenges to the nursing staff; consequently, causing potential delays in treatment or mismanagement of the patient experiencing a psychiatric emergency (Brosinksi & Riddle, 2015). Methods to improve upon potential anxiety measures for staff include providing education to lessen bias and improving outcomes.

OUTCOMES

Nursing interventions related to the at-risk individual involve care of the patient's physical needs, but also emotional needs. The prompt and accurate assessment skills of nursing are the most important intervention with respect to psychiatric emergencies. In addition, communication between nurse and patient is essential for patient–caregiver trust. In other words, the at-risk patient needs to feel safe, and trust within the health care relationship is necessary for the best outcome. Across health care settings, the goal of care is to improve the patient's health situation. This is challenging for the patient exercising a psychiatric emergency; however, usage of assessment tools, providing a safe environment for patient and staff, and nonthreatening communication can provide an atmosphere for which the patient's outcome will be improved and successful.

Summary

Emergency care settings are often used for nonemergent settings. However, due to many variables affecting the health care environment, such as lack of access to adequate care, patients seek care especially in emergent situations. Psychiatric emergencies, such as the suicidal, homicidal, and/or psychotic patient, seek or be brought for evaluation in an emergency department setting. Nursing staff should be attentive to assessment skills evaluating holistically the needs of the patient in crisis. Assessment should involve evaluating the safety of the at-risk patient, as well as the safety of team members. At the core of assessment is the need for nursing to engage in nonthreatening forms of communication to prevent escalation of crisis in order to assure improved outcomes.

American College of Emergency Physicians (2016). Wait times for care and hospital beds growing drastically for psychiatric emergency patients. Retrieved from http://newsroom .acep.org/2016-10-17-Waits-for-Care-and-Hospital-Beds-Growing-Dramatically-for -Psychiatric-Emergency-Patients

ACEP Emergency Medicine Practice Committee. (2014). Care of the psychiatric patient in the emergency department—A review of the literature. Retrieved from https:// www.acep.org

American Foundation for Suicide Prevention. (2017). Risk factors and warning signs. Retrieved from https://afsp.org/about-suicide/risk-factors-and-warning-signs

American Psychiatric Association. (2013). *Diagnostic and statistical manual of mental disorders: DSM-5*. Arlington, VA: American Psychiatric Publishing.

Brosinski, C., & Riddell, A. (2015). Mitigating nursing biases in management of intoxicated and suicidal patients. *Journal of Emergency Nursing, 41*(4), 296–299.

Centers for Disease Control and Prevention. (2011). National hospital ambulatory medical care survey: 2010 emergency department summary tables. Retrieved from http:// www.cdc.gov/nchs/data/ahcd/nhamcs_emergency/2010_ed_web_tables.pdf

Centers for Disease Control and Prevention. (2013, June). Emergency department visits by patients with mental health disorders—North Carolina, 2008–2010. *Morbidity and Mortality Weekly Report, 62*(23), 469–472.

Centers for Disease Control and Prevention. (2014). Deaths, percent of total deaths, and death rates for the 15 leading causes of death in 5-year age groups, by race and sex: United States, 2014. Retrieved from https://www.cdc.gov/nchs/data/dvs/lcwk1_2014.pdf?ncid=txtlnkusaolp00000618

Centers for Disease Control and Prevention. (2015a). Assaults or homicides. Retrieved from http://www.cdc.gov/nchs/fastats/homicide.htm

Centers for Disease Control and Prevention. (2015b). Leading causes of death. Retrieved from http://www.cdc.gov/nchs/fastats/leading-causes-of-death.htm

Centers for Disease Control and Prevention. (2016). Emergency department visits. Retrieved from http://www.cdc.gov/nchs/fastats/emergency-department.htm

Fuller Torrey, E. (2016). A dearth of psychiatric beds. Psychiatric Times. Retrieved from http://www.psychiatrictimes.com/psychiatric-emergencies/dearth-psychiatric-beds

Wright, K., & McGlen, I. (2012). Mental health emergencies: Using a structured assessment framework. *Nursing Standard, 27*(7), 48–56.

■ RESPIRATORY EMERGENCIES

Dustin Spencer

Overview

As a result of pulmonary insult or other systemic disorders, acute respiratory failure is a leading cause of emergent evaluation and treatment in the emergency department and results in a significant percentage of intensive care unit admissions (Dries, 2013). Any injury or illness that results in the inability of the respiratory system to meet the oxygenation, ventilation, or metabolic demands of the body can lead to acute respiratory failure. Acute respiratory failure from pneumonia was responsible for more than 920,000 deaths of children younger than 5 years old worldwide in 2015 (World Health Organization [WHO], 2016). Estimates of the mortality associated with acute respiratory failure approaches nearly 50% in the United States (Villar et al., 2011). Therefore, nursing care for patients with acute respiratory failure requires vigilant assessment, airway management, and urgent interventions to maintain adequate tissue respiration.

Background

Respiratory failure can result from a variety of infective, mechanical, or functional disturbances primarily within the pulmonary, neurologic, cardiovascular, or musculoskeletal system. Fundamentally, each of these cause a mismatch between the demand for oxygen and carbon dioxide exchange and the body's ability to meet these needs (Dries, 2013). In order to maintain adequate exchange of oxygen and carbon dioxide there are several requisite factors. The first factor is to ensure that there is adequate oxygen available to meet the patient's demands. The second factor is the assessment of the patient's ventilation status, in terms of adequate depth to allow for alveolar diffusion. The third factor is adequate pulmonary perfusion and impaired gas exchange. Any illness or injury that impacts one or more of these factors can lead to respiratory insufficiency and acute respiratory failure (Dries, 2013).

Although a number of chronic conditions can cause a patient to experience respiratory distress, the majority of these patients have a history of chronic obstructive pulmonary disorders (Centers for Disease Control and Prevention [CDC], n.d.). Because these patients are perpetually in a state of compensation, even typically minor illnesses can precipitate an exacerbation of their chronic condition that taxes their ability to further compensate, leading to acute respiratory failure (Dries, 2013). Although children do not typically meet criteria for a diagnosis of chronic obstructive pulmonary disorder (COPD), respiratory failure remains one of the top 10 causes of pediatric death in the United States (CDC, n.d.). The cause of death in patients with cystic fibrosis is respiratory failure in 80% of cases (Seckel, 2013).

Clinical Aspects

ASSESSMENT

Early identification of the patient with impending respiratory failure is vital to the nurse's ability to intervene and facilitate optimal outcomes. This begins with a systematic approach to the assessment process. This is most often discussed in the context of pediatric patients but applies to every patient the nurse will encounter. The assessment of patients with respiratory compromise begins as the nurse enters the patient's room. A visual inspection of the patient's condition allows the nurse to form an overall impression of the patient's appearance, circulation to the skin, and work of breathing. This general impression allows the nurse to stratify the initial urgency with which interventions need to be implemented.

Visible signs and symptoms that should signal to the nurse that emergent intervention is needed would include shallow respirations, tachypnea, bradypnea, apnea, abnormal respiratory patterns, audible breathing sounds, cyanosis, pallor, retractions, lethargy, and coma. Any of these should prompt the nurse to immediately intervene to improve oxygen ventilation and respiration while working to determine the cause of the respiratory failure. Milder symptoms in adults may be addressed less urgently; however, in children these may indicate impending collapse and should be monitored carefully.

After the initial impression, the nurse will then collect a focused history and physical exam. The nurse will be alert to items in the history that identify risk factors associated with respiratory failure such as tobacco use, occupational exposures, inhalant use, infectious disease exposure, medical history, family history of respiratory disorders. Mnemonics, such as OPQRST (onset, provocation, quality, severity, timing) or COLDSPA (character, onset, location, duration, severity, pattern and associated factors) can be beneficial in focusing the history without compromising completeness.

The focused physical exam should be done initially and then periodically throughout the course of the patient's treatment. At a minimum this should be repeated whenever there is a change in status or vital signs, after therapeutic interventions, hourly in the emergency department, and every 4 hours in the intensive care setting. The nurse should use inspection, palpation, and percussion along with auscultation to thoroughly assess the patient's respiratory system. This assessment is essential in early identification of developing or worsening respiratory distress. Although auscultation is often the hallmark assessment technique, using a combination of these techniques is required to comprehensively identify subtle changes in condition. Percussion can clue the nurse into a developing pneumothorax, hemothorax, or lung consolidation, which can be treated conservatively if addressed early and can be life-threatening if not. Palpation is often the only way to recognize subcutaneous emphysema, which may be a sign of impending fatal airway injury. Findings, especially interval changes, should be documented and addressed with the clinician(s) responsible for overseeing the patient's care.

In addition to physical and history examination, it is important to collect data on the oxygenation and perfusion status of the patient. The gold standard for assessing respiratory function is the arterial blood gas (ABG) measurement. This test quantifies the respiratory status of the patient and provides values for pH, dissolved arterial oxygen and carbon monoxide (PaO_2 and $PaCO_2$), and bicarbonate (HCO_3) in the arterial system. Other noninvasive measures of respiratory status include exhaled carbon dioxide measurement ($ETCO_2$), which is graphically represented as capnography, pulse oximetry (SpO_2), chest x-ray, or CT scan (Pierce, 2013).

NURSING INTERVENTIONS, MANAGEMENT, AND IMPLICATIONS

Management of respiratory failure focuses initially on slowing the progression of the illness rather than on correcting the underlying cause of the failure. After assisting the patient into a position that facilitates optimal air exchange, and providing airway patency through positioning or suctioning of secretions, the application of oxygen is often the first intervention (Pierce, 2013). Oxygen application often provides rapid improvement, is quick and easy to apply, easy to adjust, and can be titrated to meet the needs of the patient either through flow rate or delivery device selection. Depending on the patient's past medical history, age, and diagnosis, the oxygen level can be titrated to facilitate an SpO_2 target of as low as 90% and as high as 98% (Dries, 2013).

A number of medication classes are used to correct respiratory symptoms. Inhaled beta agonists are used in almost every case of respiratory distress associated with obstructive illness to facilitate bronchial smooth muscle relaxation. Anticholinergic agents are used in conjunction with the beta-agonists to facilitate long-term relief. There is significant data supporting the use of corticosteroids to reduce the associated inflammation in these patients as well. Antibiotic medications are used to treat infective causes using the clinician knowledge of the national, regional, and local infectious disease prevalence data (Dries, 2013).

Cardiovascular causes of respiratory failure typically are those associated with low-volume states or emboli. Treatment for these conditions remains focused on correcting the underlying cause(s). Vascular volume replacement with crystalloid solutions, blood and blood products, and vasoactive medications can correct absolute and relative low-volume states. Thrombolytic medications can be used to correct pulmonary and/or cardiac thrombosis and emboli, which are impeding the delivery of blood to the pulmonary tissues and therefore limiting alveolar gas exchange (Seckel, 2013).

Noninvasive positive pressure ventilation (NPPV) devices are used to assist patients who are in nontraumatic respiratory distress and prevent their further decline to respiratory failure. These devices deliver continuous positive pressure to the airway in a cyclical fashion allowing for inspiration and exhalation while limiting the collapse of the distal alveoli. This is a significant cause of respiratory failure in patients with COPD. Continuous pressure facilitates the movement of fluid across the alveolar membranes in pulmonary edema secondary to congestive heart failure (CHF) and other conditions (Goodacre et al., 2014).

Nurses work within the team to facilitate or perform endotracheal intubation when other measures have failed to prevent further decline or are contraindicated. Once the decision to intubate has been made, it will be vital for the nurse to be prepared to assist with not only the intubation but also with rescue airway techniques that may become necessary if complications arise. Immediately after the patient has been intubated, the nurse ensures the placement of the tube within the trachea through combination of lung assessments and chest x-ray, along with colorimetric confirmation devices and/or $ETCO_2$ measurement. Documentation of the tube size, depth, and confirmation techniques are required as they are useful during reassessments.

OUTCOMES

The inability to maintain adequate oxygenation can be a significantly frightening and anxiety-inducing state for the patient. It is important for the care team to recognize this potential complication and minimize its impact. Another potential complication that intubated patients are at risk for is that of ventilator-associated pneumonia. Each facility has prevention protocols in place that the nurse needs to follow so that the patient's risk is minimized.

Summary

Acute respiratory failure is a common condition treated in the emergent and inpatient setting. Using a systematic approach to the identification and treatment of these conditions is effective in minimizing the cascade of complications that can lead to mortality and morbidity. The main focus must always remain on correcting this underlying problem and restoring the body's ability to maintain homeostasis while addressing emergent findings.

Centers for Disease Control and Prevention. (n.d.). 10 leading causes of death by age group, United States 2014. Retrieved from https://www.cdc.gov/injury/images/lc-charts/leading_causes_of_death_age_group_2014_1050w760h.gif

Dries, D. (2013). *Fundamental critical care support*. Mount Prospect, IL: Society of Critical Care Medicine.

Goodacre, S., Stevens, J., Pandor, A., Poku, E., Ren, S., Cantrell, A., . . . Plaisance, P. (2014). Prehospital noninvasive ventilation for acute respiratory failure: systematic review, network meta-analysis, and individual patient data meta-analysis. *Academy of Emergency Medicine, 21*, 960–970.

Pierce, L. (2013). Ventilatory assistance. In M. Sole, D. Klein, & M. Moseley (Eds.), *Introduction to critical care nursing* (6th ed., pp. 170–219). St. Louis, MO: Elsevier.

Seckel, M. (2013). Acute respiratory failure. In M. Sole, D. Klein, & M. Moseley (Eds.), *Introduction to critical care nursing* (6th ed., pp. 400–431). St. Louis, MO: Elsevier.

Villar, J., Blanco, J., Santos-Bouza, A., Blanch, L., Ambros, A., Gandia, F., . . . Kacmarek, R. (2011, December). The ALIEN study: Incidence and outcome of acute respiratory distress syndrome in the are of lung protective ventilation. *Journal of Intensive Care Medicine, 37*(12), 1932–1941.

World Health Organization. (2016). Media centre: Pneumonia. Retrieved from http://www.who.int/media centre/factsheets/fs331/en

■ RETURN OF SPONTANEOUS CIRCULATION WITH HYPOTHERMIA INITIATION

Laura Stark Bai

Overview

Therapeutic hypothermia, also referred to as *targeted temperature management (TTM)*, is the intentional reduction of a patient's body temperature after return of spontaneous circulation (ROSC) after cardiac arrest (Deckard & Elbright, 2011). Although survival rates from cardiac arrest vary based on cause of arrest, setting of arrest (within or outside of a hospital), and response by bystanders or medically trained personnel, studies show that therapeutic hypothermia helps to improve survival and protect neurological function in patients with ROSC. Nursing care of patients receiving therapeutic hypothermia after ROSC is complex and requires an intensive care setting in order to manage these patients safely and effectively for optimal outcomes.

Background

More than 326,000 adult cardiac arrests and over 6,300 pediatric cardiac arrests were evaluated by emergency medical services (EMS) outside of a hospital setting in America in 2014 (Sidhu, Schulman, & McEvoy, 2016). The average survival rate to hospital discharge for these arrests was 10.6% for adults and 7.3% for pediatrics and, of these survivors, only 8.3% of adults had good neurologic function (Newman, 2014). Therapeutic hypothermia after ROSC is consistently shown to improve survival rates and outcomes for these patients.

The concept of lowering body temperature was first explored by Dr. James Currie in the 1700s. However, its use in cardiac arrest was first presented in the 1930s with the first study being published in 1958, which created a foundation for this neuroprotective treatment (Sidhu et al., 2016). In 2002, two studies were published which established that therapeutic hypothermia improves neurological outcomes and should be a standard of care in patients with ROSC after cardiac arrest due to ventricular arrhythmias, and a viable option for patients with ROSC after arrest from a nonshockable rhythm (Scirica, 2013).

The guidelines from the American Heart Association (2015) regarding TTM in postcardiac arrest care recommend that "all comatose (i.e., lacking meaningful response to verbal commands) adult patients with ROSC after cardiac arrest should have TTM, with a target temperature between 32 degrees Celsius and 36 degrees Celsius selected and achieved, then maintained constantly for at least 24 hours" (p. 15). This is an increase in targeted temperature range from the previous guideline, which was 32°C to 34°C for 12 to 24 hours. Recent studies show that there are similar outcomes for patients who are cooled to 36°C and 33°C, so clinicians can make decisions based on preference or other considerations.

There are three physiologic processes that contribute toward neurologic injury after cardiac arrest. Briefly, these phases are initial lack of tissue profusion leading to cellular death, cerebral edema, and disruption of the blood–brain barrier; injury from reprofusion with production of free radicals; and an inflammatory response, which further worsens cellular injury (Sidhu et al., 2016). Therapeutic hypothermia is effective in preventing or reducing neurologic injury by preventing or counteracting these processes. It works by stabilizing the blood–brain barrier, suppressing inflammation to reduce cerebral edema, and decreasing the brain's need for oxygen by reducing cerebral metabolism (Deckard & Ebright, 2011).

Prognosis following ROSC after cardiac arrest remains a challenge, as a majority of patients expire due to neurologic complications (Scirica, 2013). Although study results vary, the benefits of therapeutic hypothermia for patients who achieved ROSC after cardiac arrest from a shockable rhythm (ventricular tachycardia or ventricular fibrillation) are evident in the literature. It is consistently shown that there is a reduction in short-term mortality and neurologic issues in patients who receive therapeutic hypothermia. However, the evidence is still conflicting for long-term benefits of therapeutic hypothermia and for patients who receive therapeutic hypothermia after ROSC from nonshockable rhythms.

Clinical Aspects

ASSESSMENT

The care of patients undergoing therapeutic hypothermia is complex and requires intensive monitoring by nurses to assess for complications of this treatment. Nurses must closely monitor vital signs to assess for proper control over body temperature during initial cooling, the first 24 hours, and after rewarming. Electrolyte levels must also be monitored to assess for fluid and electrolyte shifts that may lead to arrhythmias. Cardiac monitoring is also important for this reason. Glucose levels must be closely checked for hyperglycemia, since therapeutic hypothermia may cause insulin resistance. Regular neurologic assessments are challenging, but are required to assess for level of sedation to control shivering and prevent rewarming. Skin integrity should be assessed regularly for breakdown. Nurses must also closely monitor for bleeding and coagulation levels, as hypothermia can lead to platelet dysfunction. Finally, nurses must closely monitor and titrate intravenous medications as needed to meet therapeutic ranges, such as vasopressors, antiarrhythmics, electrolyte replacement therapies, fluids, and insulin.

NURSING INTERVENTIONS, MANAGEMENT, AND IMPLICATIONS

Patients are at risk for multiple complications due to therapeutic hypothermia. Because this treatment suppresses the body's inflammatory response, patients are at increased risk for infection. Vigilant observation of vital signs, hand hygiene, and proper aseptic technique will help to reduce the incidence of infection. These patients are also susceptible to ventilator-acquired pneumonia due to decreased functioning of respiratory cilia and gastric hypomotility. Oral care, suctioning, and elevating the head of bed above 30° will help reduce incidence. Preventative measures should also be taken to avoid skin breakdown, such as repositioning and use of barrier products, as hypothermia may lead to vasoconstriction and reduced blood flow. Patients are at risk for bleeding due to platelet dysfunction and may require transfusion.

There are three phases of therapeutic hypothermia during which core body temperature should be closely monitored. First, the induction phase aims to quickly lower the patient's core body temperature to 32°C to 36°C through several modalities, including ice packs, noninvasive cooling devices, infusion of cooled fluids, or iced lavage. During this time, sedation and neuromuscular blockade are initiated to prevent shivering (which would cause rewarming). Next is the maintenance phase, in which the target body temperature is maintained for approximately 24 hours through use of the previously discussed cooling techniques. The rewarming phase is the final phase, during which the core body temperature is slowly increased at a rate of 0.15°C to 0.5°C per hour. This is done slowly to prevent electrolyte shifts that would cause life-threatening arrhythmias. During these three phases, nurses have the vital role of monitoring the patient's body temperature and assessing for and preventing complications.

Although therapeutic hypothermia has strong support from the research in use for patients with ROSC after cardiac arrest, this technique is only utilized 2% to 6% of the time (Sidhu et al., 2016). Consistent use of therapeutic hypothermia in patients with ROSC after cardiac arrest caused by shockable rhythms can improve neurologic functioning and short-term outcomes.

OUTCOMES

The expected outcome of evidence-based nursing care in patients receiving therapeutic hypothermia after ROSC following cardiac arrest is improved neurologic functioning and short-term outcomes from patients who had a shockable rhythm. Quick action to begin cooling after ROSC with close monitoring of vital signs, cardiac rhythm, and electrolyte levels by the nurse is a vital part of this process. Prevention of skin breakdown, bleeding, ventilator-acquired pneumonia, and bloodstream infections is also vital in the success of this treatment. Studies confirm that when this treatment is used according to the American Heart Association guidelines, there will be an improvement in mortality rates and neurologic outcomes.

Summary

Therapeutic hypothermia is the standard treatment for patients with ROSC after cardiac arrest caused by a shockable rhythm. When implemented correctly immediately after ROSC, for over 50 years studies have shown that this medical treatment improves short-term outcomes by decreasing mortality and reducing neurologic damage. Nurses play a crucial role in the success of this process through close patient monitoring, prevention and treatment of complications, and detection of alterations in patient status. Research on the effect of this treatment in patients with cardiac arrest caused by nonshockable rhythm is required.

American Heart Association. (2015). Highlights of the 2015 American Heart Association guidelines update for CPR and ECC. Retrieved from https://eccguidelines.heart.org/wp-content/uploads/2015/10/2015-AHA-Guidelines-Highlights-English.pdf

Deckard, M. E., & Ebright, P. R. (2011). Therapeutic hypothermia after cardiac arrest: What, why, who, and how. *American Nurse Today*, 6(7). Retrieved from https://www.americannursetoday.com/therapeutic-hypothermia-after-cardiac-arrest-what-why-who-and-how

Newman, M. (2014). *AHA releases 2015 heart and stroke statistics*. Wexford, PA: Sudden Cardiac Arrest Foundation.

Scirica, B. (2013). Therapeutic hypothermia after cardiac arrest. *Circulation*, 127, 244–250.

Sidhu, S. S., Schulman, S. P., & McEvoy, J. W. (2016). Therapeutic hypothermia after cardiac arrest. *Current Treatment Options in Cardiovascular Medicine*, 18(5), 30.

■ SEIZURES

Eric Roberts

Overview

A seizure is an event during which neurons of the brain discharge in an abnormal fashion causing overstimulation and involuntary change in body movement, sensation, awareness, or behavior (Kornegay, 2016). The location and the number of neurons involved produce various clinical presentations. Morbidity, mortality, quality of life, and treatment modalities vary depending on the etiology, duration, and recurrence of seizures. A classification system helps individualize the approach used to evaluate and treat seizures.

Background

Seizures are classified as provoked when a precipitating event occurs within 7 days of seizure activity such as traumatic brain injury, tumors, metabolic disorders, electrolyte disturbance, withdrawal syndromes, and illness such as meningitis or encephalitis. Primary seizures are unprovoked and when recurrent are defined as epilepsy (Kornegay, 2016). Status epilepticus is an active seizure that lasts more than 5 minutes or, when seizures are consecutive, during which the patient does not regain consciousness. Refractory status epliepticus is a persistent seizure despite intravenous (IV) administration of two antiepileptic drugs (AEDs; Kornegay, 2016).

Focal, or partial, seizures are limited to a single hemisphere of the brain. These may have motor, sensory, autonomic symptoms, or produce hallucinations depending on location of the brain affected (Institute of Medicine [IOM], 2012). Simple focal seizures occur without impaired consciousness. Mentation is not affected and may be preceded by an aura (Kornegay, 2016). Complex partial seizures present with altered consciousness and may be associated with sensations of fear, paranoia, depression, elation, or ecstasy (Kornegay, 2016). These may be confused with psychological disorders.

Generalized seizures originate from both hemispheres of the brain and may or may not be subtle (IOM, 2012). They may present with isolated tonic contraction or stiffening of the body, clonic or rhythmic contractions, or atonic state with total loss of muscle tone (IOM, 2012). A tonic–clonic seizure is a severe type of seizure that starts with sudden loss of consciousness. Distinct tonic and clonic phases follow, with a postictal period of confusion. These patients will stop breathing during seizure activity and may experience anoxia, aspiration, or physical injury. Absence seizures are a type of generalized seizure with general, brief lapses in awareness typically lasting less than 10 seconds. Atypical presentations may last longer (IOM, 2012). Myoclonic seizures are characterized by sudden and brief jerking contractions involving any group of muscles and may resemble tremors (IOM, 2012).

It is estimated that 5.1 million people in the United States were diagnosed in 2013 with a seizure disorder. This represents 1.8% of the adult population and 1% of children (Centers for Disease Control and Prevention [CDC], 2016). Between 50,000 and 150,000 of these individuals experienced an episode of status epilepticus with resulting mortality rates of less than 3% in children, but as high as 30% in adults (Glauser et al., 2016). The cost associated with seizures includes $15.5 billion annually in direct medical expenses and additional indirect costs such as community services, loss in quality of life, and productivity (CDC, 2016). Epilepsy is responsive to treatment in an estimated 60% to 70% of cases; however, many people do not have access to treatment (IOM, 2012). A higher overall prevalence of epilepsy and incidence of persistent seizures has been demonstrated in patients with lower socioeconomic status (IOM, 2012).

The impact of epilepsy extends beyond the physical seizure activity. There may be significant impact to the quality of life, including limitations on daily activities, loss of the ability to drive, a social stigma affecting personal interactions, questions about living independently, ability to have children, as well as uncertainty about social and employment situations (IOM, 2012). Medication side effects are often a concern for patients as they may cause cognitive problems, impact energy levels, school performance, motor skill coordination, and impaired sexual function (IOM, 2012). Therefore, management goals for patients with epilepsy include preventing seizures in people at risk, eliminating side effects of treatments, and helping people with epilepsy achieve a high quality of life (IOM, 2012).

Clinical Aspects

ASSESSMENT

Assessment should include a detailed history. If the patient has a known seizure disorder, inquire about recent change in medication dose. Ask whether the patient is out of or stopped taking medicines because of adverse effects. Question sleep deprivation, increase in strenuous activity, recent infection, alcohol or substance abuse, and illness that may lead to electrolyte imbalance. These may precipitate seizure activity (Kornegay, 2016). A physical exam should focus on patency of the airway, adequacy of breathing, signs of hypoxia, and adventitious lung sounds suggestive of pulmonary aspiration. Inspect for signs of injury that may have occurred during the seizure such as tongue biting and shoulder injuries. A full neurologic examination and subsequent serial exams are important in evaluating for status epilepticus (Kornegay, 2016).

NURSING INTERVENTIONS, MANAGEMENT, AND IMPLICATIONS

Interventions should address both acute and chronic needs of the patient. There are currently three generations of AEDs that focus on controlling seizure recurrence of chronic disease by decreasing brain excitation (IOM, 2012). The older generations have been associated with increased side effects. However, newer medications may come at a higher cost and be less accessible to some patients. Particular consideration should be given to women of childbearing age, as many AEDs have been associated with a risk of neurodevelopmental impairments to the unborn child (IOM, 2012).

Sudden unexpected death in epilepsy (SUDEP) has been attributed to respiratory disturbances surrounding the acute seizure (Kennedy & Seyal, 2015). Brief seizures lasting fewer than 5 minutes carry the least risk of hypoxia and should receive supportive care. Maintain the airway, apply supplemental oxygen, monitor heart rhythm with EKG monitor, consider a toxicology screen, and check blood glucose levels (Glauser et al., 2016). Status epliepticus carries a high risk of hypoxia and requires IV medication in an attempt to stop seizure activity. Benzodizepines are the initial therapy of choice (Glauser, 2016). Refractory status epilepticus should be managed with IV doses of fosphenytoin, valproic acid, or levetriacetam (Glauser, 2016). For refractory seizures that last more than 40 minutes, an anesthesiologist should be contacted for administration of thiopental, pentobarbital, or propofol (Glauser, 2016).

It is important to educate the patients and their families about seizure triggers, safety concerns, and available community resources. Topics include environmental or lifestyle factors that may precipitate seizure activity such as lack of sleep, flashing lights, high fever, or excessive alcohol consumption (IOM, 2012). Patients need to understand that concurrent medications may alter AED levels or lower the seizure threshold such as antihistamines, stimulants, tramadol, and certain antibiotics (IOM, 2012). Teach patients that physical activities may place them and others at risk for injury if they experience a seizure while biking, skiing, driving, climbing, swimming, or even bathing (IOM, 2012). Patients should be familiar with community resources such as self-management programs, counseling, school-related support, and transportation services. Patients may not be permitted to operate a motor vehicle until well controlled. This education may improve quality of life.

OUTCOMES

Because of medication side effects, noncompliance concerns, and refractory seizures, many alternative treatment modalities have been considered to treat seizures with varying degree of empirical support and clinical outcomes. There is reliable evidence to suggest that ketogenic diets, vagal nerve stimulators, and surgical interventions may reduce seizure activity in in select populations (Martin, Jackson, & Cooper, 2016; Panebianco, Rigby, Westion, & Marson, 2015; West et al., 2015). There is weak evidence to suggest that yoga, transcranial magnetic stimulation, and deep brain stimulation may have positive effects of reducing seizure activity (Chen, Spencer, Weston, & Nolan, 2016; Panebianco, Sridharan, & Ramarathnam, 2015; Sprengers, Vonck, Carrette, Marson, & Boon, 2014). Modalities that have potential application but lack empirical support and require further study include the use of melatonin, acupuncture, and cannabis (Brigo, Igwe, & Del Felice, 2016; Cheuk & Wong, 2014; Gloss & Vickrey, 2014). Applying evidence-based practice may help guide treatment plans for individuals who struggle to manage their chronic disease.

Summary

Seizures may present with a wide range of physical manifestations. A key to evaluating seizures is soliciting a detailed health history. Seizure management should focus on supportive care during self-limiting seizures, strategies to stop active seizures in status epilpeticus, and mechanisms for preventing recurrence in chronic seizure disorders. Treatment is often effective, but must be individualized to meet the unique needs of the patient, while maintaining focus on safety and quality of life.

Brigo, F., Igwe, S., Del Felice, A. (2016). Melatonin as add-on treatment for epilepsy. *Cochrane Database of Systematic Reviews, 2016*(8). doi:10.1002/14615858. CD006967

Centers for Disease Control and Prevention. (2016). Epilepsy fast facts. Retrieved from https://www.cdc.gov/epilepsy/basics/fast-facts.htm

Chen, R., Spencer, D., Weston, J., & Nolan, S. (2016). Transcranial magnetic stimulation for the treatment of epilepsy. *Cochrane Database of Systematic Reviews, 2016*(8). doi:10.1002/14615858.CD011025

Cheuk, D., & Wong, V. (2014). Accupuncture for epilepsy. *Cochrane Database of Systematic Reviews, 2014*(5). doi:10.1002/14615858.CD005062

Gloss, D., & Vickrey, B. (2014). Cannabinoids for epilepsy. *Cochrane Database of Systematic Reviews, 2014*(3). doi:10.1002/14651858.CD009270

Glauser, T., Shinnar, S., Gloss, D., Alldredge, B., Arya, R., Bainbridge, J., . . . Treiman, D. (2016). Evidence-based guideline: Treatment of convulsive status eplipticus in children and adults: Report of the Guideline Committee of the American Epilepsy Society. *Epilepsy Currents, 16*(1), 48–61.

Institute of Medicine. (2012). *Epilepsy across the spectrum: Promoting health and understanding.* Washington, DC: National Academies Press.

Kennedy, J., & Seyal, M. (2015). Respiratory pathophysiology with seizures and implications for sudden unexpected death in epilepsy. *Journal of Clinical Neurophysiology, 32*, 10–13.

Kornegay, J. (2016). Seizures. In J. Tintinalli (Ed.), *Tintinalli's emergency medicine: A comprehensive study guide* (8th ed., pp. 1173–1178). New York, NY: McGraw-Hill.

Martin, K., Jackson, C., & Cooper, P. (2016). Ketogenic diet and other dietary treatments for epilepsy. *Cochrane Database of Systematic Reviews, 2016*(2). doi: 10.1002/14651858.CD001903

Panebianco, M., Sridharan, K., & Ramarathnam, S. (2015). Yoga for epilepsy. *Cochrane Database of Systematic Reviews, 2015*(5). doi:10.1002/14651858.CD001524

Panebianco, M., Rigby, A., Weston, J., & Marson, A. (2015). Vagus nerve stimulation for partial seizures. *Cochrane Database of Systematic Reviews, 2015*(4). doi:10.1002/14615858.CD002896

Sprengers, M., Vonck, K., Carrette, E., Marson, A., & Boon, P. (2014). Deep brain stimulation for epilepsy. *Cochrane Database of Systematic Reviews, 2014*(6). doi:10.1002/14615858.CD008497

West, S., Nolan, S., Cotton, J., Gandhi, S., Weston, J., Sudan, A., . . . Newton, R. (2015). Surgery for epilepsy. *Cochrane Database of Systematic Reviews, 2015*(7). doi:10.1002/14615858.CD010541

■ SEPSIS

Ronald L. Hickman, Jr.

Overview

Sepsis is a life-threatening bloodstream infection in which an infectious pathogen overwhelms the host's immune system and an injurious systemic inflammatory response results in a chain of events that include tissue injury, end-organ failure, and death (Singer et al., 2016). Adults with sepsis can manifest physiologic derangements in cellular metabolism, hemostasis, fluid and acid–base balance, and hemodynamic stability that can rapidly worsen without exposure to effective nursing and pharmacologic interventions (De Backer, Orbegozo Cortes, Donadello, & Vincent, 2014). Nursing care for adults with sepsis is focused on the early recognition of the deleterious effects of the systemic inflammatory response and the delivery of nursing interventions that optimize the effectiveness of an individual's immune system.

Background

According to the Centers for Disease Control and Prevention, sepsis affects more than 700,000 Americans per year and the projected annual incidence rate is estimated to steadily increase with the growing prevalence of older Americans (older than 65 years; Hall, Williams, Defrances, & Golosinkiy, 2011; Mayr, Yende, & Angus, 2014). In 2013, the clinical management of hospitalized adults with sepsis accounted for nearly $24 billion of annual health care costs, which makes sepsis one of the most costly life-threatening conditions in the United States (Torio & Moore, 2016). The clinical management of an adult with sepsis has shifted from the intensive care unit and recent studies indicate that more than 50% of adults with sepsis receive care outside of the intensive care unit (Mayr et al., 2014). Despite the ability to provide sepsis care outside of the intensive care unit, adults with a diagnosis of septic shock have a 40% to 70% likelihood of a sepsis-related death and those diagnosed with severe sepsis have between a 25% and 30% chance of a sepsis-related death while hospitalized (Gauer, 2013).

Although sepsis can affect adults across the life span and occur after an infection of any tissue, there are several known risk factors that predispose adults to sepsis. The most widely accepted risk factors that enhance an individual's susceptibility to sepsis are advanced age (greater than 65 years), immune system compromise (individuals with HIV infection, transplant recipients), comorbid conditions (diabetes mellitus, high blood pressure, and obesity), recent surgical procedures, and presence of indwelling catheters (Gauer, 2013; Petäjä, 2011). In addition, there is emerging evidence that sepsis disproportionately affects males; African Americans and Hispanics; and individuals who use tobacco, consume alcohol, and have nutrient-deficient diets (Mayr et al., 2014; Petäjä, 2011). It is suspected that disparities in sepsis outcomes are the result of complex interactions among the known risk factors, as well as social determinants of health and characteristics of health care organizations (Petäjä, 2011).

Diagnosis of sepsis is predicated on the presence of an infection and a minimum of two of the following indicators of systemic inflammatory response syndrome: body temperature (less than 96.8°F or greater than 100.4°F), heart rate greater than 90 beats/min, hyperventilation (respiratory rate greater than 20 breaths per minute), arterial partial pressure carbon dioxide (less than 32 mmHg [normal 35–45 mmHg]), and leukocyte count (less than 4,000/mm³ or greater than 12,000/mm³ [normal: 5,000–10,000/mm³]; Gauer, 2013).

In approximately 80% of adults with sepsis, the common sites of the localized infections are respiratory, genitourinary, gastrointestinal, and integumentary systems. Sepsis is the result of a host's exposure to an infectious pathogen, most commonly a bacterium (*Pseudomonas aeruginosa*, *Escherichia coli*, or *Staphylococcus aureus*) that overwhelms the host's local immune defenses and incites a systemic inflammatory response. Consequently, the pathogen enters into the host's bloodstream and proinflammatory mediators (interleukin [IL]-1, IL-6, and tumor necrosis factor [TNF]-) are released to recruit macrophages and lymphocytes to aid neutralization of the pathogen (Gauer, 2013). However, the persistent release of pro-inflammatory mediators by macrophages provokes inflammation-induced tissue damage, associated hypoperfusion, and microemboli formation. Without intervention, the persistent release of proinflammatory mediators will facilitate the progression of sepsis toward *severe sepsis*, a state of diffuse tissue hypoxia and end-organ dysfunction, and *septic shock*, a state of cellular necrosis, impaired hemostasis, multiple end-organ failure, and hemodynamic instability due to hypovolemia.

Clinical Aspects

ASSESSMENT

A fundamental component of effective nursing care is an accurate record of the individual's history, physical assessment findings, and laboratory data. When obtaining a history from an adult suspected of having sepsis, the individual's age, onset of symptoms, functional status, comorbid conditions (immunosuppression, diabetes mellitus, HIV, chronic kidney disease), recent surgical or diagnostic procedures, and medications (glucocorticoids, chemotherapeutics, or antibiotics) should be documented and used to determine the individual's sepsis risk. The physical assessment should focus on changes in the following body systems: cardiovascular system (blood pressure, pulse pressure, heart rate, volume status, and cardiac output), respiratory system (tachypnea, oxygen saturation, diminished breath sounds, acid–base disturbance [metabolic acidosis in septic shock], and consolidation of the lungs on chest radiograph), renal system (oliguria with fluid intake, increased serum creatinine, and hypovolemia with edema), neurologic system (abnormal body temperature, altered mental status, and change in affect), and integumentary system (pallor, cyanosis, petechiae, or ecchymosis). Together, an accurate history and vigilant monitoring of changes in the individual's condition can result in the well-timed initiation of nursing care that can positively influence an individual's sepsis-related outcomes.

There is not a single laboratory test that confirms presence of sepsis or septic shock. To confirm the presence of an infection, cultures of the blood, urine, sputum, and any drainage should be collected to identify the causative pathogen. However, for more than one half of adults with sepsis, blood cultures are negative. In addition, assessment of the leukocyte count and differential profile of the leukocytes, thrombocyte count, hematocrit and hemoglobin levels, activated protein C levels, D-dimer levels, cytokine (IL-6) levels, chest radiographs, and arterial blood gases should be monitored (Gauer, 2013). Changes in the physical assessment findings, laboratory tests, and diagnostic data are indicative of sepsis recovery or progression.

NURSING INTERVENTIONS, MANAGEMENT, AND OUTCOMES

Nursing care of the adult with sepsis should principally focus on the prevention of the progression of sepsis to septic shock. Priority nursing-related problems include maintenance of adequate ventilation and perfusion to promote tissue respiration, fluid resuscitation to address volume contraction, identification of the causative pathogen and administration of pathogen-specific antibiotic therapy, pressure ulcer prophylaxis, and the provision of psychological support to the patient and family system.

OUTCOMES

The expected outcomes of evidence-based nursing care are centered on preventing the progression of sepsis to septic shock. Active surveillance for changes in physical assessment findings and laboratory testing can provide evidence of recovery or progression of sepsis that can alter the clinical trajectory of the adult with sepsis. Recent studies confirm that routine screening of high-risk adults for sepsis has resulted in the early identification and initiation of empiric antibiotic therapy that attenuated the injurious effects associated with a systemic inflammatory response. The implementation of fluid resuscitation bundles, supplemental oxygen or mechanical ventilation, inotropic or vasopressor drug therapy, and hemodynamic monitoring have been shown to improve tissue perfusion and maintain adequate cellular respiration (Gauer, 2013). The expected outcomes of effective nursing care should attenuate the effects of the systemic inflammatory response associated with sepsis and prevent end-organ dysfunction related to severe sepsis or septic shock.

Summary

Adults diagnosed with sepsis can progress rapidly from sepsis to septic shock in a matter of hours if they do not receive appropriate nursing care and pharmacotherapy. Early recognition of sepsis and initiation of evidence-based nursing care and pharmacologic therapy are crucial to derailing the vicious chain of events associated with sepsis in adults.

De Backer, D., Orbegozo Cortes, D., Donadello, K., & Vincent, J. L. (2014). Pathophysiology of microcirculatory dysfunction and the pathogenesis of septic shock. *Virulence, 5*(1), 73–79. doi:10.4161/viru.26482

Gauer, R. L. (2013). Early recognition and management of sepsis in adults: The first six hours. *American Family Physician, 88*(1), 44–53.

Hall, M., Williams, S., Defrances, C., & Golosinkiy, A. (2011). Inpatient care for septicemia or sepsis: A challenge for patients and hospitals. *NCHS Data Brief, 62*, 1–8.

Mayr, F. B., Yende, S., & Angus, D. C. (2014). Epidemiology of severe sepsis. *Virulence, 5*(1), 4–11. doi:10.4161/viru.27372

Petäjä, J. (2011). Inflammation and coagulation. An overview. *Thrombosis Research, 127*, S34–S37. doi:10.1016/S0049-3848(10)70153-5

Singer, M., Deutschman, C. S., Seymour, C., Shankar-Hari, M., Annane, D., Bauer, M., . . . Angus, D.C. (2016). The third international consensus definitions for sepsis and septic shock (sepsis-3). *Journal of the American Medical Association, 315*(8), 801–810. doi:10.1001/jama.2016.0287

Torio, C., & Moore, B. (2016, May). *National inpatient hospital costs: The most expensive condition by payer, 2013* (HCUP Statistical Brief No. 5). Rockville, MD: Agency for Healthcare Research and Quality.

■ SEXUAL ASSAULT

Patricia M. Speck
Diana K. Faugno
Rachell A. Ekroos
Melanie Gibbons Hallman
Sallie J. Shipman
Martha B. Dodd
Qiana A. Johnson
Stacey A. Mitchell

Overview

"Rape is a legal term . . . [referring] to any penetration of a body orifice (mouth, vagina, or anus) involving force or the threat of force or incapacity (i.e., associated with young or old age, cognitive or physical disability, or drug or alcohol intoxication) and non-consent" (Linden, 2011, p. 834). Sexual assault and rape are violent intrusions toward an individual or group of individuals (usually female) that are intentional and harmful, perpetrated by individuals or groups with preferential paraphilias toward victims and type of sexual offense, but variable with multiple modus operandi (Lasher, McGrath, & Cumming, 2014). Rape is also a weapon of war (United Nations News Centre, 2017). Effects of rape have lifelong consequences for the victim that deny the person quality of life, and place the victim(s) at increased risk of "unwanted pregnancy, sexually transmitted infections, sleep and eating disorders, and other emotional and physical problems" (Kruttschnitt, Kalsbeek, & House, 2014, para 2). In ancient times, virginity or chastity had value as property, hence laws were enacted that paid the owner for damage or access to (consortium) property (family or husband), but these laws also punish the victim for adultery (Conley, 2014). The social construct that places value on virginity persists in trafficking slaves today (Joffres et al., 2008; McAlpine, Hossain, & Zimmerman, 2016). In the United States, persons charged with sexual crimes publicly support their acts with justifications for forcing sex on another; misperceptions of victim behavior, including alcohol consumption; and numbers of contacts with the victim (Abbey & Jacques-Tiura, 2011; Wegner, Abbey, Pierce, Pegram, & Woerner, 2015). When alcohol exposure includes justification for force or opportunity (victim did not say "no"), or when the rapist lacks insight about the victim's view of the event, the rapist is likely to repeat the behavior (Abbey, 2011; Wegner et al., 2015). When rapists are publicly charged with a crime, their marginal logic may blame the victim, say it was consensual, or that the suspect cries "foul" because there was no "intent" to harm, which is a new defense for crimes. Understanding the victim's reactions, and the rapist's proclivity toward a specific victim, helps nursing communities plan evidence-based prevention programs, interventions, and mitigation strategies for improving a patient's predictable negative health outcomes.

Background

Sexual assault is a life-altering event, undermining an individual's confidence and perception of safety. For many, the acute traumatic reaction and allostatic load are the beginning of diminished physical and mental health (McEwen, 1998; McEwen & Seeman, 1999; Schafran, 1996; Stein et al., 2004). To date, for those surviving the rape, posttraumatic stress disorder is a primary outcome (Jaycox, Zoellner, & Foa, 2002; Krakow et al., 2002; Zoellner, Goodwin, & Foa, 2000). For others, exposure to violence and rape increase somatic symptoms of anxiety and mood disorders in which their behavior increases the risk of sexually transmitted diseases and requests for therapeutic abortion (Tinglof, Hogberg, Lundell, & Svanberg, 2015). Although medication is available to minimize symptoms of anxiety and other mood disorders, the side effects of the medication, the person's age or gender, and having to pay for the medication may prevent many from completing the regimen, which is an opportunity for registered nurse anticipatory guidance intervention (Bogoch et al., 2014; Krause et al., 2014).

The Centers for Disease Control and Prevention is a leader in understanding sexual violence. The current understanding about sexual violence is divided into the following types:

- Completed or attempted forced penetration of a victim
- Completed or attempted alcohol/drug-facilitated penetration of a victim
- Completed or attempted forced acts in which a victim is made to penetrate a perpetrator or someone else
- Completed or attempted alcohol/drug-facilitated acts in which a victim is made to penetrate a perpetrator or someone else
- Nonphysically forced penetration that occurs after a person is pressured verbally or through intimidation or misuse of authority to consent or acquiesce
- Unwanted sexual contact
- Does not include physical contact of a sexual nature between the perpetrator and the victim; this occurs against a person without his or her consent, or against a person who is unable to consent or refuse (Basile et al., 2016, para 1)

The incidence of sexual assault and rape types in populations varies according to family dynamics, culture, and community tolerance for violence, but the primary reason for inconsistencies between statistical reports is that victims do not report (DuMont, Miller, & Myhr, 2003). One reason victims do not report is they do not know whether their experiences meet the legal definition of rape or sexual assault. They self-blame, have guilt, shame, and embarrassment, which leads to the desire to keep the assault a private matter, fearing humiliation or complicity, fear of not being believed, and lack of trust in the criminal justice system (Boykins & Mynatt, 2007; Darnell et al., 2015; DuMont et al., 2003). Even if victims did report, the definition of rape and combining sexual crimes with other types of crimes (Kruttschnitt et al., 2014) diminishes accuracy of data. Strikingly, 37.4% of females reported their first rape occurred between the ages of 18 and 24 years (Black et al., 2011) and 12.3% of female rape victims and 27.8% of male rape victims were first raped when they were age 10 or younger (National Center for Injury Prevention and Control Division of Violence Prevention, 2012). Individuals committing sexual offenses rarely do so spontaneously and there is a significant level of planning that leads up to the offense (Lasher et al., 2014; Mitchell, Angelone, Kohlberger, & Hirschman, 2009; Terry & Freilich, 2012). Grooming is a process by which an offender draws a victim into a relationship that becomes sexual and is maintained in secrecy by using authority and supervision to delay and sustain the deception (Terry & Freilich, 2012). The outcomes of long-term predatory sexual violence promote victim risk for subsequent rape (Sadler, Booth, Mengeling, & Doebbeling, 2004) and risk behaviors (early sexual activity, sexually transmitted infections, smoking, drug and alcohol abuse, obesity, etc.), subsequent poor health (e.g., hypertension, diabetes, heart disease, stroke, and lung disease), and ultimately early death by as much as 20 years (Acierno, Resnick, Flood, & Holmes, 2003; Adams et al., 2016; Anda et al., 2009; Armstrong, 1997; R. B. Baker, 2006; Campbell, Sefl, & Ahrens, 2004; Draucker, 1999; Hillis et al., 2004; Zinzow et al., 2012). Understanding rape incidence, particularly against children, and offender methods provides nurses opportunity to screen and identify patients early, mitigating the impact by using trauma-informed and patient-centered care in all nursing settings.

In some cases, there are instances in which sexual violence results in death, particularly in domestic violence. Violent behavior during a sexual assault may escalate and the victim may be killed; older victims with frail health are at higher risk of death (Safarik, Jarvis, & Nussbaum, 2002). In 1997, male-perpetrated domestic violence caused 1,830 deaths, in which 73% of victims were women (Gilliland, Spence, & Spence, 2000). Blaming the victim is a frequent reaction to persons with trauma sequelae and manifests in a variety of negative behaviors by health care system providers (Marantz, 1990) and criminal justice responders (Venema, 2016). Questions about violent experiences *in all care settings* provide nurses the opportunity to mitigate lethal outcomes.

Clinical Aspects

ASSESSMENT

Rarely does sexual assault create visible injury requiring treatment in urgent or emergent settings (Gaffney, 2003; Jones, Rossman, Diegel, Van Order, & Wynn, 2009; Jones, Rossman, Wynn, Dunnuck, & Schwartz, 2003). The offender's modus operandi and paraphilias influence offender's choice to injure (Lasher et al., 2014), but victim responses to the capture and awareness of situation always mitigate injury, which may include the inability to act or address a threat, which is involuntary associated with postevent anxiety and posttraumatic stress disorder (PTSD; Abrams, Carleton, Taylor, & Asmundson, 2009), or surrender, which is a voluntary decision to not resist and stay alive, but not well studied (Speck, Ropero-Miller, & McCullough, 2010). Regardless, victim response is influenced by alcohol and drug use (Anderson, Flynn, & Pilgrim, 2017) as well as previous trauma reactions. Nurses are the key to providing trauma-informed and patient-centered care to support reporting victims, explaining processes, and facilitating a coordinated community response.

To date, there is no consistent education about sexual assault across curricula in basic RN or graduate programs, or the health (mental and physical), or legal outcomes following rape or sexual assault, or about the expected toll of the vicarious trauma experience from caring for victims of crimes. For RNs wanting to care for victims of sexual assault, there is education offered by the International Association of Forensic Nurses (IAFN), translated into a 40-hour training seminar for the sexual assault nurse examiner (SANE)—adolescent and adult role (International Association of Forensic Nurses, 2015). Other organizations offer continuing-education units in training to meet state board of nursing rules or regulations (Maryland Board of Nursing, n.d.; Texas Board of Nursing, 2013). Many RNs return to schools offering graduate education hours toward certificates or graduate/doctoral degrees, where online-blended graduate programs require face-to-face clinical practicums for competency demonstrations (J. Baker et al., 2016; Metcalfe, Hall, & Carpenter, 2007). Advanced Forensic Nursing Board Certification requires significant advanced forensic nursing practice hours and continuing education (American Nurses Credentialing Center, n.d.).

In a trauma-informed care environment, each patient should be screened for a history of violence and sexual assault. However, in the acute assessment of a patient with a suspicion or complaint of rape or sexual assault, the coordinated community response includes a sexual assault response team (SART) with members having unique roles and role limitations. There are tools in the literature to guide the focus on the type of assault and the developmental age, and this may include the age of the first assault, the relationship of the assailant(s), and what the patients think the impact is on their lives (Basile, Hertz, & Back, 2007). The screening tools provide the nurse insight into the patient's vulnerabilities, including risk behaviors. In addition, when there is therapeutic screening, this is the best hope for patient engagement in the health care system. The RN implements the nursing role as a gatherer of health and medical information, including medical history and conditions or what is seen and heard, objectively documenting injury, treatments, and recommendations and referrals. The nurse uses the nursing process to ensure comfort and care and forensic science to avoid contamination during sample collection, which is used to further assess the patients, their responses to the intervention, and their needs. The RN who is SANE-trained is answerable to the board of nursing under the RN licensed authority, and never becomes a law enforcement investigator (evidence collector). Samples, as well as nursing assessment documentation, are useful to the prosecution (or not), when helping either law enforcement or prosecution introduces significant RN bias and undermines the comprehensive scope and standards of the forensic nurse role in sexual assault care.

OUTCOMES

Victims of rape and sexual assault experience risk of transmission of sexually transmitted diseases, in which follow-up with sexual assault victims is poor

(Ackerman, Sugar, Fine, & Eckert, 2006; Boykins & Mynatt, 2007; Parekh & Brown, 2003). Therefore, the recommendation is *treatment at point of care* by the nurse, which includes "an empiric antimicrobial regimen for chlamydia, gonorrhea, and trichomonas; emergency contraception...; post-exposure hepatitis B vaccination...; HPV vaccination is recommended for female survivors aged 9–26 years and male survivors aged 9–21 years; [and] recommendations for HIV PEP are individualized according to risk" (Centers for Disease Control and Prevention, 2017, section 3). With newer technology, nurses have opportunity to improve victim follow-up with health care systems.

Summary

Sexual assault is an intentional trauma that alters the victim's biophysiology. When one in four women and one in six men are victims of sexual assault and rape, many before age 18, it is likely that nurses will care for patients with a sexual assault history. When systems lack preparation for care of rape victims seeking treatment, the system becomes the problem and results in failed justice; the failure occurs not only in meeting the needs of the patient, but also in meeting the needs of the community at large. The libelous burden on the health system occurs when systems deny or delay treatment, when there are untoward outcomes contributing to increasing risk for mental and physical health sequelae. Eventually, these patients become high users of the systems, which began when their needs went unmet after victimization.

The SANE responds to the acute victim of sexual assault. This role, in existence since 1973 in Memphis, Tennessee, expanded in the 1990s with the advent of IAFN and its membership of mainly SANEs. The growing trend is to offer comprehensive graduate education in forensic nursing and accomplish this with integration of forensic nursing exemplars in concept-based basic and advanced nursing curricula with simulation (for instance, intentional injury as a concept in an acute care nurse practitioner curriculum). Colleges and schools now offer graduate and doctoral practice and research degrees, with paths in the specialty of forensic nursing, which guarantees an ample supply of expert forensic nurse leaders able to navigate complex medical–forensic patient presentations in a variety of hospital, community, and entrepreneurial systems.

Abbey, A. (2011). Alcohol's role in sexual violence perpetration: Theoretical explanations, existing evidence and future directions. *Drug and Alcohol Review*, 30(5), 481–489. doi:10.1111/j.1465-3362.2011.00296.x

Abbey, A., & Jacques-Tiura, A. J. (2011). Sexual assault perpetrators' tactics: Associations with their personal characteristics and aspects of the incident. *Journal of Interpersonal Violence*, 26(14), 2866–2889. doi:10.1177/0886260510390955

Abrams, M. P., Carleton, R. N., Taylor, S., & Asmundson, G. J. (2009). Human tonic immobility: Measurement and correlates. *Depression and Anxiety*, 26(6), 550–556. doi:10.1002/da.20462

Acierno, R., Resnick, H. S., Flood, A., & Holmes, M. (2003). An acute post-rape intervention to prevent substance use and abuse. *Addictive Behaviors, 28*(9), 1701–1715.

Ackerman, D. R., Sugar, N. F., Fine, D. N., & Eckert, L. O. (2006). Sexual assault victims: Factors associated with follow-up care. *American Journal of Obstetrics and Gynecology, 194*(6), 1653–1659. doi:10.1016/j.ajog.2006.03.014

Adams, Z. W., Moreland, A., Cohen, J. R., Lee, R. C., Hanson, R. F., Danielson, C. K., . . . Briggs, E. C. (2016). Polyvictimization: Latent profiles and mental health outcomes in a clinical sample of adolescents. *Psychology of Violence, 6*(1), 145–155. doi:10.1037/a0039713

American Nurses Credentialing Center. (n.d.). Advanced forensic nursing certification eligibility criteria. Retrieved from http://www.nursecredentialing.org/AdvForensicNursing-Eligibility.aspx

Anda, R. F., Dong, M., Brown, D. W., Felitti, V. J., Giles, W. H., Perry, B. D., . . . Dube, S. R. (2009). The relationship of adverse childhood experiences to a history of premature death of family members. *BMC Public Health, 9*(106). Retrieved from http://www.biomedcentral.com/1471-2458/9/106

Anderson, L. J., Flynn, A., & Pilgrim, J. L. (2017). A global epidemiological perspective on the toxicology of drug-facilitated sexual assault: A systematic review. *Journal of Forensic and Legal Medicine, 47*, 46–54. doi:10.1016/j.jflm.2017.02.005

Armstrong, R. (1997). Sexual assault: Clinical issues. When drugs are used for rape. *Journal of Emergency Nursing, 23*(4), 378–381.

Baker, J., Kelly, P. J., Carlson, K., Colbert, S., Cordle, C., & Witt, J. S. (2016). SANE-A-PALOOZA: Logistical development and implementation of a clinical immersion course for sexual assault nurse examiners. *Journal of Forensic Nursing, 12*(4), 176–182. doi:10.1097/jfn.0000000000000133

Baker, R. B. (2006). Genital injuries in adolescents after rape. Retrieved from http://search.ebscohost.com/login.aspx?direct=true&db=rzh&AN=109847295&site=ehost-live

Basile, K. C., DeGue, S., Jones, K., Freire, K., Dills, J., Smith, S. G., & Raiford, J. L. (2016). *STOP SV: A technical package to prevent sexual violence.* Atlanta, GA: Centers for Disease Control and Prevention, National Center for Injury Prevention and Control. Retrieved from https://www.cdc.gov/violenceprevention/sexualviolence/definitions.html

Basile, K. C., Hertz, M. F., & Back, S. E. (2007). *Intimate partner violence and sexual violence victimization assessment instruments for use in healthcare settings: Version 1.* Atlanta, GA: Centers for Disease Control and Prevention, National Center for Injury Prevention and Control. Retrieved from https://www.cdc.gov/violenceprevention/pdf/ipv/ipvandsvscreening.pdf

Black, M. C., Basile, K. C., Breiding, M. J., Smith, S. G., Walters, M. L., Merrick, M. T., . . . Stevens, M. R. (2011). *The National Intimate Partner and Sexual Violence Survey (NISVS): 2010 summary report.* Atlanta, GA: National Center for Injury Prevention and Control, Centers for Disease Control and Prevention.

Bogoch, I. I., Scully, E. P., Zachary, K. C., Yawetz, S., Mayer, K. H., Bell, C. M., & Andrews, J. R. (2014). Patient attrition between the emergency department and clinic among individuals presenting for HIV nonoccupational postexposure prophylaxis. *Clinical Infectious Diseases, 58*(11), 1618–1624. doi:10.1093/cid/ciu118

Boykins, A. D., & Mynatt, S. (2007). Assault history and follow-up contact of women survivors of recent sexual assault. *Issues in Mental Health Nursing, 28*(8), 867–881. doi:10.1080/01612840701493394

Campbell, R., Sefl, T., & Ahrens, C. E. (2004). The impact of rape on women's sexual health risk behaviors. *Health Psychology, 23*(1), 67–74. doi:10.1037/0278-6133.23.1.67

Centers for Disease Control and Prevention. (2017). 2015 sexually transmitted diseases treatment guidelines: Sexual assault and abuse and STDs: Adolescents and adults. Retrieved from https://www.cdc.gov/std/tg2015/sexual-assault.htm

Conley, C. A. (2014). *Sexual violence in historical perspective.* In R. Gartner, B. McCarthy, & C. A. Conley (Eds.), *The Oxford handbook of gender, sex, and crime.* New York, NY: Oxford University Press. Retrieved from http://www.oxfordhandbooks.com/view/10.1093/oxfordhb/9780199838707.001.0001/oxfordhb-9780199838707-e-012

Darnell, D., Peterson, R., Berliner, L., Stewart, T., Russo, J., Whiteside, L., & Zatzick, D. (2015). Factors associated with follow-up attendance among rape victims seen in acute medical care. *Psychiatry, 78*(1), 89–101. doi:10.1080/00332747.2015.1015901

Draucker, C. B. (1999). The psychotherapeutic needs of women who have been sexually assaulted. *Perspectives in Psychiatric Care, 35*(1), 18–28.

DuMont, J., Miller, K. D., & Myhr, T. L. (2003). The role of "real rape" and "real victim" stereotypes in the police reporting practices of sexually assaulted women. *Violence Against Women, 9*(4), 466–486.

Gaffney, D. (Ed.). (2003). *Genital injury and sexual assault.* St. Louis, MO: G. W. Medical.

Gilliland, M. G., Spence, P. R., & Spence, R. L. (2000). Lethal domestic violence in eastern North Carolina. *North Carolina Medical Journal, 61*(5), 287–290.

Hillis, S. D., Anda, R. F., Dube, S. R., Felitti, V. J., Marchbanks, P. A., & Marks, J. S. (2004). The association between adverse childhood experiences and adolescent pregnancy, long-term psychosocial consequences, and fetal death. *Pediatrics, 113*(2), 320–327.

International Association of Forensic Nurses. (2015). *Sexual assault nurse examiner adult/adolescent and pediatric education.* Arnold, MD: Forensics Nurses.

Jaycox, L. H., Zoellner, L., & Foa, E. B. (2002). Cognitive-behavior therapy for PTSD in rape survivors. *Journal of Clinical Psychology, 58*(8), 891–906. doi:10.1002/jclp.10065

Joffres, C., Mills, E., Joffres, M., Khanna, T., Walia, H., & Grund, D. (2008). Sexual slavery without borders: Trafficking for commercial sexual exploitation in India. *International Journal for Equity in Health, 7,* 22. doi:10.1186/1475-9276-7-22

Jones, J. S., Rossman, L., Diegel, R., Van Order, P., & Wynn, B. N. (2009). Sexual assault in postmenopausal women: Epidemiology and patterns of genital injury. *American Journal of Emergency Medicine, 27*(8), 922–929. doi:10.1016/j.ajem.2008.07.010

Jones, J. S., Rossman, L., Wynn, B. N., Dunnuck, C., & Schwartz, N. (2003). Comparative analysis of adult versus adolescent sexual assault: Epidemiology and patterns of anogenital injury. *Academic Emergency Medicine, 10*(8), 872–877.

Krakow, B., Schrader, R., Tandberg, D., Hollifield, M., Koss, M. P., Yau, C. L., & Cheng, D. T. (2002). Nightmare frequency in sexual assault survivors with PTSD. *Journal of Anxiety Disorders*, 16(2), 175–190.

Krause, K. H., Lewis-O'Connor, A., Berger, A., Votto, T., Yawetz, S., Pallin, D. J., & Baden, L. R. (2014). Current practice of HIV postexposure prophylaxis treatment for sexual assault patients in an emergency department. *Women's Health Issues*, 24(4), e407–e412. doi:10.1016/j.whi.2014.04.003

Kruttschnitt, C., Kalsbeek, W. D., House, C. C. & Panel on Measuring Rape and Sexual Assault in Bureau of Justice Statistics Household Surveys. (2014). *Estimating the incidence of rape and sexual assault*. Washington, DC: National Academies Press.

Lasher, M. P., McGrath, R. J., & Cumming, G. F. (2014). Sex offender modus operandi stability and relationship with actuarial risk assessment. *Journal of Interpersonal Violence*, 30(6), 911–927. doi:10.1177/0886260514539757

Linden, J. A. (2011). Clinical practice. Care of the adult patient after sexual assault. *New England Journal of Medicine*, 365(9), 834–841. doi:10.1056/NEJMcp 1102869

Marantz, P. R. (1990). Blaming the victim: The negative consequence of preventive medicine. *American Journal of Public Health*, 80(10), 1186–1187.

Maryland Board of Nursing. (n.d.). Forensic nurse examiner. Retrieved from http://mbon.maryland.gov/Pages/forensic-nurse-examiner.aspx

McAlpine, A., Hossain, M., & Zimmerman, C. (2016). Sex trafficking and sexual exploitation in settings affected by armed conflicts in Africa, Asia and the Middle East: Systematic review. *BMC International Health and Human Rights*, 16(1), 34. doi:10.1186/s12914-016-0107-x

McEwen, B. S. (1998). Stress, adaptation, and disease: Allostasis and allostatic load. *Annals of the New York Academy of Sciences*, 840, 33–44. doi:10.1111/j.1749-6632.1998.5b09546.x

McEwen, B. S., & Seeman, T. (1999). Protective and damaging effects of mediators of stress. Elaborating and testing the concepts of allostasis and allostatic load. *Annals of the New York Academy of Sciences*, 896, 30–47.

Metcalfe, S. E., Hall, V. P., & Carpenter, A. (2007). Promoting collaboration in nursing education: The development of a regional simulation laboratory. *Journal of Professional Nursing*, 23(3), 180–183. doi:10.1016/j.profnurs.2007.01.017

Mitchell, D., Angelone, D. J., Kohlberger, B., & Hirschman, R. (2009). Effects of offender motivation, victim gender, and participant gender on perceptions of rape victims and offenders. *Journal of Interpersonal Violence*, 24(9), 1564–1578. doi:10.1177/0886260508323662

National Center for Injury Prevention and Control Division of Violence Prevention. (2012). Sexual violence: Facts at a glance. Retrieved from https://www.cdc.gov/violence prevention/pdf/sv-datasheet-a.pdf

Parekh, V., & Brown, C. B. (2003). Follow up of patients who have been recently sexually assaulted. *Sexually Transmitted Infections*, 79(4), 349.

Sadler, A. G., Booth, B. M., Mengeling, M. A., & Doebbeling, B. N. (2004). Life span and repeated violence against women during military service: Effects on health status and outpatient utilization. *Journal of Women's Health*, 13(7), 799–811.

Safarik, M. E., Jarvis, J. P., & Nussbaum, K. E. (2002). Sexual homicide of elderly females: Linking offender characteristics to victim and crime scene attributes. *Journal of Interpersonal Violence, 17*(5), 500–525. doi:10.1177/0886260502017005002

Schafran, L. H. (1996). Topics for our times: Rape is a major public health issue. *American Journal of Public Health, 86*(1), 15–17.

Speck, P. M., Ropero-Miller, J. R., & McCullough, T. (2010). *An overview of DFSA SANE/SAFE/SART Protocol 1: Surrendered rape defined* [Webinar slide 14]. Research Triangle Park, NC: Research Triangle Institute and Department of Justice Office of Victims of Crime.

Stein, M. B., Lang, A. J., Laffaye, C., Satz, L. E., Lenox, R. J., & Dresselhaus, T. R. (2004). Relationship of sexual assault history to somatic symptoms and health anxiety in women. *General Hospital Psychiatry, 26*(3), 178–183. doi:10.1016/j.genhosppsych.2003.11.003

Terry, K. J., & Freilich, J. D. (2012). Understanding child sexual abuse by Catholic priests from a situational perspective. *Journal of Child Sexual Abuse, 21*(4), 437–455. doi:10.1080/10538712.2012.693579

Texas Board of Nursing. (2013). Education—Continuing nursing education & competency. Retrieved from https://www.bon.texas.gov/education_continuing_education.asp

Tinglof, S., Hogberg, U., Lundell, I. W., & Svanberg, A. S. (2015). Exposure to violence among women with unwanted pregnancies and the association with post-traumatic stress disorder, symptoms of anxiety and depression. *Sexual & Reproductive Healthcare, 6*(2), 50–53. doi:10.1016/j.srhc.2014.08.003

United Nations News Centre. (2017). Perpetrators, not victims, should be shamed for conflict-related sexual violence—UN report [Press release]. Retrieved from http://www.un.org/apps/news/story.asp?NewsID=56675#.WSHynmjyuMp

Venema, R. M. (2016). Making judgments: How blame mediates the influence of rape myth acceptance in police response to sexual assault. *Journal of Interpersonal Violence.* doi:10.1177/0886260516662437

Wegner, R., Abbey, A., Pierce, J., Pegram, S. E., & Woerner, J. (2015). Sexual assault perpetrators' justifications for their actions: Relationships to rape supportive attitudes, incident characteristics, and future perpetration. *Violence Against Women, 21*(8), 1018–1037. doi:10.1177/1077801215589380

Zinzow, H. M., Resnick, H. S., McCauley, J. L., Amstadter, A. B., Ruggiero, K. J., & Kilpatrick, D. G. (2012). Prevalence and risk of psychiatric disorders as a function of variant rape histories: Results from a national survey of women. *Social Psychiatry and Psychiatric Epidemiology, 47*(6), 893–902. doi:10.1007/s00127-011-0397-1

Zoellner, L. A., Goodwin, M. L., & Foa, E. B. (2000). PTSD severity and health perceptions in female victims of sexual assault. *Journal of Traumatic Stress, 13*(4), 635–649. doi:10.1023/a:1007810200460

■ SHOCK AND MULTIPLE ORGAN DYSFUNCTION SYNDROME

Jennifer Wilbeck

Overview

Most often shock is a secondary set of physiological processes resulting from a primary insult or injury. As such, emergency department (ED) and critical care nurses may encounter patients both at risk for, or are experiencing shock with multiple organ dysfunction. Early recognition, combined with targeted supportive therapies, is essential to restoration of the patient's health and prevention of end-stage organ dysfunction. Without prompt and aggressive interventions, shock and multiple organ dysfunction syndrome (MODS) lead to death.

Background

Shock is an acute, generalized process of inadequate tissue perfusion resulting in cellular, metabolic, and hemodynamic alterations (Carlson & Fitzsimmons, 2014). Imbalances of cellular oxygen supply and demand occur for a variety of reasons, and are classified into four broad types of shock: hypovolemic, obstructive, cardiogenic, and distributive (Carlson & Fitzsimmons, 2014; Shapiro & Fischer, 2015).

Hypovolemic shock results from the loss or redistribution of volume (blood, plasma, or other body fluids) leading to decreased intravascular volume. Etiologies may include acute blood loss or ongoing hemorrhage, gastrointestinal (GI) losses such as vomiting and diarrhea, burns, polyuria, excess pharmaceutical diuresis, or insensible losses. The loss of vascular volume leads to inadequate preload, followed by decreased diastolic filling and ultimately a decreased cardiac output.

Obstructive shock occurs secondary to mechanical obstruction that decreases ventricular filling and/or emptying, ultimately resulting in decreases in cardiac output, tissue perfusion, and oxygen delivery. Causes of obstructive shock include cardiac tamponade, tension pneumothorax, vena cava compression or thrombus, atrial mass or thrombus, and pulmonary embolism.

Cardiogenic shock occurs when the heart fails as a pump; decreased contractility leads to decreased stroke volume, cardiac output, and blood pressure, resulting in decreased tissue perfusion. Common causes of cardiogenic shock include myocardial infarction, heart failure exacerbations, dysrhythmias, and left ventricular outflow tract obstructions.

Distributive shock results in massive vasodilation and loss of vasomotor tone from three etiologies: anaphylactic (allergic-mediated), septic (infectious etiology), and neurogenic shock. Anaphylactic and septic shock are also associated with increased capillary permeability. Spinal cord injuries above the T4 level may result in sympathetic pathway damage and lead to decreased sympathetic tone to innervated organs distal to the level of the injury, leaving them stimulated by parasympathetic tone and causing bradycardia, massive vasodilatation, and inability to regulate body temperature. As a general rule, the higher the injury, the more severe the symptoms.

Regardless of the type of shock, resulting cellular hypoxia and subsequent vital organ dysfunction progress across a continuum of decline. The four stages of shock progression are initial, compensatory, progressive (or uncompensated), and refractory (Carlson & Fitzsimmons, 2014). Left untreated, shock ultimately leads to the development of multiple organ dysfunction and/or failure. MODS is the failure of more than one organ system in acutely ill patients, which requires intervention to maintain homeostasis (Carlson & Fitzsimmons, 2014; Kaml & Davis, 2016) and its severity can be measured by any of three standardized scoring systems (Frohlich et al., 2016).

Clinical Aspects

ASSESSMENT

Although the underlying processes are the same, the development, compensation, and timing of progression may vary based on a patient's age, prior health, initial insult, and treatment. Within the geriatric population, shock progression is rapid due to reduced compensatory mechanisms and preexisting comorbidities. Changes of decreased cardiac output and perhaps slight anxiety that are seen with initial shock are discrete; clinical signs and symptoms do not appear until the intravascular volume is reduced by greater than 15%. Compensated shock may be easily overlooked as the clinical presentation is relatively stable due to compensatory mechanisms from the renin–angiotensin–aldosterone system and stimulation of the central nervous system resulting in peripheral vasoconstriction, sodium reabsorption, and water retention. Early signs and symptoms of shock include tachycardia, borderline hypotension, tachypnea, nausea, oliguria, hyperglycemia, and extremities that are cool to the touch. During compensated shock, rapid correction of underlying etiologies increases the likelihood of minimal residual effects.

If not corrected, progressive (or uncompensated shock) develops with rapid patient deterioration and ensuing failure of compensatory mechanisms, which results in cellular hypoxia. Decreased cellular perfusion exacerbates anaerobic metabolism processes due to the lack of oxygen delivery to distal tissues, which can be indirectly measured by serum lactate levels. Anaerobic metabolism produces metabolic acidosis, resulting in hyperkalemia, cellular death, and both generalized and interstitial edema (including pulmonary edema). Increased vascular permeability and vasodilation also occur at this stage. Clinically, the nurse may identify the following findings in uncompensated shock: altered mentation/decreased responsiveness, tachycardia and arrhythmias, weak thready pulses and delayed capillary refill, hypoxia, absent or hypoactive bowel sounds, oliguria/anuria, hypoglycemia, and cold extremities. If not corrected at this point, refractory shock that is unresponsive to treatment and irreversible will ensue.

MODS then develops as individual organ systems die from tissue ischemia. MODS represents a complex physiologic process wherein uncontrolled inflammatory responses, in conjunction with changes of the vascular endothelium, immune function, metabolism and circulatory system, become a self-perpetuating process that leads to organ dysfunction and failure. Mortality rates increase with the number of failed organ systems; for patients with failure of two or more organs, estimated mortality rate is 54% (Carlson & Fitzsimmons, 2014).

Although shock presentations vary, shock should be suspected in patients with a mean arterial pressure (MAP) less than 60 mmHg, or in the presence of tissue hypoperfusion. Elevated lactic acid levels serve as a surrogate marker. Both physical assessments and diagnostic testing seek to identify the underlying etiology of shock and MODS. Standardized diagnostic criteria are available for each of these processes (Kaml & Davis, 2016; Vogel et al., 2016).

NURSING INTERVENTIONS, MANAGEMENT, AND IMPLICATIONS

Progression of shock through stages to the point of MODS allows ongoing opportunities to identify and intervene to halt further deterioration. Regardless of where the patient falls within the continuum of shock and/or MODS, goals of management are to provide supportive therapy to affected body systems while identifying, managing, and treating the initial source. This is accomplished by optimizing oxygen delivery and tissue perfusion, establishment of intravenous (IV) access, preferably central access, volume resuscitation, and vasopressor support. As adequate oxygenation requires a secure and patent airway, supplemental oxygen and mechanical ventilation are often required. Appropriate volume resuscitation may be achieved using crystalloid boluses with continuous fluid infusion and, if appropriate, blood product administration. Vasopressors are utilized once any volume deficits are replaced. Ultrasound evaluation of inferior vena cava (IVC) responsiveness, echocardiogram and central venous pressure (CVP) measurements provide diagnostic options and ability to evaluate treatment efficacy.

Targeted treatments for shock states may be added to the mainstay treatment noted previously:

- Hypovolemic shock requires targeted volume resuscitation to replace lost fluids (and/or blood). Bleeding or GI losses to vomiting or diarrhea must also be resolved.
- Treatment of obstructive shock requires resolution of the underlying structural occlusion.
- For cardiogenic shock due to myocardial infarction (MI), restoration of coronary artery perfusion and anticoagulation are needed. If due to heart failure, inotropic support, afterload reduction, and diuresis are utilized. Antiarrhythmic drugs and/or defibrillation are indicated for dysrhythmias.
- Neurogenic shock requires spinal stabilization, emergency neurosurgery consult, and surgical decompression. Vasopressors are used to provide chronotropic and blood pressure support. Activities that trigger vagal responses must be avoided.
- Anaphylactic shock requires aggressive airway management, adrenergic agonists, H1 & H2 receptor antagonists, bronchodilators, corticosteroids, and often vasopressors.

- Septic shock treatment follows the Surviving Sepsis Campaign clinical guidelines, which outline the timed treatment goals, including early antibiotics for infectious etiology in addition to fluid replacement and vasopressors (Dellinger et al., 2013).

OUTCOMES

Promoting positive outcomes can be achieved through a detailed nursing health history and physical examination identifying risk factors, mechanisms, and early signs of shock and multiple organ dysfunction. Nurses must understand the normal physiology and pathophysiology of these disorders to prevent complications. Working as a team with other health professionals and providers is important to ensure high-quality care in these patients as well as any others.

Summary

Shock states are dynamic; nurses must stay vigilant and utilize a collaborative team for the required complex care to ensure best outcomes. Regardless of the advances in care, basic ABCs (airway, breathing, and circulation) remain the mainstay of treatment. Optimal patient outcomes are recognized with early recognition of shock and aggressive intervention.

Carlson, B. & Fitzsimmons, L. (2014). Shock, sepsis, and multiple organ dysfunction syndrome. In L. D. Urden, K. M. Stacy, & M. E. Lough (Eds.), *Critical care nursing* (7th ed., pp. 887–925). St. Louis, MO: Elsevier.

Dellinger, R. P., Levy, M. M., Rhodes, A., Annane, D., Gerlach, H., Opal, S. M., . . . Moreno, R. (2013). Surviving sepsis campaign: International guidelines for management of severe sepsis and septic shock, 2012. *Intensive Care Medicine, 39*, 165–228.

Frohlich, M., Wafaisade, A., Mansuri, A., Koenen, P., Probst, C., Maegele, M., . . . Sakka, S. (2016). Which score should be used for posttraumatic multiple organ failure?—Comparison of the MODS, Denver, and SOFA Scores. *Scandainavian Journal of Trauma, Resuscitation & Emergency Medicine, 24*, 130. doi:10.1186/s13049-016-0321-5

Kaml, G. J., & Davis, K. A. (2016). Surgical critical care for the patient with sepsis and multiple organ dysfunction. *Anesthesiology Clinics, 34*, 681–696.

Shapiro, N., & Fischer, C. M. (2015). Shock. In J. J. Schaider, R. M. Barkin, S. R. Hayden, R. E. Wolfe, A. Z. Barkin, P. Shayne, & P. Rosen (Eds.), *Rosen & Barkin's 5-minute emergency medicine consult* (pp. 1026–1027). Philadelphia, PA: Wolters Kluwer.

Vogel, J. A., Newgard, C. D., Holmes, J. F., Diercks, D. B., Arens, A. M., Boatright, D. H., . . . Haukoos, J. S. (2016). Validation of the Denver emergency department trauma organ failure score to predict post-injury multiple organ failure. *Journal of the American College of Surgeons, 222*, 73–82.

■ SOLID ORGAN TRANSPLANTATION

Marcia Johansson

Overview

Solid organ transplantation has become widely accepted as a treatment for end-stage organ failure. With the use of immunosuppressive medications, the organs that can now be transplanted have expanded and include liver, kidney, pancreas, small bowel, and thoracic organs. All organs remain in short supply with increased waiting times for potential recipients (HRSA, 2017). Despite the many advances in treatment, appropriate critical care management is required to support prompt graft recovery and prevent systemic complications. Immunosuppressive medications, graft rejection (acute and chronic), and specific long-term complications have a direct effect on morbidity and mortality for the organ and recipient, and will be the focus of this chapter.

Background

There is no single consensus definition that can be applied to all organ transplants but each organ has specific criterion. The overall clinical problems in solid organ transplant are availability of organs and the prevention of complications and rejection. Despite advances in medicine and knowledge as well as increased awareness of organ donation and transplantation, there continues to be a gap between supply and demand. More progress is necessary to ensure that all individuals with end-stage organ failure have a chance to receive a transplant (Health Resources and Services Administration [HRSA], 2017).

According to the Organ Procurement Transplant Network (OPTN) current statistics, there are 118,278 people on the list in need of a lifesaving organ transplant. Of those, 75,857 people are active candidates on the waiting list. In the first quarter of 2017, 5,367 organ transplants were performed. There were only 2,554 donors during that same time period (HRSA, 2017). Living-related organ transplants continue to increase for both kidney and partial liver transplant.

Evaluation of an individual for organ transplant includes identifying the cause of organ failure, comorbid conditions, social and financial support, treatment before transplant, specific laboratory values that support organ failure, human leukocyte antigen (HLA) typing, ABO compatibility with the donor, and immune response testing to the proposed donors. For orthotopic liver transplant patients (OLT), calculation of the Model for End-Stage Liver Disease (MELD) scores is necessary. The range is from 6 (less ill) to 40 (gravely ill; Klein & Miller, 2014). The individual score establishes the severity of illness and is useful in determining the urgency of an individual's need to receive a liver transplant.

There have been significant strides in overcoming immunologic barriers through the use of desensitization techniques. The pretransplant evaluation identifies opportunities to assess the risks for common posttransplant infections and to develop individualized preventive strategies.

Cardiovascular morbidity and mortality complicate the progress of a significant proportion of renal transplant recipients and have an increased prevalence among recipients of other solid organ transplants. Early transplant complications include infection and rejection. Long-term risk factors include metabolic and cardiovascular disease, which pose the most serious risk factors impacting patient survival. Significant advances in immunosuppressive therapy have prolonged the allograft and patient survival in solid organ transplant.

Clinical Aspects

ASSESSMENT

Assessment and care of the transplant patient in the immediate postoperative period is organ specific and is also dependent on the patient's preoperative clinical status and comorbidities. Determination of postoperative disposition of the patient is based on the surgeon preference, hospital protocols, and intraoperative concerns of both the surgeon and anesthesiologist.

Evaluation and care of the OLT patient is the most complex. These patients are usually admitted to the intensive care unit (ICU) for at least 24 hours. Assessment begins with the handoff of the operating room (OR) team to the bedside nurse. Hemodynamic bedside monitoring includes electrocardiogram tracing, continuous blood pressure via arterial line, and continuous cardiac output monitoring. Depending on the length of the surgical procedure, OLT patients usually remain intubated for the first 4 to 6 hours and are then weaned off the ventilator and extubated.

NURSING INTERVENTIONS, MANAGEMENT, AND IMPLICATIONS

The initial evaluation of all posttransplant patients includes monitoring electrolytes, blood count, coagulation panel, and urine output. For OLT patients, it is vital to evaluate liver function tests that include total bilirubin, aspartate transaminase (AST), gamma-glutamyltransferase (GGT), alkaline phosphatase, and surgical drain output (Klein & Miller, 2014). Surgical drains are placed in strategic areas and if there is an anastomosis leak or bleeding, it is usually visible in the drain. Elevation in transaminases can indicate acute rejection or graft thrombosis. Renal orthotopic kidney transplantation (OKT) and pancreatic transplants do not always require admission to the ICU; however, monitoring is similar and is based on the organ transplanted. OKT patients require focused attention to electrolytes, blood urea nitrogen (BUN), creatinine, and urine output. A decreased urine output can indicate graft dysfunction or dehydration. Pancreas transplant patients require focused attention to blood glucose, amylase, lipase, hemoglobin A1c (HbA1c), and C-peptide levels. Elevations in blood glucose are indicative of graft dysfunction. These are all indicators specific to graft function and patients will need ongoing surveillance throughout their hospital stay as well as during follow-up clinic visits. All transplants require routine postoperative care, including monitoring of the surgical site for integrity and infection, early ambulation, aggressive pulmonary hygiene to prevent respiratory complications, and instruction regarding medication use and compliance, signs of rejection, and postoperative protocols.

Immunosuppression is the mainstay of organ transplantation. Immunosuppressive medications are used to prevent acute and chronic rejection and are normally continued for the life of the functioning transplant. Many variables are considered in the choice of the drug and dose as well as monitoring of the level. Guidelines for dosing for each specific organ are different. OLT patients may need a lower dose of immunosuppression based on the blood levels than an OKT patient who is experiencing acute rejection. The guidelines are national but have been modified to make them center specific.

Glucocorticoids, such as prednisone, have both immunosuppressive and anti-inflammatory properties. Side effects are well known and are associated with increased morbidity for the patient.

Antiproliferative agents include azathioprine and mycophenolic acid also known as *mycophenolate mofetil*, inhibit the steps in de novo purine synthesis (Klein & Miller, 2014, p. 609). Side effects include gastrointestinal disturbances, such as nausea, diarrhea and abdominal pain, as well as hematologic disturbances such as leukopenia and thrombocytopenia. Assessing white blood cell (WBC) and platelet counts is extremely important for any patient receiving these medications.

Mammalian target of rapamycin (mTOR) inhibitors include sirolimus and everolimus. They inhibit the activation of a regulatory kinase and prohibit T-cell progression. Side effects include hyperlipidemia, proteinuria, and difficulty with wound healing. These medications should not be used in moderate to severe kidney disease, hepatic artery thrombosis and immediately postoperative due to poor wound healing.

Calcineurin inhibitors include cyclosporin and tacrolimus. The mechanism of action is inhibition of T-lymphocyte activation and proliferation. Both calcineurin inhibitors are nephrotoxic, but cyclosporin is less neurotoxic and diabetogenic than tacrolimus. There is a narrow therapeutic window and doses are adjusted based on blood levels (Klein & Miller, 2014).

Biologic agents include polyclonal antibodies (ATGAM [lymphocyte immune globulin] and thymoglobulin) and monoclonal antibodies (daclizumab and basiliximab). These drugs can be utilized at the time of transplantation to promote engraftment and as a subsequent treatment for acute rejection. Thymoglobulin is given to reduce the damage that can occur during the storage and transplant procedure. The long-term risk of malignancy remains a concern with these agents (Klein & Miller, 2014).

OUTCOMES

Infection prophylaxis includes keeping current with immunization schedules and prophylactic antibiotics to prevent opportunistic infections, such as cytomegalovirus (CMV) infections, herpes simplex virus (HSV) infections, systemic fungal infections, respiratory, and urinary tract infections. The key to preventing infections and rejection episodes includes early recognition of symptoms, close monitoring of laboratory values, and basic infection-control principles like handwashing to promote positive health care outcomes.

Summary

Prolonged allograft survival, decreased morbidity from comorbid conditions, decreased medication side effects, and decreased mortality remain the goals for posttransplant care. Education of the patient and family, vigilance with nursing care, open communication with the medical team, and attention to laboratory values produce early interventions and promote the best outcomes for a transplant program. Research is ongoing to improve the care of the transplant patient and formulation of new targets for future research to deal with this ever-increasing population of high-risk patients remains a priority for the "transplant team," which includes nurses, advanced practice providers, and physicians.

Health Resources and Services Administration. (2017). Organ procurement & transplantation network [Data file]. Retrieved from https://optn.transplant.hrsa.gov

Klein, C. L., & Miller, B. W. (2014). *The Washington manual of medical therapeutics* (34th ed.). Philadelphia, PA: Wolters Kluwer/Lippincott Williams & Wilkins.

■ SPINAL CORD INJURY

Lamon Norton
Melanie Gibbons Hallman

Overview

Spinal cord injuries (SCIs) arise from both traumatic and nontraumatic origins. Spinal injuries incurred from trauma include motor vehicle crashes; sports injuries; blast injuries; acts of violence, including stabbing and gunshot wounds; and falls. Common causes of nontraumatic SCIs include tumors, birth defects, infection, and neurodegenerative diseases. It has been estimated that as many as 337,000 patients are currently living with SCIs (National Spinal Cord Injury Statistical Center [NSCISC], 2015). SCIs may present acutely and resolve with time and treatment; but many persist, becoming chronic conditions requiring ongoing care. Nurses play an imperative role in triage and management of SCIs. Urgent identification of acute spinal injury and potential physical or structural instability are crucial to achieving quality patient outcomes. Nurses provide essential clinical care by conducting strategic triage activities that include acquisition of pertinent history, focused physical assessment, initiation of definitive care, and early prevention of complications. Evidence-based education for patients diagnosed with SCIs, including known or potential sequelae, is paramount and a key responsibility of nurses.

Background

SCIs are often permanent and debilitating. Treatment is largely palliative. National incidence of SCI estimations range between 12,000 and 20,000 new cases per year (Ma, Chan, & Carruthers, 2014). Motor vehicles accidents are the source of SCIs in the majority of cases nationwide; and over 80% of patients sustaining injury are male. Risk-taking behaviors and heavy involvement in sporting pursuits impact the incidence with regard to age and gender. Falls are the primary cause of SCIs affecting the elder population. In a study conducted by Crutcher, Ugiliweneza, Hodes, Kong, and Boakye (2014), the presence of alcohol was noted in 20% of all SCI cases regardless of age and was associated with increased hospital complications and morbidity. SCIs range from simple cord contusions with minimal symptomology, to complete transaction of the cord with potential for physiologic instability.

Long-term management of SCI is costly to patients, the health care system, and society in general. These costs are not only reflected in monetary losses, but also in potential loss of contribution to family and community dynamics. The estimated average expense for a young person who sustains complete quadriplegic injury exceeds $4.5 million (NSCISC, 2015). Financial impact is dependent on the severity of injury and disability that is sustained (Ma et al., 2015). Typically, the higher the level of injury is anatomically located within the spine, the more intense the requirement for physical support of activities of daily living will be. Patients may be relatively independent if the injury is at the level of the first thoracic vertebra or lower. Higher cervical injury necessitates more dependency and support for daily life. National education initiatives and prevention programs, such as vehicle restraint use, firearms safety, and sports injury safety, are designed to be preemptive deterrents to traumatic SCI. These strategies have proven to be successful in reducing preventable spine trauma.

Mechanisms of injury for patients seeking care in emergency departments typically include trauma related to accidents, athletics, and violence. Acute complications of chronic SCIs are another reason that patients require emergency services care. Acute SCIs have both a primary and secondary component. A primary injury is the initial injury to the cord and/or spinal column. The secondary injury is caused by bleeding, swelling, and ischemia. The majority of cord injuries are cervical, with the fewest injuries being thoracic-level injuries. Approximately 20% of traumatic cervical injuries results in complete quadriplegia. Common SCI complications consist of autonomic dysreflexia, bladder infection, respiratory dysfunction, and problematic sequelae related to sensory loss (Hagan, 2015; Silva, Sousa, Reis, & Salgado, 2014).

Clinical Aspects

ASSESSMENT

Rapid baseline clinical assessment coupled with expeditious verbal and written communication that documents evolving physical improvement or deterioration are key components to providing safe and effective care for patients presenting with SCIs. Until now, communicating changes specific to SCIs has been historically problematic; likely due to the absence of validated tools for such an assessment (Battistuzzo et al., 2016). Obtaining a clear history of the mechanism of injury is important to determining potential unappreciated injuries. It is crucial to monitor temperature, blood pressure, ventilation, and other real or potential complications when caring for a spinal cord–injured patient. Interventions to prevent infection and monitoring for early indications of infection are also important. Providing support to SCI patients in acute psychosocial distress is paramount to future psychosocial outcomes. Secondary cord injuries can precipitate worsening symptoms rapidly or over a period of weeks (Silva et al., 2014).

NURSING INTERVENTIONS, MANAGEMENT, AND IMPLICATIONS

Stabilization of the spinal column and cord is one of the highest patient care priorities if not already accomplished before triage. The only treatments currently available for SCI are stabilization and/or decompression of the spinal cord by either surgical or pharmacologic means. Neither of these interventions have been conclusively determined to be more preferential than the other. Methylprednisolone is the most commonly prescribed medication for acute SCIs in clinical practice, but this corticosteroid therapy is also highly controversial (Silva et al., 2014). There are multiple drug studies in progress to investigate the effects of medications, such as naloxone, monosialotetrahexosylganglioside (GM-1), minocycline, and thyrotropin-releasing hormone (TRH), on SCI treatment outcomes.

Serial recording of assessments, occurring hourly at a minimum during the acute phase, and additional assessments if deterioration is suspected, or the patient has been moved substantially (i.e., transported, rolled) are imperative to patient safety. Close scrutiny of vital signs is crucial since symptoms of autonomic dysreflexia are common in SCIs and can be fatal. Severe respiratory complications, such as atelectasis, pneumonia, and respiratory failure, are evidenced in 67% of acute SCI patients (Hagan, 2015). Pulmonary toileting and bronchodilator administration are common orders requiring nursing intervention for SCI patients. The goal of these interventions is to prevent respiratory insufficiency or failure. Cardiovascular assessment is necessary as the spinal cord-injured patient is predisposed to hypotension. The nurse should anticipate managing hypotension with volume resuscitation and administration of vasopressors. Increased predisposition to thromboembolism due to venous stasis and physical inactivity is also a concern for these patients. Deep vein thrombosis (DVT) prophylaxis measures should be anticipated. Bradycardia is sometimes present in the acute phase, but most patients adapt over time. Poikilothermia is more commonly noted with cervical level injuries and complete motor loss injuries (Hagan, 2015). Monitor and adjust environmental temperature as needed to stabilize core temperatures. Core temperature measurement may be accomplished by obtaining rectal temperatures unless continuous core temperature monitoring has been instituted. Bladder decompression is necessary to prevent urinary retention, thus requiring early Foley catheter insertion during the acute phase. Abdominal assessment for distention, and bowel elimination monitoring are necessary to detect development of an ileus or constipation. Distention of the bladder or bowel may result in acute autonomic dysreflexia. Frequent range-of-motion exercises and antispasmodic administration help to prevent contractures. Dermatologic problems associated with skin breakdown may be prevented by providing frequent, thorough skin care and assessment. Repositioning every 2 hours, weight shifting every 30 minutes whenever the patient is upright; and paying particular attention to bony prominences and areas beneath splints or braces are imperative to skin protection (Hagan, 2015). Psychological stress, depression, and anxiety are all commonly associated with this stressful life event. Current life situations, including social stability, employment status, social and family support availability, and financial security, are variables that warrant consideration while evaluating the level of stress response in individual patients. Facilitating therapeutic engagements that include all members of the patient's professional team may prove to assist the patients in their psychological rehabilitation (Hagan, 2015).

Autonomic dysreflexia (AD) or hyperreflexia is a medical emergency and one that is not uncommon in SCIs at the level of T6 and higher. It is a serious complication affecting both acute and long-term spinal cord-injured patients. Complications of this phenomena include stroke, seizures, myocardial infarction, and possible death (Hagan, 2015; Wan & Krassioukov, 2014). Autonomic dysreflexia causes a sudden onset of blood pressure elevation. In the setting of a spinal cord-injured patient and the typically lower normal blood pressure to which they adapt, it is important to consider AD even in the case of a "normal" blood pressure. This response may provide early evidence of an underlying instigating problem. Comparing an elevation in blood pressure to a patient's typical baseline blood pressure is the best method to identify early onset of AD. The clinical syndrome of AD is precipitated by a stimulus lower than the level of cord injury. Overfull bladder, constipation, pressure sores, other musculoskeletal injuries, tight clothing or device pressure, and sexual stimulation are all examples of possible precipitating circumstances.

OUTCOMES

It is not common for a patient with acute SCI to have concomitant injuries that require urgent attention. If not addressed, these injuries may have synergistic negative impact on ultimate rehabilitation. Traumatic brain injury, extremity fractures, and pneumohemothorax are often companion injuries of SCI. Timely interventions and expedited transfer to a specialty medical center are associated with better long-term outcomes for the patients (Hagan, 2015).

Summary

Patients sustaining SCIs are common presentations in emergency departments. Nurses play a vital role in close assessment with particular attention to early identification of potential complications, care, and treatment for these patients. Providing skillful nursing interventions with caring compassion creates optimal conditions for the transitional life experience for SCI patients.

Battistuzzo, C., Smith, K., Skeers, P., Armstrong, A., Clark, J., Agostinello, J., . . . Batchelor, P. (2016). Early rapid neurological assessment for acute spinal cord injury trials. *Journal of Neurotrauma, 33*(21), 1936–1945.

Crutcher, C., Ugiliweneza, B., Hodes, J., Kong, M., & Boakye, M. (2014). Alcohol intoxication and its effect on spinal cord injury outcomes. *Journal of Neurotrauma, 31*(9), 798–802.

Hagan, E. (2015). Acute complications of spinal cord injuries. *World Journal of Orthopedics, 18*(6), 17–23.

Ma, V., Chan, L., & Carruthers, K. (2014). Incidence, prevalence, costs, and impact on disability of common conditions requiring rehabilitation in the United States: Stroke, spinal cord injury, traumatic brain injury, multiple sclerosis, osteoarthritis, rheumatoid arthritis, limb loss, and back pain. *Archives of Physical Medicine and Rehabilitation, 95*, 986–995.

National Spinal Cord Injury Statistical Center. (2015). *Facts and figures at a glance.* Birmingham, AL: National Spinal Cord Injury Statistical Center, University of Alabama at Birmingham.

Silva, N., Sousa, N., Reis, R., & Salgado, A. (2014). From basics to clinical: A comprehensive review on spinal cord injury. *Progress in Neurobiology, 114,* 25–57.

Wan, D., & Krassioukov, A. (2014). Life-threatening outcomes associated with autonomic dysreflexia: A clinical review. *Journal of Spinal Cord Medicine, 37*(1), 2–10.

■ SUBSTANCE USE DISORDERS AND TOXICOLOGICAL AGENTS

Al Rundio

Overview

The purpose of this entry is to discuss the major substances of abuse, common street names of substances that are abused, and the most prevailing clinical effects. Common toxidromes encountered in emergency situations are also described.

Background

Substance use disorders have been a problem in the U.S. society for some time now. Under President Richard Nixon the Controlled Substances Act of 1970 was enacted, which established the Drug Enforcement Agency (DEA), as an attempt to control substance abuse in the United States (Van Dusen & Spies, 2007). Despite such efforts, the problem continues to grow at an alarming rate.

The United States is dealing with an opiate epidemic. Provider prescribing of opiates for pain control is one of the major factors that contributes to this epidemic. Pain as the fifth vital sign and accrediting bodies' focus on pain control is now being questioned (Rundio, 2013).

The use of benzodiazepines has also increased and many substance users abuse benzodiazepines along with opiates. This synergistic effect is most pronounced on the respiratory system most often causing respiratory depression with resultant cardiac arrest and death.

It has been estimated that the total economic cost of substance use disorders (alcohol, tobacco, and illicit drugs) in the United States exceeds $700 billion annually (National Institute of Drug Abuse [NIDA], 2017). This dollar amount is inclusive of costs related to crime, lost work productivity, and the cost of health care.

The anxiolytic class of substances is becoming more popular among young adults. Alcohol falls in this class as well as benzodiazepines, barbiturates, rohypnol, and GHB (gamma hydroxybutyrate). The common names for these substances include *beer, wine, distilled spirits, Xanax, Valium, roofies,* and *Liquid X.* These substances can be ingested or snorted. The effects from the use of these substances include disorientation, poor coordination, slurred speech, headache, nausea, vomiting, diarrhea, decreased mental alertness, miosis, hyporeflexia, decreased bowel sounds, hypothermia, hypotension, bradycardia, respiratory depression, and unconsciousness.

The opiate class of drugs are derived directly from the opium poppy and also can be semisynthetic or synthetic in nature. The drugs in this class are morphine and codeine. The semisynthetic opioids are heroin (diacetylmorphine), hydromorphone (Dilaudid), oxycodone (Percocet, OxyContin) and hydrocodone (Loricet, Vicodin). The synthetic opioids are methadone, fentanyl, meperidine (Demerol), and propoxyphene (Darvocet). Common street names for these drugs are *junk, H, dope, smack, chiba, tar, brown sugar, chiva, white horse, skag, dragon*, and *white*. These drugs are primarily used via nasal insufflation and direct intravenous injection. Medically, they are used as pain killers with the exception of heroin. The drugs block pain and produce euphoria. They are highly addictive.

The effects of use of these drugs include decreased mental alertness, miosis, hyporeflexia, hypothermia, hypotension, bradycardia, decreased bowel sounds, respiratory depression, and death.

Overdoses may result from variability in the potency of the heroin purchased on the street, rapid loss of tolerance after abstinence, and concurrent use of other central nervous system depressants, for example, heroin is now being laced with fentanyl, which is responsible for many deaths.

The stimulant class of drugs includes cocaine, crack cocaine, amphetamines, methamphetamine, and MDMA (methylene dioxymethamphetamine). Common names are *coke, blow, crack, rock, speed, uppers, cross tops, ectasy, XTC, X, club drug, rolls, love drug*, and *Adam*. These drugs can be snorted, smoked, injected, or ingested.

The effects of use of these drugs are alertness, a false sense of power, tachycardia, elevated blood pressure (BP), itchy skin, compulsive tooth grinding, tachycardia, weight loss, hallucinations, nausea, insomnia, and an elevated body temperature.

The common names for tetrahydrocannabinol (THC) or cannabis is marijuana or hashish. Street names include *weed, pot, grass, bud, joints, bong hits, hash*, and *hash oil*. This class of drugs is usually smoked. The effects of use of cannabis include poor concentration, short-term memory loss, anxiety, and increased appetite. Although many individuals feel that THC should be legalized for use, it causes profound effects most noted on the adolescent brain. This class of drugs is often used by adolescents as well as others in society.

One of the more common toxidromes are the anticholinergics (antimuscarinics). This class of drugs include antihistamines, antiparkinsonian agents, antipsychotics, tricycle antidepressants, mydriatics, antispasmodics, and plants with atropine, for example, *Datura stramonium* (malpitte).

These drugs are primarily ingested.

The effects of use of these substances include delirium, dilated pupils, seizures, elevated temperature, tachycardia, urinary retention, decreased bowel movements, dry skin, flushed skin, myclonus, cardiac dysrhythmias (van Hoving, Veale, & Müller, 2011).

The other common toxidromes are the cholinergics (muscarinic and nicotine receptor stimulation). Common agents are organophosphate and carbamate pesticides (e.g., household, garden, and farm insecticides). These drugs are primarily ingested. The effects include confusion, central nervous system (CNS) depression, miosis, seizures, muscle fasiculations, muscle weakness (including respiratory muscles), diaphoresis, salivation, lacrimation, bronchorrhoea, and pulmonary edema (Hoving et al., 2011).

Clinical Aspects

ASSESSMENT

Assessment of substance use disorders follows general assessment guidelines for nursing with additional key components. These components include obtaining an accurate history on the type of substance used, the method of use, the frequency of use, and the last time used. It is also important to assess whether the patient is sharing needles and other paraphernalia as such behaviors may lead to other types of illnesses such as HIV, hepatitis A, B, and C. As substance abusers also present with other comorbidities (psychological and/or medical) assessing for such comorbidities is critical. Many substance abusers have an underlying depression and may be suicidal. Assessment of suicide ideation and plan are necessary in the initial assessment and ongoing assessments.

NURSING INTERVENTIONS, MANAGEMENT, AND IMPLICATIONS

Nursing must complete accurate and timely ongoing assessment especially when one is in the detoxification stage of treatment. Accurately recording vital signs with specific attention to alertness and respirations is essential. Use of clinical withdrawal scales, such as the COWS (Clinical Opiate Withdrawal Scale) for opiates and the CIWA (Clinical Institute Withdrawal Alcohol Scale) for alcohol and benzodiazepines is necessary. These scales rate objective criteria for how symptomatic a patient is. The administering of detoxification medications is based on defined parameters from these scales and approved by the treatment facility's medical staff.

Benzodiazepines are generally prescribed for detoxification from alcohol and benzodiazepines. Such medications include Librium, Ativan, Serax, or Valium. Buprenorphine or a combination of buprenorphine with naloxone (Suboxone) is used for opiate withdrawal. Naloxone is administered for opiate overdose situations. Cannabis (THC) and the stimulant class of drugs generally do not require specific detoxification medications.

OUTCOMES

The ability of the nurse to not only identify persons potentially or actually abusing substances but also have an understanding of the effects the substances have on the body is beneficial for assisting the patient to be successful with interventions and rehabilitation. It can be difficult to manage a person using substances that can be lethal and toxic but the nurse needs to do his or her best to assist the patient through the process. Advocating for patients through interdisciplinary team approached care is optimal for positive patient outcomes.

Summary

The goal of treatment is to have the patient detox safely and engage in other necessary treatment modalities such as individual and group counseling, psychotherapy and attendance at 12-step meetings. As substance use disorders are considered chronic illnesses, monitoring the patient's recovery for long-term maintenance of sobriety is necessary. Recovery systems of care must be implemented.

National Institute of Drug Abuse. (2017). Trends and statistics. Retrieved from https://www.drugabuse.gov/related-topics/trends-statistics.

Van Dusen, V., & Spies, A. R. (2007). An overview and update of the controlled substances act of 1970. *Pharmacy Times*. Retrieved from http://www.pharmacytimes.com/publications/issue/2007/2007-02/2007-02-6309

van Hoving, D. J., Veale, D. J. H. & Müller, G. F. (2011). Clinical review: Emergency management of acute poisoning. *African Journal of Emergency Medicine*, 1(2), 69–78.

■ THORACIC AORTIC ANEURYSM

Megan M. Shifrin
Ronald L. Hickman, Jr.

Overview

Thoracic aortic aneurysms (TAAs) remain one of the most life-threatening conditions in adult patients with atherosclerosis. Prompt preoperative diagnosis of expanding or ruptured aortic aneurysms is critical to improving patient morbidity and mortality. High-quality nursing care across the perioperative continuum is critical to ensure optimal outcomes in patients living with a TAA.

Background

Aortic aneurysms have been traditionally defined as permanent, localized dilation of at least 50% of the expected diameter of the aortic artery (Abraha, Romagnoli, Montedori, & Cirocchi, 2016). However, several organizations have favored using objective numerical measurements to standardize criteria for evaluation and intervention (Erbel et al., 2014; Hiratzka et al., 2010). Aortic aneurysms can be broadly divided into two separate categories based on location: TAA and abdominal aortic aneurysm (AAA). Major morbidity and mortality associated with both TAAs and AAAs stems from aortic dissection and aortic rupture (Abraha et al., 2016; Erbel et al., 2014; Hiratzka et al., 2010; Vapnik et al., 2016).

TAAs are typically associated medial degeneration along with a host of acute and chronic conditions that affect the integrity of the vessel wall of the thoracic aorta. Medial degeneration is an inflammatory process that results in the production of free oxygen radicals and proinflammatory cytokines that contribute to the degradation of proteins and smooth muscle apoptosis. The end result of medial degeneration is the loss of the medial elastic lamellae and thinning of the tunica media of the aortic arterial wall. These pathophysiologic alterations in the integrity of the ascending aortic arterial wall make the affected area susceptible to the wall strain due to the velocity and hydrostatic pressure of the blood flowing through the thoracic aorta. Chronic hypertension creates higher than normal mechanical and shear forces that contribute to the weakening of the thoracic aortic vessel wall. In addition to medial degeneration and chronic hypertension, other processes that weaken and cause damage to the vessel are atherosclerosis of the thoracic aortic vessel, infections (e.g., syphilis), collagen disorders (e.g., Marfan syndrome), and traumatic injury to the chest. There is also emerging evidence of the gene polymorphisms that enhance an individual's susceptibility to the development of a TAA.

TAAs encompass aneurysms that occur in the ascending aorta, aortic arch, and descending aorta to the level of the diaphragm. Risk factors for TAAs include hypertension, Marfan syndrome, bicuspid aortic valve, genetic predisposition, and atherosclerosis (Abraha et al., 2016). TAAs have an incidence of 10.4

per 100,000 (Abraha et al., 2016). Patients with a TAA diameter greater than 50 mm who also have preexisting risk factors and a rapid aneurysmal expansion should be considered for surgical intervention (Erbel et al., 2014; Hiratzka et al., 2010). The reported 5-year mortality risk for patients with TAAs greater than 60 mm ranges from 38% to 64%. However, once a TAA has ruptured, reported mortality rates have been reported as high as 97% (Abraha et al., 2016). Acutely symptomatic patients with a history of TAA should undergo expedited radiographic imaging to assess the need for emergent surgical intervention to lower their morbidity and mortality risk.

Clinical Aspects

ASSESSMENT

Patients who present with a TAA should be carefully assessed for neurovascular, cardiac, and pulmonary complications. In particular, the nurse should assess for the presence or absence of pain or chest pressure. From a neurovascular standpoint, patients with a TAA are at a risk for neuralgic pain and ipsilateral dilation of the pain, which may result in nerve compression. In addition, patients may experience dyspnea, cough, hoarseness, and dysphagia due to aneurysmal compression on the laryngeal nerve and esophagus, or displacement of the trachea, which should be assessed. Given the pathophysiology of the TAA, nurses should assess for blood pressure variations between arms and dilated superficial veins of the chest wall, which are indicators of compromised systemic circulation.

There are several diagnostic tests that can help the nurse and the health care team inform the care of the patient with a TAA. An initial workup for a patient suspected to have a TAA may include chest radiographs, which indicate calcification of the affected aorta and establish the presence of an aneurysm. A CT scan or magnetic resonance angiography (MRA) are often used to monitor the size of the aneurysm and evaluate the arterial circulation, respectively.

NURSING INTERVENTIONS, MANAGEMENT, AND IMPLICATIONS

Patients who have a TAA are at high risk for developing neurovascular complications in the postoperative period. Maintaining meticulous care of patients with lumbar drains and maintaining hemodynamic goals may help prevent neurovascular complications. For patients with a TAA repair, neurological status and extremity sensation, movement, and strength should be assessed hourly in the immediate postoperative period (Cronenwett & Johnston, 2014). Change in a patient's neurological exam, paresthesia, or paralysis may be indicative of a compromise in vascular perfusion. Immediate notification of the vascular surgical team is warranted in these circumstances (Cronenwett & Johnston, 2014).

Patients with a TAA frequently vacillate between hypotensive to hypertensive states, and thus, should be monitored closely. Patients with hypotension tend to be at higher risk for end-organ ischemia and vascular occlusion. Volume resuscitation with crystalloid intravenous fluids combined intravenous vasopressors remains a mainstay of treatment (Chen & Crozier, 2014; Cronenwett & Johnston, 2014). For patients with hypertension, intravenous beta-1 agonists and calcium channel blockers may be administered. If a patient is also at high risk for developing a postoperative myocardial infarction or has objective findings indicative of an evolving myocardial infarction, nitrates may also be considered for hypertensive management (Chen & Crozier, 2014; Cronenwett & Johnston, 2014).

Following either open or endovascular repair of a TAA, acute blood loss anemia and coagulopathy are common. Potential coagulopathies should be quickly evaluated by assessing a patient's prothrombin time (PT)/international normalized ratio (INR), activated partial thromboplastin time (aPTT), fibrinogen, platelet count, and platelet function; the administration of products, such as fresh frozen plasma, cryoprecipitate, and pooled platelets, should also be considered (Cronenwett & Johnston, 2014). Packed red blood cells should be administered to patients with a hemoglobin level less than 7 mg/dL who also have signs and symptoms of hemodynamic instability and/or ischemia. Noncoagulopathic causes of acute postoperative anemia include bleeding from the surgical anastomosis site or endovascular leak. Ongoing postoperative bleeding that is not associated with coagulopathy may warrant surgical reexploration (Cronenwett & Johnston, 2014).

In preoperative care settings, the nurses should prioritize their neurovascular, cardiac, and respiratory assessments of patients with acute symptoms of a TAA. Specifically, nurses should monitor for signs and symptoms of worsening chest pain, paresthesia, stroke, dyspnea, and cardiac tamponade. Frequent monitoring of neurologic status, blood pressure, peripheral pulses, respiratory rate, pulse oximetry, and capillary refill is recommended and changes reported.

OUTCOMES

For patients who require a surgical intervention for a repair of a TAA, the nurse should continue to be vigilant in the assessment of the patient's neurovascular, cardiac, and respiratory status. During the immediate postoperative period, monitoring for signs of blood loss and anemia (e.g., hypotension, tachycardia, urine output, and pallor) is recommended. Similar to other populations of surgical patients, the nurse should aim to provide adequate pain management, assess for signs of surgical site infection, and administer prescribed antibiotics in a timely fashion to optimize the patient's postoperative outcomes.

Summary

Expanding and ruptured TAAs are associated with extensive morbidity and mortality. However, prompt diagnosis, surgical and endovascular management, and vigilant critical care nursing management can improve patient outcomes. Ongoing cardiovascular, neurological, and abdominal assessments are of particular importance given the postoperative complications that may occur. Hemodynamic management, coagulopathy evaluation and correction, and volume resuscitation are also mainstays of effective postoperative treatment.

Abraha, I., Romagnoli, C., Montedori, A., & Cirocchi, R. (2016). Thoracic stent graft versus surgery for thoracic aneurysm. *Cochrane Database of Systematic Reviews, 2016*(6). doi:10.1002/14651858.CD006796.pub4

Chen, T., & Crozier, J. A. (2014). Endovascular repair of thoracic aortic pathologies: Postoperative nursing implications. *Journal of Vascular Nursing, 32*(2), 63–69. doi:10.1016/j.jvn.2013.07.001

Cronenwett, J. L., & Johnston, K. W. (2014). *Rutherford's vascular surgery* (8th ed.). Philadelphia, PA: Elsevier Saunders.

Erbel, R., Aboyans, V., Boileau, C., Bossone, E., Di Bartolomeo, R., Eggebrecht, H., . . . Vlachopoulos, C. (2014). 2014 ESC guidelines on the diagnosis and treatment of aortic diseases. *European Heart Journal, 35*(41), 2873–2926. doi:10.1093/eurheartj/ehu281

Hiratzka, L. F., Bakris, G. L., Beckman, J. A., Bersin, R. M., Carr, V. F., Casey, D. E., . . . Williams, D. M. (2010). 2010 ACCF/AHA/AATS/ACR/ASA/SCA/SCAI/SIR/STS/SVM guidelines for the diagnosis and management of patients with thoracic aortic disease: Executive summary. *Journal of the American College of Cardiology, 55*(14), 1509–1544. doi:10.1016/j.jacc.2010.02.010

Vapnik, J. S., Kim, J. B., Isselbacher, E. M., Ghoshhajra, B. B., Cheng, Y., Sundt, T. M., . . . Lindsay, M. E. (2016). Characteristics and outcomes of ascending versus descending thoracic aortic aneurysms. *American Journal of Cardiology, 117*(10), 1683–1690. doi:10.1016/j.amjcard.2016.02.048

■ THROMBOCYTOPENIA IN ADULTS

Khoa (Joey) Dang

Overview

Thrombocytopenia is a common and potentially life-threatening condition in which there is a decrease in platelet count within the circulating blood volume. Adults can develop thrombocytopenia from various causes, including bone marrow suppression from radiation or chemotherapy, liver failure, disseminated intravascular coagulation, bacterial or viral infections, autoimmune disorders, and various medication effects (Chavan, Chauhan, Joshi, Ojha, & Bhat, 2014; Hunt, 2014).

Background

Thrombocytopenia is identified as a platelet count below the lower limit of normal of 150,000/μL (normal range 150,000–450,000/μL), based on most laboratory standards (Sekhon & Roy, 2006). Platelets are developed from the fragmentation of megakaryocytes and circulate in the blood for a week to 10 days. Thrombocytopenia can be caused from various conditions and can be associated with different degrees of risk from life-threatening bleeding to no risk of complications.

Thrombocytopenia can result from pathophysiologic mechanisms of platelet destruction and consumption, bone marrow disease, dilutional processes, and splenic disorders. Patients who present without symptoms are more likely to have immune thrombocytopenia, also known as *idiopathic thrombocytopenic purpura (ITP)*. However, patients who are acutely ill with symptoms of thrombocytopenia typically have multisystem involvement with etiologies of infection/sepsis, nutritional deficiencies, autoimmune disease, drug-induced thrombocytopenia (such as in heparin-induced thrombocytopenia) or platelet destruction.

In children with thrombocytopenia, the causes can generally be categorized by either platelet-destructive mechanisms or by decreased production of platelets. Platelet-destruction disorders include immune-mediated destruction (such as immune thrombocytopenia), platelet activation and consumption (such as in disseminated intravascular coagulation and thrombotic thrombocytopenic purpura), drug-induced thrombocytopenia, mechanical destruction (from the use of extracorporeal therapies), and sequestration and trapping (such as with hypersplenism). Thrombocytopenia caused from decreased platelet production can occur with infection (usually from suppression of bone marrow or immune mediated process), bone marrow disorders, deficiencies from poor nutrition, and genetic conditions.

The prevalence of thrombocytopenia is determined based on the underlying etiology causing the low platelet count. The most recent estimates of ITP show a prevalence exceeding incidence and that ITP affects all ages, with approximately eight per 100,000 cases in children and 12 in 100,000 in adults (Terrell et al., 2008). With drug-induced immune thrombocytopenia, the estimated incidence is 10 cases per million population per year and accounts for approximately 20% to 25% (when combined with ITP and TTP) of all blood disorders (Kam & Alexander, 2014). Thrombocytopenia occurrence in pregnancy is common with many etiologies and not always clinically relevant. The most common cause of thrombocytopenia during pregnancy, with rates as high as 5% of all pregnant women, is gestational thrombocytopenia (Kasai et al., 2015).

Bleeding risk is the main concern with patients who have thrombocytopenia and spontaneous hemorrhage is considered when other factors exist, such as previous history of bleeding, other coagulopathies, and platelet-function defects. Although there are no evidence-based recommendations on what is considered a safe platelet count, clinical judgment and history of prior bleeding should be evaluated to determine bleeding risk. There appears to be no correlation between the risk of spontaneous bleeding and specific platelet counts.

Clinical Aspects

ASSESSMENT

A thorough patient history is crucial in determining other conditions that may explain thrombocytopenia in both inpatient and outpatient settings. Individualized, patient-centered nursing care begins with obtaining a complete history, performing a full physical assessment/exam, and evaluating pertinent laboratory data. The history data should be obtained from sources, including the patient, other medical records, family members of the patient, and other clinicians who have cared for the patient. Important historical data helpful in managing the patient include prior platelet counts, history of bleeding or blood dyscrasias, infectious exposures (viral, bacterial, rickettsial) or recent travel to endemic areas, dietary practices, medication exposures (such as heparin, aspirin, anticoagulants, sulfa-containing medications, etc.), family history of bleeding disorders or thrombocytopenia, and other medical conditions (such as auto-immune disorders, rheumatological diseases, malignancies, blood transfusions, etc.). A thorough physical exam can provide important information on potential causes of the thrombocytopenia (such as hepatomegaly and lymphadenopathy) and should be focused on identifying signs of bleeding. Bleeding-related changes in the skin and other sites of bleeding include purpura (bleeding into skin), petechiae, or ecchymosis. Marking the skin bleeding by circumscribing the area is helpful to assess and document the extent of bleeding and determine the persistence or worsening of thrombocytopenia. The liver, spleen, and lymph nodes should be palpated for enlargement and pain; these signs can denote a specific etiology of thrombocytopenia. Additional physical assessments in the following areas can evaluate new-onset or worsening of bleeding: cardiovascular (hypotension, tachycardia, dizziness or epistaxis), pulmonary (tachypnea, hemoptysis or respiratory distress), gastrointestinal (hematemesis, abdominal discomfort or distension, rectal bleeding), genitourinary (vaginal or urethral bleeding), and neurological (headache, changes in vision, altered level of consciousness). The full nursing assessment/exam must be performed every shift with focused bleeding risk assessments throughout the shift to determine worsening physical status and to evaluate any new onset of bleeding.

Laboratory monitoring of a complete blood count (CBC) with an emphasis on the platelet count, hemoglobin and hematocrit, and white blood count (WBC) is important to determine bleeding risks, severity of acute bleeding, acute infections, and the possibility of systemic disorders. Blood crossmatch and typing are recommended if a blood transfusion is anticipated in the setting of severe anemia secondary to acute blood loss. Testing of urine, stool, and emesis for occult blood is advised to evaluate for systemic bleeding from thrombocytopenia.

NURSING INTERVENTIONS, MANAGEMENT, AND IMPLICATIONS

The nursing care of a patient with thrombocytopenia should be focused on decreasing the risk of bleeding and reducing complications of active bleeding. Additional responsibilities should include managing underlying conditions attributed to thrombocytopenia and providing support to the systems affected by thrombocytopenia.

The nursing care interventions are aimed at decreasing bleeding complications of thrombocytopenia. Performing physical assessments and reassessments at regular intervals allows for early identification of hemorrhaging and alerts providers to initiate appropriate medical management. Other interventions to prevent complications include avoiding medications that worsen bleeding (such as anticoagulants), avoiding certain routes of medication administration (such as intramuscular injections and suppositories), using stool softeners or laxatives to prevent constipation, applying direct pressure to venipuncture sites for at least 5 minutes or until the bleeding ceases, avoiding unnecessary suctioning (oral, nasotracheal, and endotracheal), preventing falls by ambulatory patients, and administering blood products (such as platelets, packed red blood cells, and fresh frozen plasma) as prescribed (Winkeljohn, 2013).

OUTCOMES

A nursing evaluation for risk of bleeding from activity should be also be included in the nursing interventions. Health education and patient teaching should address signs and symptoms of disease exacerbation, medication therapy, activity restrictions (if applicable), diet selection that does not contribute to platelet reduction, and routine monitoring of platelet count. Careful evaluation, interventions, and education promote positive outcomes in these patients.

Summary

Nursing care for thrombocytopenia should coordinate medical management with nursing interventions to decrease morbidity and mortality. General management principles apply to all patients with thrombocytopenia, regardless of etiology: activity restrictions in moderate to severe thrombocytopenia (less than 50,000/µL), antiplatelet medication avoidance, avoiding invasive procedures if platelet count is low, and management of bleeding. Nursing management of thrombocytopenia requires performing accurate assessment and evaluation of severity of disease, developing nursing care objectives, implementing timely treatment strategies and nursing interventions, and ongoing appraisal and revision of nursing care goals.

Chavan, P., Chauhan, B., Joshi, A., Ojha, S., & Bhat, V. (2014). Differential diagnosis of thrombocytopenia in hematopoietic stem cell transplant patients. *Journal of Hematology & Thromboembolic Diseases, 2*, 168. doi:10.4172/2329–8790.1000168

Hunt, B. J. (2014). Bleeding and coagulopathies in critical care. *New England Journal of Medicine, 370*(22), 2153. doi:10.1056/NEJMc1403768

Kam, T., & Alexander, M. (2014). Drug-induced immune thrombocytopenia. *Journal of Pharmacy Practice, 27*(5), 430–439. doi:10.1177/0897190014546099

Kasai, J., Aoki, S., Kamiya, N., Hasegawa, Y., Kurasawa, K., Takahashi, T., & Hirahara, F. (2015). Clinical features of gestational thrombocytopenia difficult to differentiate from immune thrombocytopenia diagnosed during pregnancy. *Journal of Obstetrics and Gynaecology Research, 41*(1), 44–49. doi:10.1111/jog.12496

Sekhon, S. S., & Roy, V. (2006). Thrombocytopenia in adults: A practical approach to evaluation and management. *Southern Medical Journal, 99*(5), 491–498; quiz 499. doi:10.1097/01.smj.0000209275.75045.d4

Terrell, D., Beebe, L. A., George, J., Neas, B. R., Vesely, S. K., & Segal, J. (2008). The prevalence of immune thrombocytopenic purpura (ITP). *Blood, 112*(11), 1277–1277.

Winkeljohn, D. (2013). Diagnosis, treatment, and management of immune thrombocytopenia. *Clinical Journal of Oncology Nursing, 17*(6), 664–666. doi:10.1188/13.CJON.664-666

■ THYROID CRISIS

Cynthia Ann Leaver

Overview

Thyroid crisis, also known as *thyrotoxic crisis, thyroid storm,* or *hyperthyroid storm,* is an acute, life-threatening exacerbation of thyrotoxicosis (De Groot & Bartalena, 2015; Ross et al., 2016). Thyroid crisis occurs in the presence of thyrotoxicosis, in which an individual's ability to maintain adequate metabolic, thermoregulatory, and cardiovascular compensatory mechanism is surpassed (Warnock, Cooper, & Burch, 2014). Thyroid crisis ranks as one of the most critical endocrine emergencies and requires immediate recognition and steadfast commitment to an aggressive, therapeutic, and multifaceted intervention to prevent the high morbidity and mortality associated with the disorder (Angell et al., 2015; Ross et al., 2016; Warnock et al., 2014). It is noteworthy that the American Thyroid Association recommends the diagnosis of thyroid storm as a clinical diagnosis that is augmented by the use of sensitive empiric diagnostic systems (Burch-Wartofsky Point Scale [BWPS] or the Japanese Thyroid Association criteria). Nursing care of the patient with thyroid crisis requires rapid assessment and intervention for multisystem decompensation (Ross et al., 2016).

Background

Thyroid crisis is one on the most critical endocrine emergencies; incidence for patients hospitalized for thyrotoxicosis, progressing to thyroid crisis, is identified to be less than 10% (Warnock et al., 2014). However, the mortality rate due to thyroid crisis ranges from 8% to 25% (De Leo, Lee, & Braverman, 2016; Ross et al., 2016). An apparent trigger of thyroid crisis can be identified in up to 70% of cases (De Leo et al., 2016). In the past, thyroid crisis most frequently occurred after surgery for thyrotoxicosis. Today, with earlier diagnosis and treatment of thyrotoxicosis, and improvement in pre- and postoperative medical management, postoperative thyroid crisis is now a rare occurrence (De Groot & Bartalena, 2015). Currently, the most common underlying cause of thyrotoxicosis progression to thyroid crisis is Graves' disease (80%), and it is notable that Graves' disease occurs most frequently in young women, but can occur in either gender and any age group (Carroll & Matfin, 2010).

Thyroid crisis represents the extreme manifestations of thyrotoxicosis, in which factors have provoked progression on the thyrotoxic continuum (De Groot & Bartalena, 2015; Warnock et al., 2014). The spectrum of thyrotoxicosis ranges from asymptomatic, subclinical, to life-threatening thyroid crisis. *Hyperthyroidism* refers to disorders that result from overproduction of hormone from the thyroid gland, *thyrotoxicosis* refers to any case of excessive thyroid hormone concentration, and *thyroid crisis* is the severely thyrotoxic patient with systemic decompensation. The factors impacting thyrotoxicity include age, comorbidities, rapid onset of hormone excess, and presence or absence of precipitating event (Warnock et al., 2014). Therefore, management of thyroid storm is broadly divided into therapy directed against thyroid hormone secretion, synthesis, and action at the tissue level; reversal of systemic decompensation, and treatment of the precipitating event (Ross et al., 2016).

Normal thyroid function is maintained by endocrine interactions among the hypothalamus, anterior pituitary, and thyroid gland (Carroll & Matfin, 2010). Iodide is transported across the basement membrane of the thyroid cells by an intrinsic membrane protein (Na/I symporter). Then, at the apical boarder, a second iodide transport protein (pendirin) moves iodide into the colloid, where iodide is involved in hormonogenesis of thyroxine (T4) and triiodothyronine (T3). Thyroxine (T4) is the major thyroid hormone secreted into the circulation. Circulating thyroid hormone consists of 90% T4, and 10% T3. (Carroll & Matfin, 2010). There is evidence that T4 is converted to T3 before it can act physiologically, therefore making T3 the active form of circulating thyroid hormone.

The precise pathogenesis of thyroid crisis is still poorly understood (De Leo et al., 2016). One hypothesis to explain the pathogenesis of thyroid crisis is an increase in the amount of free thyroid hormones. One study found mean T4 concentration was higher in subjects with thyroid crisis, whereas the total T4 concentration was similar in both study groups (De Groot & Bartalena, 2015). Another theory that may explain the pathogenesis of thyroid crisis is a possible increase in target cell beta-adrenergic receptor density or postreceptor modification in signaling pathways (Nayak & Burman, 2006).

Ross et al. (2016) identified general impetuses for thyrotoxicosis to be excessive thyroid stimulation by trophic factors; thyroid hormone synthesis and secretion, leading to autonomous release of excess thyroid hormone; thyroid stores of performed hormone are passively released in excessive amounts owing to autoimmune, infectious, chemical, or mechanical insult; or exposure to extrathyroidal sources of thyroid hormone, which may be either endogenous (struma ovarii, metastatic differentiated thyroid cancer) or exogenous (factitious thyrotoxicosis). Consequently, thyrotoxicosis provoked by age, comorbidities, rapid onset of hormone excess, and presence or absence of precipitating event may lead to thyroid crisis (Carroll & Matfin, 2010; Warnock et al., 2014).

Clinical Aspects

ASSESSMENT

The important clinical point in effective nursing care of a patient considered for potential thyroid crisis is to assess and treat in an active, preemptory fashion when possible. The distinction between severe thyrotoxicosis and thyroid crisis is a matter of clinical judgment.

Nursing care of thyroid crisis is to include history, physical assessment, and laboratory data. Accurate history of an individual who is suspected to have thyroid crisis must include query into any condition predisposing the individual to risk of thyrotoxicosis and reported for medical treatment.

The physical assessment should focus on general organ decompensation and changes in the following body systems should include fever 102.2°F or higher; respiratory system (tachypnea greater than 20 breaths/minute, breath sounds reveal signs and symptoms consistent with congestive heart failure to include bibasilar rales and crackles); cardiovascular system (systolic hypertension or hypotension; tachycardia and disproportionate to the degree of fever; bounding pulses, systolic murmur, widening pulse or weak thready pulses; peripheral edema); neurologic system (agitation, delirium, psychosis, tremors, seizures, extreme lethargy, or coma); gastrointestinal system (increase in bowel sounds, diarrhea, nausea/vomiting, or abdominal pain, and possible jaundice); and endocrine system (enlarged or nodular thyroid). Assessment of diagnostic data is to be followed astutely for indications of progression or recovery of thyroid crises.

NURSING INTERVENTIONS, MANAGEMENT, AND IMPLICATIONS

Nursing care of the patient with possible thyroid crisis should principally focus on management of the ABCDEs (i.e., airway, breathing, circulation; disability, i.e., level of consciousness; and examination). Priority nursing-related issues include decreased cardiac output related to increased cardiac work secondary to increased adrenergic activity and deficient fluid volume secondary to increased metabolism and diaphoresis.

Nursing management of the patient with thyroid crisis consists of dextrose-containing intravenous fluids as ordered to correct fluid and glucose deficits, assessment for heart failure or pulmonary edema, dopamine may be used to support blood pressure, and supplemental oxygen as ordered to help meet increased metabolic demands.

Once the patient is hemodynamically stable, nursing management comprises pulmonary hygiene to reduce pulmonary complications. If the patient is in heart failure, typical pharmacologic agents for treatment of heart failure may also be indicated. Nursing management must include strategies to reduce oxygen demands by decreasing anxiety, reduce fever, decrease pain, and limit visitors if necessary. Nursing care must anticipate aggressive treatment of precipitating factors and institute pressure ulcer strategies.

OUTCOMES

The expected outcomes of evidence-based nursing care are focused on preventing progression of thyroid crisis. Nursing outcome criteria include continuous monitoring of oxygen saturation with pulse oximetry, lung sounds clear to auscultation, level of consciousness, peripheral pulses palpable and presence of peripheral edema, continuous EKG monitoring for dysthymias or heart rate greater than 140 beats/minute that can adversely affect cardiac output, life-threatening dysrhythmias, ST segment changes indicative of myocardial ischemia, continuous monitoring of pulmonary artery pressure, urine output 30 mL/hr, fluid volume status with hourly urine output and determination of fluid balance every 8 hours, and serial ABGs for hypoxemia and acid–base imbalance.

Summary

Thyroid crisis, also known as *thyrotoxic crisis, thyroid storm,* or *hyperthyroid storm,* is a life-threatening exacerbation of thyrotoxicosis, in the presence of a precipitating factor, and results when an individual's ability to maintain adequate metabolic, thermoregulatory, and cardiovascular compensatory mechanism is surpassed. Immediate recognition and aggressive, therapeutic, and multifaceted intervention to prevent the high morbidity and mortality associated with the disorder are required. Nursing care of patients with thyroid crisis is principally focused on management of ABCDEs, with vigilant assessment for factor precipitating the thyroid crisis.

Angell, T., Lehner, M. G., Nguyen, C. T., Salvato, V. L., Nicoloff, J. T., & LoPtesti, J. S. (2015). Clinical features and hospital outcomes in thyroid storm: A retrospective cohort study. *Journal of Clinical Endocrinology and Metabolism, 100*(2), 451–459. doi:10.1210/jc.2014-2850

Carroll, R., & Matfin, G. (2010). Endocrine and metabolic emergencies: Thyroid storm. *Therapeutic Advances in Endocrinology and Metabolism, 1*(3), 139–145. doi:10.1177/2042018810382481

De Groot L. J., & Bartalena L. (2015). Thyroid storm. In L. J. De Groot, G. Chrousos, K. Dungan, K. R. Feingold, A. Grossman, J. M. Hershman, . . . A. Vinik (Eds.), *Endotext* [Online]. South Dartmouth, MA: MDText. Retrieved from https://www.ncbi.nlm .nih.gov/books/NBK278927

De Leo, S., Lee, S. Y., & Braverman, L. E. (2016). Hyperthyroidism. *Lancet, 27*(388), 906–918. doi:10.1016/S0140-6736(16)00278-6

Nayak, B., & Burnam, K. (2006). Thyrotoxicosis and thyroid storm. *Endocrinology and Metabolism Clinics of North America, 35,* 663–686. doi:10.1016/j.ecl.2006.09.008

Ross, D. S., Burch, H. B., Cooper, M., Greenlee, C., Laurberg, P., Mala, A. L., . . . Walter, M. A. (2016). 2016 American thyroid association guidelines for diagnosis and management of hyperthyroidism and other causes of thyrotoxicosis. *Thyroid, 26*(10), 1343–1422. doi:10.1089/thy.2016.0229

Warnock, A. L., Cooper, D. S., & Burch, H.B. (2014). Life-threatening thyrotoxicosis: Thyroid storm and adverse effects of antithyroid drugs. In G. Matfin (Ed.), *Endocrine and metabolic medical emergencies: Thyroid disorders* (pp. 110–126). Washington, DC: Endocrine Society/Endocrine Press. Retrieved from http://press .endocrine.org/doi/pdf/10.1210/EME.9781936704811.ch11

■ TRAUMATIC BRAIN INJURY

Elizabeth Wirth-Tomaszewski

Overview

Traumatic brain injury (TBI) is the leading cause of trauma-related death and disability worldwide, affecting both adult and pediatric populations significantly. The incidence in the United States is estimated at 1.36 million cases with 52,000 deaths, as well as 275,000 hospitalizations annually (Centers for Disease Control and Prevention [CDC], 2016). Worldwide, TBI remains the leading cause of morbidity and mortality in those aged younger than 45 years (Andersen, Gazmuri, Marin, Regueira, & Rovegno, 2015). TBI encompasses a wide variety of conditions, ranging from mild to life-threatening, and can best be described as an alteration in brain function and/or structure due to external forces such as blunt or penetrating trauma or acceleration/deceleration forces (White & Venkatesh, 2016). Many types of TBI exist, such as concussions, hemorrhages, axonal injuries, and skull fractures, to name a few. These injuries may further be designated as acute, subacute, chronic, or acute on chronic. TBIs also include primary and secondary injury classifications. Nursing implications include the assessment, identification of nursing problems, interventions, evaluation, and prevention of these injuries.

Background

TBIs are defined as a pathological alteration in the function or structure of the brain by way of external forces. These forces can cause friction of the tissue, tearing of the vessels, or axonal injuries at the cellular level that cause impairment of function. Initial injuries are capable of causing secondary injuries, usually due to cerebral edema, increased intracranial pressure (ICP; intracranial hypertension), oxidative stress, excitotoxicity, and seizures. Performing a thorough assessment and performing appropriate intervention, the incidence of secondary brain injuries can be reduced (Andersen et al., 2015).

PREVALENCE OF TBI VARIES BY AGE

Children younger than 4 years of age, adolescents between 15 and 19 years of age, and adults older than the age of 65 years are most often diagnosed with TBI. Children under 14 years of age constitute approximately half of a million emergency department visits annually. Those aged 75 years and older are most likely to incur TBI-related hospitalization and death. TBI is a contributing factor to one third of all injury-related deaths in the United States. Mild TBIs constitute a majority of the reported injuries, with no available data on those who suffer mild TBI and do not seek care. TBI is a costly public health issue, totaling approximately $60 billion per year when accounting for the direct and indirect costs (CDC, 2016).

Mild TBIs, such as concussions, are most prominent and are responsible for 80% of all TBIs. The leading cause of severe TBI is motor vehicle collisions, accounting for 30% to 50% of head injuries, with males aged 15 to 24 years being the demographic most affected. Other risk factors include participation in contact sports, falls, advanced age (due to polypharmacy and sensory losses related to age), and failure to use safety devices, such as helmets, seat belts, and handrails (Garton & Lehmann, 2015). The structural pathology in TBI includes primary and secondary causes, as well as Monro–Kellie hypothesis (equilibrium of pressure and volume of brain structures inside the skull), and Cushing's triad phenomena (irregular respirations, bradycardia, and widening pulse pressure).

Primary TBIs include skull fractures, hemorrhages, contusions, and diffuse axonal injury (DAI). Due to the extreme forces required, there exists high suspicion for concomitant cervical spine injury, and care should be taken to immobilize the spine. Skull fractures may require surgery to repair, or may be medically managed by observation. Hemorrhages are treated differently, depending on type and severity. Epidural hemorrhages are arterial in nature, usually arising from a torn temporal artery and usually require surgical intervention. Subdural hemorrhages are venous in origin, and may require evacuation if there is significant mass effect or deficits noted. Traumatic subarachnoid hemorrhages may require an external ventricular drain (EVD) to be placed to monitor bleeding and ICP. Contusions and DAI are medically monitored (Garton & Lehmann, 2015).

SECONDARY TBI

Secondary TBI includes cytotoxic and/or vasogenic cerebral edema, cellular ischemic injury, and loss of cerebral blood flow regulation, which occurs in response to the primary brain injury. Mechanisms include apoptosis, calcium-dependent cascades, and oxidative stress creating damage at the cellular level. Prevention of hypoperfusion of the brain and increased metabolic demands are key to limiting secondary brain injuries (Andersen et al., 2015; Garton & Lehmann, 2015).

ICP is the result of three components within the skull: the brain tissue, cerebrospinal fluid, and blood. The brain is able to compensate for a small amount of tissue swelling, with displacement of the cerebrospinal fluid (CSF) and blood. When the brain tissue becomes compressed related to its own edema or mass effect from hematomas, blood supply is reduced leading to cerebral hypoperfusion and secondary brain injury. Untreated, this may lead to herniation through foramen magnum (tonsillar herniation) or skull fractures (Garton & Lehmann, 2015).

The constellation of symptoms that many times accompanies herniation is known as *Cushing's triad*. This includes bradycardia, hypertension, and respiratory irregularities. If the patient is intubated and on mechanical ventilation, many times the respiratory pattern goes unnoticed. The presence of Cushing's triad is ominous, and requires immediate attention by the neurosurgical provider. In severe cases of TBI with high ICPs and danger of herniation, decompressive craniectomy (removal of skull bone flap) may be required to allow expansion of the tissue in an effort to preserve life (Garton & Lehmann, 2015).

Clinical Aspects

ASSESSMENT

Obtaining an accurate history of the injury is important, as injury patterns may be identified. For instance, epidural hemorrhages are suspected when there is an initial loss of consciousness, a period of lucidity, and then loss of consciousness once again. Amnesia, nausea, vomiting, headache, vertigo, nuchal rigidity, and vision disturbances are examples of significant findings in those with TBI (Garton & Lehmann, 2015).

In terms of physical assessment, frequent serial neurological exams are key in those diagnosed with TBI. Consistency of those exams between providers is extremely important, and should be performed with both receiving and departing providers present to ensure continuity in method and examination findings. Components of the assessment should include airway patency, adequacy of breathing, blood pressure monitoring parameters, Glasgow Coma Scale scoring, protective reflexes (cough, gag, corneal), pupillary size, equality and reaction, level of consciousness, as well as any focal deficits identified. Changes in exam should promptly be reported to the attending provider or neurosurgeon. Any impairment in airway patency (including loss of gag or cough reflex), ventilation, and/or depression in level of consciousness with a Glasgow Coma Scale score less than 8 requires emergency intervention for airway protection and mechanical ventilation (Garton & Lehmann, 2015).

Nursing problems associated with TBI include alteration in tissue perfusion, potential for alteration in airway patency, potential for seizures, potential for infection (related to monitoring/drainage devices), malnutrition, alteration in skin integrity related to immobility, and alteration in mental status related to acute TBI.

NURSING INTERVENTIONS, MANAGEMENT, AND IMPLICATIONS

Nursing interventions for TBI center on supportive care, prevention of secondary brain injuries, and restoration of homeostasis. For those diagnosed with mild TBI, serial neurological exams may be required for the first few days, with neurology follow-up. In moderate TBI, serial exams and cardiovascular monitoring may be required for close observation. In severe TBI, serial exams and cardiovascular monitoring are required, along with other possible modalities. Intracranial monitoring may be initiated by neurosurgery to facilitate monitoring of cerebral perfusion pressures (CPP) or EVDs employed to monitor and treat elevated ICPs by way of removal of CSF through a conduit placed in the ventricle. EEG may be used if seizures are suspected. Seizure precautions should be instituted by nursing, and antiepileptic drugs may be ordered by neurology on a prophylactic basis (Carney et al., 2016).

Maintenance of normal ventilation is essential in patients mechanically ventilated with severe TBI. Ventilation strategies are aimed at maintaining a normal level of carbon dioxide (CO_2; 35–45 mmHg). Lower CO_2 levels cause cerebral perfusion and ischemia, and higher CO_2 levels cause vasoconstriction and increased ICP.

Temperature-targeted therapy (therapeutic hypothermia) may be instituted to decrease metabolic demands and reduce cytotoxic events associated with cerebral edema. This type of therapy requires the critical care environment and is reserved for those with severe TBI. These patients are intubated, mechanically ventilated, and may require vasopressors to support a blood pressure sufficient enough to maintain cerebral perfusion (Andersen et al., 2015; Carney et al., 2016).

Cerebral edema may also be treated with hyperosmolar therapy in the form of mannitol or hypertonic saline. Both modalities employ osmolar pull to reduce edema in the brain by increasing the osmolality of the serum to pull fluid from this tissue. Mannitol has an additional diuretic component, which can ultimately affect blood pressure and reduce CPP. Hypertonic (3%) saline has been employed for the same osmotic effect, without diuretic properties (Carney et al., 2016).

Central diabetes insipidus is a condition related to antidiuretic hormone deficiency, characterized with large amounts of dilute urine output with low-specific gravity, and high serum osmolality is noted. This condition leads to hypernatremia, and is the body's attempt at hyperosmolar treatment. Desmopressin acetate may be required to control this phenomenon (Fitzgerald, 2017).

OUTCOMES

Goals of therapy include stabilization of primary injury, minimization of secondary injury, and return of homeostasis. Targets should include protecting airway patency and optimal ventilation, minimizing metabolic demands, providing nutrition support, and seizure precautions/prophylaxis. Measureable outcomes include maintaining a mean arterial pressure sufficient to provide cerebral perfusion (CPP = 60–70 mmHg), measureable with monitoring devices such as intracranial bolts or EVDs. ICPs should ideally be maintained at 0 to 10 mmHg. Normoglycemia, fever prevention, and normocarbia are also measureable outcomes that benefit those diagnosed with TBI (Carney et al., 2016).

Prevention is the most valuable of all interventions. Nurses are at the forefront of public health, and are in a position to provide assessment and education to those identified at risk. Nurses should encourage the use of concussion guidelines in sports, promote the use of helmets and other safety devices, and assist in the provision of home safety, medication reconciliation, and sensory screening for elders.

Summary

TBI is a prevalent world health issue and carries significant financial cost, as well as the morbidity and mortality associated with head injuries in many demographics. The long-term sequelae of TBI can last a lifetime, and prevention is the key. The utilization of safety devices and established guidelines in contact sports should be encouraged for all age groups.

TBI can be characterized as primary or secondary, by the acuity, and also by severity. Concussions, contusion, hemorrhages, and cellular injuries are some examples. Maintenance of cerebral perfusion and prevention of secondary injury are paramount in those with TBI. The goals of care are supportive and restorative, with guidelines in place by the Brain Trauma Foundation to guide providers in the care of these very complex patients. An ever-expanding wealth of knowledge is being gained in the area of TBI, and updates to these guidelines occur regularly.

Andersen, M., Gazmuri, J. T., Marin, A., Regueira, T., & Rovegno, M. (2015). Therapeutic hypothermia for acute brain injuries. *Scandinavian Journal of Trauma, Resuscitation, and Emergency Medicine, 23*(42), 1. doi:10.1186/s13049-015-0121-3

Carney, N., Totten, A. M., O'Reilly, C., Ullman, J. S., Hawryluk, G. W. J., Bell, M. J., . . . Ghajar, J. (2016). *Guidelines for management of traumatic brain injury* (4th ed.). Retrieved from https://braintrauma.org/uploads/03/12/Guidelines_for_Management_of_Severe_TBI_4th_Edition.pdf

Centers for Disease Control and Prevention. (2016). Get the stats of traumatic brain injury in the United States. Retrieved from https://www.cdc.gov/traumaticbrain injury/pdf/BlueBook_factsheet-a.pdf

Fitzgerald, P. A. (2017). Endocrine disorders. In M. A. Papadakis & S. J. McPhee (Eds.), *Current medical diagnosis and treatment* (56th ed., pp. 1113–1114). New York, NY: McGraw-Hill.

Garton, H., & Lehmann, E. (2015). Neurosurgery. In G. M. Doherty (Ed.), *Current diagnosis and treatment: Surgery* (14th ed., pp. 863–874). New York, NY: McGraw-Hill.

White, H., & Venkatesh, B. (2016). Traumatic brain injury. In W. Kolka, M. Smith, & G. Citerio (Eds.), *Oxford textbook of neuro critical care* (p. 210). Oxford, UK: Oxford University Press.

■ TRAUMATIC INJURY

Dustin Spencer

Overview

Traumatic injury is a significant cause of morbidity and mortality for people worldwide. Trauma is a frequent cause for patients across the life span to receive medical treatment in the outpatient, emergency, or inpatient setting. The sudden application of external force to tissues, whether intentional or unintentionally inflicted, results in traumatic injuries (American College of Surgeons Committee on Trauma, 2012). These injuries can range from relatively minor cutaneous contusions and abrasion to immediately life-threatening internal organ damage. Because of this, a deliberate and systematic approach to the trauma patient is required to identify injuries early in the treatment of the patient so that they can be addressed with the goal of achieving optimal short- and long-term outcomes (American College of Surgeons Committee on Trauma, 2012). This approach is applied across the trauma continuum: from public health prevention efforts to the prehospital phase through initial resuscitation, hospital admission, discharge, and postdischarge follow-up.

Background

Traumatic injury is a leading cause of disability worldwide. Globally, nearly 970 million people required some sort of medical attention due to a traumatic injury in 2013, of these nearly 5 million people died from their injuries (Haagsma et al., 2015). In the United States, unintentional injury remains the number one cause of death in the 1- to 44-year-old age group and is in the top 10 for every other age group (Centers for Disease Control and Prevention, n.d.). Of the nearly 27 million people treated in the emergency department for traumatic injuries in 2014, approximately 10% were hospitalized, leading to a total medical cost of over $80 million and work loss costs of over $150 million (CDC, 2017). Annually nearly 10 million people in the United States suffer disabling injuries and of these 3 million will experience some sort of permanent disability. In the United States, traumatic injuries cost upwards of $400 billion annually (CDC, 2017).

Common mechanisms of injury include motor vehicle collisions, falls, firearms, and burns. Of these, falls are the most common with approximately 9 million falls annually. Serious injury can result from falling from even relatively low-level heights, especially in the very young and very old. Motor vehicle injuries are the second most common and result in over 36,000 deaths per year (CDC, 2017). These deaths are predominately related to blunt trauma of the thorax, abdomen, pelvis, and head. These injuries can present as obvious initially or delayed by hours or days (American College of Surgeons Committee on Trauma, 2012).

Due to a direct blow, concussive transfer of energy, or the forces of inertia contribute to internal injuries that may not be notable without radiographic imaging or ultrasonography. Blunt trauma to the thorax can result in injury to great vessels leading to hemothorax and/or cardiac tamponade. Injury to the pulmonary tissue can lead to pulmonary contusion, pneumothorax, or tension pneumothorax (American College of Surgeons Committee on Trauma, 2012). Blunt trauma to the abdomen and pelvis can result in injury to the hollow organs (urinary bladder, stomach, intestines), solids organs (liver, spleen, kidneys, pancreas), genitourinary tract, diaphragm, aorta, or bony pelvis.

Traumatic injury to the musculoskeletal system occurs in far greater frequency than either thoracic or abdominal trauma. Although these injuries typically are less likely to be fatal, they can lead to significant disability and morbidity if potential sequelae are not prevented and identified early. A single-closed femur fracture can lead to significant blood loss and put the patient at risk for developing a fat embolus, both of which are potentially fatal conditions. An open fracture of any bone creates the potential for potentially serious infection to develop (American College of Surgeons Committee on Trauma, 2012). Injured muscle tissue can lead to an overwhelming demand on the kidneys, causing rhabdomyolysis. Penetrating trauma from a stab wound, impaled object, or a projectile, such as shrapnel or a bullet, results in similar injuries to these systems but with an added component of unpredictability associated with the movement of the penetrating object once it enters the cavity and travels to nearby cavities and organs (American College of Surgeons Committee on Trauma, 2012).

Clinical Aspects

ASSESSMENT

Each of these potential injuries has a unique presentation and associated interventions that are necessary to facilitate immediate, short-term and long-term survivability and limit disability. The single most important intervention is the application of a systematic process for assessment and management of the trauma patient. This process begins in the prehospital setting and follows the patient through the hospital stay until discharge. For this reason, trauma patients are best cared for in hospitals designated as trauma treatment centers. These facilities have verified that they have the specialized services, staff education, and follow-up procedures in place to achieve the best possible outcomes for trauma patients.

Early recognition of these injuries is paramount to determining the treatment priorities that are unique to the presenting case. The American College of Surgeons Committee on Trauma (2012) recommends an initial assessment and management phase followed by a secondary survey and management phase. During the initial assessment and management phase, the nurse should focus on the assessment and management of life-threatening compromise of a patient's airway, breathing, circulation, disability, and environment. In this order deficits are identified and corrected before moving to the next assessment. Only after airway, breathing and circulation have been stabilized can the secondary survey begin to help identify radiographic studies, laboratory studies, and diagnostic or treatment interventions that are necessary to further stabilize the patient before transfer to definitive care (American College of Surgeons Committee on Trauma, 2012).

During the secondary survey, assessment of the trauma patient's abdomen, thorax, and musculoskeletal system consists of the common skills of inspection, auscultation, and palpation. Inspection and palpation of the entire patient from head to toe allow the nurse to find occult injuries that may not be evident otherwise. These findings assist in the identification of further diagnostic testing considerations.

NURSING INTERVENTIONS, MANAGEMENT, AND IMPLICATIONS

The nursing focus during the care of trauma patients should be three pronged. First nurses should ensure that there are no subtle or overt changes in the patient's condition (vital signs, pain level, perfusion status, bowel sounds, etc.) that could indicate a change in hemodynamic stability. As noted earlier, trauma patients can have multisystem injuries, some of which may not present for a significant amount of time after the initial insult (American College of Surgeons Committee on Trauma, 2012). An astute nurse should be aware of these potentials and recognize these early signs. The second focus is on prevention of further injury. Trauma patients are often a fall risk at baseline and once given pain medications this risk increases. Many of these patients are admitted to the nursing unit following surgical procedures and as such they are prone to confusion and potentially may be unsteady on their feet. The third focus of the nurse should be on ensuring that an adequate postdischarge rehabilitation plan is in place. This should include not just follow-up with the appropriate medical and rehabilitation specialist, but also resources for nutritional support, psychosocial support, environmental accommodations, and prevention of further injury (Worsowicz, Hwang, & Dawson, 2015).

OUTCOMES

The care of trauma patients is focused on facilitating survival with the least amount of residual disability. To meet these outcomes, trauma systems have dedicated resources to creating an infrastructure that supports the training, treatment, evaluation, and follow-up of patients who experience traumatic injuries (American College of Surgeons Committee on Trauma, 2012). Using a centralized data-collection tool, data are collected on trauma patients across the trauma continuum. This data is used to establish the evidence-based practice guidelines necessary for greater achievement of these outcome goals (American College of Surgeon, 2017).

Summary

Nurses across the trauma continuum have a direct impact on the outcomes their patients achieve. Using a systematic approach, the health care team can achieve the highest quality, evidence-based care for patients who have experienced a traumatic injury. This approach is based on an extensive analysis of the available data and designed to rapidly identify and proficiently intervene to address the apparent and occult injuries resulting from the traumatic event.

American College of Surgeons. (2017). National trauma data bank (NTDB). Retrieved from https://www.facs.org/quality-programs/trauma/ntdb

American College of Surgeons Committee on Trauma. (2012). *Advanced trauma life support* (9th ed.). Chicago, IL: Author.

Centers for Disease Control and Prevention. (n.d.). 10 leading causes of death by age group, United States 2014. Retrieved from https://www.cdc.gov/injury/images/lc-charts/leading_causes_of_death_age_group_2014_1050w760h.gif

Centers for Disease Control and Prevention. (2017). Welcome to WISQARS: Cost of injury data. Retrieved from https://wisqars.cdc.gov:8443/costT

Haagsma, J., Graetz, N., Bolliger, I., Naghavi, M., Higashi, H., Mullany, E., . . . Vos, T. (2015). The global burden of injury: Incidence, mortality, disability-adjusted life years and time trends from the Global Burden of Disease study 2013. *Injury Prevention, 22*(1), 3–18.

Worsowicz, G., Hwang, S., & Dawson, P. (2015). Trauma Rehabilitation. In I. Maitin & E. Cruz (Eds.), *Current diagnosis & treatment*. New York, NY: McGraw-Hill.

■ UROLOGIC EMERGENCIES

Kelley Toffoli

Overview

Several urologic conditions warrant prompt diagnosis and treatment. Urinary tract infection, pyelonephritis, renal calculi, acute urinary retention, acute kidney injury, and testicular torsion necessitate emergent treatment. This section provides a meaningful overview of these urologic disorders that may manifest as a urological emergency.

Urinary Tract Infection

Background

Urinary tract infection (UTI) is a common urologic problem. In the United States, UTI is one of the most prevalent infections (Lingenfelter et al., 2016). UTIs occur throughout all age groups. UTI occurs more often in females than in males. It is estimated that 50% of females will experience at least one UTI in their lifetime (Barber, Norton, Spivak, & Mulvey, 2013).

Clinical Aspects

A UTI is defined as microbial infiltration of an otherwise sterile urinary tract (Barber et al., 2013). UTI can occur within the urethra, bladder, ureters, and kidney. *Escherichia coli* is the most common bacterial cause of UTI, estimated to be responsible for infection 54% to 90% of the time (Traisman, 2016). A UTI is considered to be complicated in patients with pregnancy, neurogenic dysfunction, bladder outlet obstruction, obstructive uropathy, bladder catheterization, urologic instrumentation, indwelling stent, urinary tract surgery, chemotherapy, radiation injury, renal impairment, diabetes, and immunodeficiency (Tonolini & Ippolito, 2016).

ASSESSMENT

Diagnosis of UTI should be based on clinical symptoms and confirmed by positive urine microscopy and culture (Schulz, Hoffman, Pothof, & Fox, 2016). Clinical symptoms of UTI may include acute dysuria or burning with urination, fever, urinary urgency, urinary frequency, urinary incontinence, suprapubic pain, gross hematuria or obvious blood in the urine, costovertebral angle tenderness or flank pain, shaking, chills, change in mental status, or change in functional status (Eke-Usim, Rogers, Gibson, Crnich, & Mody, 2016). UTI diagnosis is made from a midstream clean-catch urine specimen, urinary catheter specimen, or urine specimen from suprapubic aspiration. A quality urine specimen has fewer than five epithelial cells in urinalysis (Schulz et al., 2016). Diagnosis of UTI should be made in patients with elevated urine nitrate, and/or elevated leukocyte esterase with greater than five white blood cells in the presence of clinical signs and symptoms of UTI.

Pyelonephritis

Background

Acute pyelonephritis is less common than acute cystitis or infection of the bladder. Pyelonephritis can occur in all individuals of all ages. The estimated annual incidence per 10,000 people is 27.6 cases in the United States (Neumann & Moore, 2014). Pyelonephritis is more common in women. Women are approximately five times more likely than men to be hospitalized with acute pyelonephritis (Neumann & Moore, 2014).

Clinical Aspects

Acute pyelonephritis, or upper UTI, is caused by bacterial infiltration of the renal pelvis and sometimes the renal parenchyma. Pyelonephritis is potentially an organ-threatening and life-threatening infection. Infection can be a result of an infection of the bladder or lower urinary tract, and sometimes from infection of the bloodstream. Most cases of pyelonephritis are caused by a gram-negative bacterial infection, usually *Escherichia coli*, but like UTI, may be caused by other organisms (Neumann & Moore, 2014).

Mortality with pyelonephritis is greater in those individuals older than 65 years, with concomitant septic shock, those who are immobilized or bedridden, and those with immunosuppression. Individuals with pyelonephritis who have underlying renal disease, diabetes mellitus, and/or immunosuppression may have a poor prognosis (Neumann & Moore, 2014).

ASSESSMENT

Acute pyelonephritis is defined by the following criteria: fever (temperature greater than 100.4°F or 38.0°C), or a history of chills within 24 hours of initial presentation, and at least one symptom associated with a UTI (i.e., dysuria, frequency, urgency, perineal pain, flank pain, or tenderness of the costovertebral angle), and a positive UTI based on a urinalysis (Park et al., 2016). Renal ultrasound or CT scan may be utilized to assess for the presence of pyelonephritis and affected structures.

Renal Calculi

Background

A renal calculus, or nephrolithiasis, can occur in individuals across the life span. Ingimarsson, Krambeck, and Pais (2016) found that nephrolithiasis affects approximately 10% of adults. Male gender, Caucasian race, lower socioeconomic status, obesity, diabetes, and gout have been associated with a higher incidence of nephrolithiasis (Ingimarsson et al., 2016).

Clinical Aspects

Renal calculi are usually composed of salts, commonly calcium and urate. Dietary intake, endocrine factors, and malabsorptive intestinal disorders, such as ulcerative colitis, pancreatitis, and short gut syndromes, have all been associated with the development of renal calculi (Ingimarsson et al., 2016). Renal calculi can be found throughout the urinary tract. Renal calculi can cause ureteral scar, ureteral stricture, and obstruction of the urinary tract (Ingimarsson et al., 2016). Hydronephrosis, or fluid within or surrounding the kidney, is a complication associated with obstructive renal calculi. Sepsis is a severe complication of nephrolithiasis.

ASSESSMENT

Renal calculi present in the ureter are often painful, leading to a condition known as *renal colic*. Pressure in the ureter stimulates nerve endings in the urothelium to spasm, which causes a colicky pain, thus the term *renal colic* is used to describe this phenomenon (Ingimarsson et al., 2016). Individuals may present with pain in the flank region, also known as the *costovertebral angle region*, or pain in the abdomen and/or nausea and vomiting (Ingimarsson et al., 2016). Hematuria, gross or microscopic, may be present in the urine. Absence of hematuria does not exclude the presence of renal calculi; hematuria is only accurate for predicting renal calculi 62% of the time (Ingimarsson et al., 2016). Individuals with renal calculi and renal colic may or may not have associated UTI.

Acute Urinary Retention

Background

Acute urinary retention (AUR) is typically found in men older than 60 years of age (Sliwinski, D'Arcy, Sultana, & Lawrentschuk, 2016). AUR can also occur in women and children. The overall AUR incidence in the general male population varies between 2.2 and 8.5 of 1,000 man-years without known risk factors or previous history of AUR (Oelke, Speakman, Desgrandchamps, & Mamoulakis, 2015).

Clinical Aspects

AUR is a urologic emergency. AUR is most commonly a result of benign prostatic hyperplasia (BPH) in men (Sliwinski et al., 2016). AUR in men and women can be caused by renal calculi or other obstructive pathology. AUR in children is uncommon, but can be a result of constipation.

ASSESSMENT

AUR is characterized by the painful inability to void. Pain or discomfort and bloating in the lower abdomen along with a painful urgent feeling of need to urinate are common symptoms of AUR.

Acute Kidney Injury

Background

Acute kidney injury (AKI) is characterized by an abrupt decline in renal function. AKI can affect individuals of all ages. AKI was previously referred to as *acute renal failure*. AKI is associated with a great risk for morbidity and mortality (Yang, Zhang, Wu, Zou, & Du, 2014).

Clinical Aspects

An intact renal system is essential in order to maintain homeostasis. The renal system regulates the body's fluid volume, maintains electrolyte balance, and excretes toxic metabolic agents through glomerular filtration, tubular reabsorption, and tubular secretion via the formation and excretion of urine (Yang et al., 2014).

AKI is most often due to infection, obstruction, renal ischemia, and/or nephrotoxic drugs (Yang et al., 2014). AKI has clinical manifestations ranging from a small elevation in serum creatinine levels to anuric renal failure (Yang et al., 2014). AKI is classified into three groups: prerenal, renal, and postrenal. Recovery of AKI is based on improvement of renal function measured by serum creatinine levels and urine output.

ASSESSMENT

Clinical presentation of AKI may be retention of fluid or swelling. Individuals may report decreased urine output. Symptoms of electrolyte imbalance associated with AKI may include nausea, vomiting, muscle aches, fatigue, seizure, tachycardia, irregular heartbeat, diarrhea, and/or constipation.

Testicular Torsion

Background

Testicular torsion (TT) is one of the most common urologic emergencies. It is estimated that one in 1,500 males under the age of 18 years will suffer from TT (Afsarlar et al., 2016). TT is most common in neonates, children, and adolescents.

Those at greatest risk for TT are African American, of younger age (12–18 years), and lacking private insurance (American Urological Association, 2016). Rate of testis loss with TT has been estimated to be as high as 42% (Afsarlar et al., 2016).

Clinical Aspects

In TT, the spermatic cord is twisted, which can cause decreased blood supply to the testis. Scrotal ultrasound (US) is highly sensitive in the diagnosis of TT, reported to be over 90% sensitive (Yagil et al., 2010). Early presentation, accurate diagnosis, and prompt treatment are essential for the best outcome. TT can lead to infarction of the testicle, loss of testicle, infertility, infection, and cosmetic deformity.

ASSESSMENT

Individuals with TT often present with severe sudden onset of testicular pain and/or pain in the abdomen, nausea or vomiting, high-rising testicle, and sometimes swelling of the scrotum. Individuals may have a diminished cremasteric reflex. Assessment of positive Prehn's sign is indicative of TT. Prehn's sign is relief of pain with elevation of the scrotum. Emergent manual detorsion may be indicated.

NURSING INTERVENTIONS, MANAGEMENT, AND IMPLICATIONS

It is essential for nurses to understand and recognize various serious urologic conditions. Nursing education and guidance related to prevention of infection are essential. Regular voiding and stooling, perineal hygiene, use of probiotics, polyethylene glycol as needed for constipation, regular physical activity, increased intake of oral fluids, consumption of fresh or dried cranberries, prevention of perineal irritation, avoiding tight clothing, avoiding bubble bath, avoiding pools, encouraging the use of condoms, encouraging voiding after sexual intercourse, and the use of oxybutynin for bladder spasticity may reduce incidence of UTI (Traisman, 2016).

If obstructive uropathy is present, nursing must implement measures to relieve obstruction as quickly as possible to prevent AKI. In the case of urinary obstruction, placement of an indwelling urinary catheter may be need. Nursing should carefully consider need before placing an indwelling urinary catheter. Catheter-acquired urinary tract infection (CAUTI) is one of the most common preventable health care-associated infections (Flanders, 2014).

OUTCOMES

Treatment of urologic infection is essential. Prompt identification of the offending bacterial pathogen and antimicrobial susceptibility testing via urine culture for effective treatment may limit complications. Complications may include renal abscess, renal impairment, and septic shock (Neumann & Moore, 2014). Individuals with tachycardia and hypotension may indicate more severe diseases such AKI and/or sepsis.

Nursing care related to urologic emergencies includes management of pain, management of electrolyte imbalances, acidosis, focus on restoring renal profusion and fluid balance, providing nutritional support, avoiding nephrotoxic drugs, and providing necessary pharmacological intervention if appropriate. Individuals may need to be prepared for renal dialysis in severe cases.

Summary

Nurses are challenged to provide the most effective, evidence-based care in order to treat and limit the progression and severity of urologic disease. Early presentation, accurate diagnosis, and prompt treatment are essential for the best patient-centered outcomes.

Afsarlar, C., Ryan, S., Donel, E., Baccam, T., Jones, B., Chandwani, B., . . . Chester, K. (2016). Standardized process to improve patient flow from the emergency room to the operating room for pediatric patients with testicular torsion. *Journal of Pediatric Urology*, *12*(4), 233.e1–233.e4.

American Urological Association. (2016). Acute scrotum. Retrieved from https://www .auanet.org/education/acute-scrotum.cfm

Barber, A., Norton, P., Spivak, A., & Mulvey M. (2013). Urinary tract infections: Current and emerging management strategies. *Clinical Infectious Diseases*, *57*(5), 719–724.

Eke-Usim, A., Rogers, M., Gibson, K., Crnich, C., & Mody, L. (2016). Constitutional symptoms trigger diagnostic testing before antibiotic prescribing in high-risk nursing home residents. *Journal of the American Geriatrics Society*, *64*(10), 1975–1980.

Flanders, K. (2014). Rounding to reduce CAUTI. *Nursing Management*, *45*(11), 21–23.

Ingimarsson, J., Krambeck, A., & Pais, V. (2016). Diagnosis and management of nephrolithiasis. *Surgical Clinics of North America*, *96*(3), 517–532.

Lingenfelter, E., Drapkin, Z., Fritz, K., Youngquist, S., Madsen, T., & Fix, M. (2016). ED pharmacist monitoring of provider antibiotic selection aids appropriate treatment for outpatient UTI. *American Journal of Emergency Medicine*, *34*(8), 1600–1603.

Neumann, I., & Moore, P. (2014). Clinical evidence: Pyelonephritis in non-pregnant women. *BMJ Clinical Evidence*, *807*. Retrieved from https://www.ncbi.nlm.nih.gov/ pmc/articles/PMC4220693

Oelke, M., Speakman, M., Desgrandchamps, F., & Mamoulakis, C. (2015). Acute urinary retention rates in the general male population and in adult men with lower urinary tract symptoms participating in pharmacotherapy trails: A literature review. *Urology*, *86*(4), 654–665.

Park, S., Oh, W., Kim, Y., Yeom, J., Choi, H., Kwak, Y., . . . Kim, B. (2016). Health care-associated acute pyelonephritis is associated with inappropriate empiric antibiotic therapy in the ED. *American Journal of Emergency Medicine*, *34*(8), 1415–1420.

Schulz, L., Hoffman, R., Pothof, J., & Fox, B. (2016). Top ten myths regarding the diagnosis and treatment of urinary tract infections. *Journal of Emergency Medicine*, *51*(1), 25–30.

Sliwinski, A., D'Arcy, F., Sultana, R., & Lawrentschuk, N. (2016). Acute urinary reten-tion and the difficult catheterization: Current emergency management. *European Journal of Emergency Medicine, 23*(2), 80–88.

Tonolini, M., & Ippolito, S. (2016). Cross-sectional imaging of complicated urinary infections affecting the lower tract and male genital organs. *Insights into Imaging, 7*(5), 689–711.

Traisman, E. (2016). Clinical management of urinary tract infections. *Pediatric Annals, 45*(5), e108–e111.

Yagil, Y., Naroditsky, I., Milhem, J., Leiba, R., Leiderman, M., Badaan, S., & Gaitini, D. (2010). Role of Doppler ultrasonography in the triage of acute scrotum in the emer-gency department. *Journal of Ultrasound Medicine, 29*(1), 11–21.

Yang, F., Zhang, L., Wu, H., Zou, H., & Du, Y. (2014). Clinical analysis of cause, treat-ment and prognosis in acute kidney injury patients. *PLOS ONE.* doi:10.1371/journal.pone.0085214

■ VENTILATOR-ASSOCIATED PNEUMONIA

Nancy Jaskowak Cresse

Overview

Pneumonia is an infection in the lungs that can vary from mild to severe. Caused by bacteria, viruses, or fungi, pneumonia can be acquired in the community, or associated with contact with the health care system (Centers for Disease Control and Prevention [CDC], 2017). Health care-associated conditions are also referred to as *nosocomial*. The most serious of health care-associated infections is ventilator-associated pneumonia (VAP), impacting patient mortality, ventilator days, and costs (CDC, 2017; Lim et al., 2015). As science is evolving the current definition and reportable event protocol to improve sensitivity and specificity of VAP, the focus of nursing care is on reduction of incidence, and prevention of VAP through the use of a set of interventions called a *care bundle* that reduces the incidence of VAP thereby reducing patient length of stay, cost, and mortality (Alcan, Kormaz, & Uyar, 2016; CDC, 2017).

Background

VAP is a lung infection that develops in a person who is on a ventilator. A ventilator is a machine that helps a patient breathe by giving breaths, providing oxygen, and it can administer a varying depth of each breath. To accomplish patient oxygenation, a tube is placed in the patient's nose or mouth (endotracheal), or through a hole that is placed in the front of the patient's neck (tracheostomy; CDC, 2017).

Mechanical ventilation is a necessary, life-sustaining therapy for many patients with critical injury or illness. Ventilated patients are a vulnerable population at increased risk for complications, poor outcomes, and death. Complications of receiving mechanical ventilation include VAP, acute respiratory distress syndrome (ARDS), pulmonary embolism, and pulmonary edema. If a patient were to develop a complication, it can lead to additional time on the ventilator, longer stays in intensive care and the hospital, increased costs, and increased risk of disability and death (CDC, 2017). National surveillance and data collection before 2013 was limited to VAP and the incidence ranged from 0.0 to 4.4 per 1,000 ventilator days in medical–surgical intensive care units (ICUs) in the United States, and in developing countries it ranged from 10 to 41.7 cases per 1,000 ventilator days (CDC, 2017; Lim et al., 2015). Between 10% and 20% of patients receive mechanical ventilation for a duration more than 48 hours develop VAP (Speck et al., 2016). In 2013, the CDC proposed new surveillance categories capturing ventilator-associated events (VAE), infectious ventilator-associated events (IVAC), and then possible ventilator-associated pneumonia (PVAP; CDC, 2017; Nair & Niederman, 2015). It is not certain that these newer surveillance designations, although broader in scope, will support the efficacy of the care bundles for VAP (Nair & Neiderman, 2015; O'Horo et al., 2016).

Although there is no standard definition, VAP has been defined as a lower respiratory tract infection developed after 48 hours of intubation with mechanical ventilation, or within 48 hours after disconnecting the ventilator (CDC, 2017; Lim et al., 2015). Clinically, VAP can be divided into early onset (less than 5 days) or late onset (longer than 5 days after hospitalization), but some studies vary that parameter (Nair & Niederman, 2015). And although there were practice guidelines used to prevent VAP, several studies from 1999 to 2009 identified approximately 50% of patients received evidence-based care (Alcan et al., 2016). For this reason, the Institute for Healthcare Improvement (IHI) introduced a care bundle, a set of evidence-based practices that, when executed together, improves the patient recovery process and outcomes better than when implemented separately (Alcan et al., 2016).

Clinical Aspects

ASSESSMENT

A critical component of nursing care is accurate assessment and documentation. Identifying a patient who requires increased oxygen concentrations from the ventilator, or increased positive pressure from the ventilator to deliver the oxygen (as in use of positive end-expiratory pressure [PEEP]) is a primary function of the nurse in acute care and is pivotal in identifying early VAE. Monitoring patient temperature to identify a temperature above 38°C, as well as documenting increased frequency of suctioning and/or change in the purulent appearance of endotracheal or tracheal secretions will capture the data consistent with VAE or IVAE.

NURSING INTERVENTIONS, MANAGEMENT, AND IMPLICATIONS

Nursing care of the adult on a ventilator or who has recently been on a ventilator and who is at risk for VAP should center around maintaining patent airway and adequate patient oxygenation. Caring for the patient holistically, using priority nursing-related problems/diagnoses includes maintaining adequate ventilation (ineffective airway clearance, ineffective breathing pattern), noting imbalanced nutrition, immobility, hyperthermia, risk for infection, risk of fluid volume deficit, and disturbed sleep pattern.

The commonly used ventilator bundle developed by the IHI identifies five elements to reduce the rate of VAP. These measures include (a) head of the bed (HOB) elevation 30° to 45°, (b) daily sedation vacation and patient assessment for readiness to wean, (c) peptic ulcer disease prevention, (d) deep vein thrombosis prophylaxis, and (e) daily oral care with chlorhexidine (Lim et al., 2015). In addition to the HOB elevation, and daily oral care by nursing, several other elements have evidence-based support to include in a *customized* bundle of care interventions, including hand hygiene before and after patient contact and endotracheal tube cuff pressure monitoring (greater than 20–25 cm H_2O; Alcan et al., 2016; Lim et al., 2015). Standardizing nursing interventions also has a positive impact on VAP rates, such as oral cavity secretion clearance before changing position or supination (every 2–4 hours), and oral care with chlorhexidine every 8 hours.

OUTCOMES

Ventilator care bundle implementation in clinical practice has exposed barriers, and compliance in some centers remain modest (Nair & Niederman, 2015). Lim et al. (2015) identified keys to success in care bundle implementation and nurse efficacy through the development and use of nursing checklists, staff education, posters, and standardizing interventions that will contribute to a reduction in VAP rates. It was also noted that nurse compliance rates in applying the ventilator care bundle improved when staff is observed and compliance is recorded (Alcan et al., 2016).

Efforts to continually improve clinical care quality and patient safety are important, as is clinician involvement and buy-in (Speck et al., 2016). Obtaining clinician input on what interventions to include, and the supporting processes necessary for the implementation, increases the likelihood that caregivers and providers adhere to the intervention bundle.

Summary

VAP is the most common and serious type of health care infection in the ICU, and is associated with significant mortality, morbidity, and cost. Ventilator care bundles include nursing care interventions that have shown to reduce the incidence of VAP. New knowledge supports customizing the care bundle to maximize the effect of reducing incidence of VAP and improving patient outcomes.

Alcans, A. O., Korkmaz, F. D., & Uyar, M. (2016). Prevention of ventilator-associated pneumonia: Use of the care bundle approach. *American Journal of Infection Control,* 44, 173–176. doi:10.1016/j.ajic.2016.04.237

Centers for Disease Control and Prevention. (2017). *Ventilator-associated event (VAE)* (pp. 1–44). Retrieved from https://www.cdc.gov/nhsn/pdfs/pscmanual/10-vae_final .pdf

Lim, K. P., Kuo, S. W., Ko, W. J., Sheng, W. H., Chang, Y. Y., Hong, M. C., . . . Chang, S. C. (2015). Efficacy of ventilator-associated pneumonia care bundle for prevention of ventilator-associated pneumonia in the surgical intensive care units of a medical center. *Journal of Microbiology, Immunology and Infection,* 48, 316–321. doi:10.1016/ j.jmii.2013.09.007

Nair, G. B., & Niederman, M. S. (2015). Ventilator-associated pneumonia: Present understanding and ongoing debate. *Intensive Care Medicine,* 41, 34–48. doi:10.1007/ s00134-3564-5

O'Horo, J. C., Lan, H., Thongprayoon, C., Schenck, L., Ahmed, A., & Dziadzko, M. (2016). "Bundle" practices and ventilator-associated events: Not enough. *Infection Control & Hospital Epidemiology, 37*(12), 1453–1457. doi:10.1017/ice.2016.207

Speck, K., Rawat, N., Weiner, N. C., Tujuba, H. G., Farley, D., & Berenholtz, S. (2016). A systematic approach for developing a ventilator-associated pneumonia prevention bundle. *American Journal of Infection Control, 44,* 652–656. doi:10.1016/j.ajic.2015.12.020

■ VENTRICULAR ASSIST DEVICES

S. Brian Widmar

Overview

A ventricular assist device (VAD) is a mechanical pump that is surgically implanted and assists the failing ventricle by increasing cardiac output (Chmielinski & Koons, 2017). The VAD is most often used to support the failing left ventricle (LVAD), but the right ventricle (RVAD) or both ventricles (BIVAD) can also be supported. The LVAD can be used as a bridge to transplantation (BTT), supporting the patient until a heart transplant is received, or as destination therapy (DT), supporting the patient as a permanent therapy for heart failure (Chmielinski & Koons, 2017; O'Shea, 2012). In addition, the LVAD can be used as a bridge to decision, when ventricular support is required before a determination of eligibility for transplant can be made, or as a bridge to recovery, in which the LVAD supports the patient while the heart recovers from injury and can eventually be removed, or explanted, as myocardial function recovers (Chmielinski & Koons, 2017).

Background

Approximately 6.5 million Americans are living with heart failure, and 960,000 new heart failure cases are diagnosed annually (Writing Group Members et al., 2016). Heart failure is a progressive and chronic condition, and is categorized in stages, by both the severity of presenting signs and symptoms and by the goal-directed therapies aimed at relieving them (Hunt et al., 2001a). Stage D heart failure is seen in patients with advanced structural heart disease who have symptoms of heart failure at rest or refractory to optimized medical therapy, and these patients require specialized treatments or interventions in order to survive (Hunt et al., 2001b). Interventions for patients with stage D heart failure include optimized and maximal medical therapies, continuous intravenous (IV) inotropes, heart transplantation, mechanical circulatory support device therapy, or palliative or hospice care (Fang et al., 2015).

Limited data are available regarding stage D heart failure, but despite advances in medical management and technology, prognosis for end-stage heart failure patients remains poor. From 1987 until 2012, 40,253 people were waiting for heart transplant, whereas only 26,943 received a transplant, which highlights the clinical impact of VADs as a strategy to prolong the life of patients living with end-stage heart failure (Writing Group Members et al., 2016). In the Randomized Evaluation of Mechanical Assistance for the Treatment of Congestive Heart Failure (REMATCH) trial, end-stage heart failure patients who were managed medically had a 75% mortality rate at 1 year (Fang et al., 2015; Rose et al., 2001). From 2006 until 2016, the Interagency Registry for Mechanically Assisted Circulatory Support (INTERMACS) database reports a total of 19,013 VAD implants, with 2,480 VAD implants in 2016 alone; survival at 1 year was 80%, and 70% at 2 years (INTERMACS, 2017). Patients receiving VAD support have reported an improvement in quality of life (Grady et al., 2004; Maciver & Ross, 2012). VAD therapy has not proven to be a cost-effective solution compared to heart transplantation, possibly due to issues such as equipment costs, hospital length of stay, and hospital readmissions. The most commonly reported causes of hospital readmissions include device malfunction, cardiac arrhythmia, infection, gastrointestinal (GI) bleeding, and stroke (Writing Group Members et al., 2016).

VADs vary by type of support offered (LVAD, RVAD, BIVAD), by anatomical position (internal or "intracorporeal"; external or "extracorporeal"), and by the duration of time support can be maintained. Some devices are designed to provide temporary support, permitting recovery from cardiogenic shock or from high-risk cardiac surgery, whereas others offer a longer duration of support, such as a bridge to transplant or as a destination therapy (Chilcott & Hazard, 2017). Examples of long-term or durable VADs include the Heartmate II, the HeartWare HVAD, and the Thoratec paracorporeal VAD. Short-term support VADs include intra-aortic balloon pumps (IABPs), Tandem Heart, Impella, CentriMag, Maquet, and Medtronic VADs (Chilcott & Hazard, 2017). The IABP, Tandem Heart, and Impella devices can be placed percutaneously (Hollenberg & Parrillo, 2014). In addition, VADs can be further categorized by the type of flow generated by the device. Pulsatile-flow VADs generate a pulsation of blood through sequential filling and emptying, similar to normal cardiac function. Continuous-flow VADs deliver a continuous flow of blood throughout systole and diastole; these include axial and centrifugal flow pumps (Chilcott & Hazard, 2017; O'Shea, 2012). One important variant of continuous flow pumps is that patients with continuous flow devices have lower systolic blood pressures and elevated diastolic pressures, resulting in a greatly diminished pulse pressure. At normal settings, the patient with a continuous-flow VAD may not have a palpable pulse (Chilcott & Hazard, 2017; O'Shea, 2012).

Clinical Aspects

Immediate postoperative monitoring and care is similar despite the type of VAD implanted (Grady & Shinn, 2008). VADs are preload sensitive, and pump flow relies on adequate filling of the pump chamber. Vital signs, fluid volume status, pump settings and function, anticoagulation, maintaining adequate end-organ perfusion, and reducing risk of infection are all important considerations in the postoperative setting (Chilcott & Hazard, 2017).

ASSESSMENT

Close monitoring for cardiac arrhythmias is important, and any arrhythmias should be promptly reported. VAD patients are at high risk for atrial and ventricular arrhythmias. Alterations in cardiac rate and rhythm can decrease cardiac and pump filling, ultimately reducing pump flow (Chmielinski & Koons, 2017). Blood pressure should be closely monitored, as hypertension can increase resistance to pump flow (Chilcott & Hazard, 2017). Mean arterial pressure (MAP) between 70 and 80 mmHg should be maintained to ensure adequate end-organ perfusion while decreasing resistance to pump flow. Due to the very narrow pulse pressure noted in continuous-flow VADs, noninvasive blood pressure cuff monitoring can prove especially difficult; blood pressure measurements may be obtained using Doppler (Chmielinski & Koons, 2017; O'Shea, 2012). Secondary organ dysfunction may occur due to hypoperfusion during surgery. In addition to maintaining an acceptable MAP between 70 and 80 mmHg, close monitoring of urine output, blood urea nitrogen (BUN) and creatinine, as well as liver function test (LFT) is important in identifying hepatic or renal dysfunction postoperatively (Chilcott & Hazard, 2017).

NURSING INTERVENTIONS, MANAGEMENT, AND IMPLICATIONS

VAD pump settings should be confirmed with the physician or provider. Continuous-flow VADs have one setting that is ordered by the provider: the pump speed, which is noted on the VAD device as revolutions per minute (RPM). Blood flow through the pump and pump power are approximations: Pump power is the amount of energy needed to generate the set RPM, and flow is calculated from pump speed and power (Chilcott & Hazard, 2017).

Close monitoring of clotting times and anticoagulation therapy is crucial to the prevention of complications related to bleeding or thromboembolism, both of which are known adverse events after VAD implantation (Chmielinski & Koons, 2017). All VAD pumps include an artificial chamber that comes into direct contact with the patient's blood, increasing the potential for thrombus formation. Ischemic strokes occur in roughly 8% to 10% of VAD patients, most commonly due to pump thrombosis or subtherapeutic anticoagulation. Hemorrhagic strokes may occur from a previous ischemic stroke, from supra-therapeutic anticoagulation, or infection (Chmielinski & Koons, 2017). In the absence of postoperative bleeding, the International Society for Heart and Lung Transplantation supports an international normalized ratio (INR) of 2.0 to 3.0 in continuous-flow VAD devices (Chilcott & Hazard, 2017). GI bleeding is another known adverse effect in VAD patients, and may be due to anticoagulation therapy, or the development of acquired von Willebrand disease, or GI tract angiodysplasia, both of which are thought to be due to the decreased pulsatility seen in continuous-flow VAD devices (Chmielinski & Koons, 2017). Melena, or frank blood from stools, should be reported, as anticoagulation reversal and blood volume replacement could be required (Chilcott & Hazard, 2017; Chmielinski & Koons, 2017).

Postoperative infection is one of the more common complications of VAD therapy and can develop at multiple sites, including the VAD driveline exit site, pump pocket, sternal incision, invasive lines, or bloodstream (O'Shea, 2012). Nurses must closely follow VAD program protocols for site care and immobilization of the VAD exit site as well as site care of invasive lines, and antibiotic prophylaxis must be given to reduce the risk of surgical wound infections (Druss, Rohrbaugh, Levinson, & Rosenheck, 2001; O'Shea, 2012). Timely extubation and pulmonary hygiene; removal of vascular access catheters, indwelling urinary catheters, and chest tube drains as soon as clinically appropriate; and early mobilization are essential to reducing postoperative infection risk (Chilcott & Hazard, 2017; O'Shea, 2012).

OUTCOMES

VAD device malfunction is rare, but is possible. Health care providers caring for VAD patients must understand the critical alarms associated with the specific device supporting the patient. In the event of VAD alarms, the patient's VAD coordinator or physician should be notified immediately (Chmielinski & Koons, 2017). Critical alarms are due to either pump failure, low power, or controller failure (Chmielinski & Koons, 2017). Patients and their caregivers are instructed to carry spare power sources, such as additional batteries, and a spare device controller that is programmed to the same settings the primary controller is set to (O'Shea, 2012). In the event of a critical alarm, nurses should assess the patient, and then the connection from the driveline, controller, and VAD power source. The VAD coordinator or provider should be contacted immediately to assist if correct connections do not alleviate critical alarms, or if controller exchange is required (Chmielinski & Koons, 2017; O'Shea, 2012). In the event of patient arrest, device malfunction should be suspected and the cardiac surgeon, VAD coordinator, and cardiologist should be notified immediately. Advanced cardiac life support protocols should be followed, but the care team must be aware of the risk of internal bleeding from cardiopulmonary resuscitation (CPR) should dislodgement of the device occur (Chmielinski & Koons, 2017). VAD centers have protocols in place for responding to VAD patient arrest situations, and CPR is generally avoided (Lala & Mehra, 2013).

Summary

VADs are indicated for patients in stage D heart failure as either a BTT; bridge to decision; bridge to recovery; or as a chronic, destination therapy for heart failure. VADs may provide short-term or long-term support, depending upon the clinical indication for therapy. VADs can support the failing left ventricle, a failing right ventricle, or can provide biventricular support. VADs may be pulsatile- or continuous-flow devices; in continuous-flow devices, a pulse may not be palpable. Due to numerous types of VADs used, nurses should understand the type of device used and its settings. Monitoring of heart rate and blood pressure, filling pressures, pump settings and function, and anticoagulation are crucial to maintaining adequate MAP for end-organ perfusion and reducing the likelihood of device-related adverse events. Nurses should closely follow hospital protocols for device wound-site care, and monitor and report any signs of infection. Lastly, nurses must be aware of potential device-related complications, and signs and symptoms of device malfunction and should seek assistance immediately should a critical alarm or patient arrest situation occur.

Chilcott, S. R., & Hazard, L. (2017). Mechanical circulatory support. In S. Cupples, S. Lerret, V. McCalmont, & L. Ohler (Eds.), *Core curriculum for transplant nurses* (pp. 414–452). Philadelphia, PA: Mosby.

Chmielinski, A., & Koons, B. (2017). Nursing care for the patient with a left ventricular assist device. *Nursing, 47*(5), 34–40. doi:10.1097/01.NURSE.0000515503.80037.07

Druss, B. G., Rohrbaugh, R. M., Levinson, C. M., & Rosenheck, R. A. (2001). Integrated medical care for patients with serious psychiatric illness: A randomized trial. *Archives of General Psychiatry, 58*(9), 861–868.

Fang, J. C., Ewald, G. A., Allen, L. A., Butler, J., Westlake Canary, C. A., & Colvin-Adams, M. (2015). Advanced (stage D) heart failure: A statement from the Heart Failure Society of America Guidelines Committee. *Journal of Cardiac Failure, 21*(6), 519–534. doi:10.1016/j.cardfail.2015.04.013

Grady, K. L., Meyer, P. M., Dressler, D., Mattea, A., Chillcott, S., Loo, A., . . . Piccione, W. (2004). Longitudinal change in quality of life and impact on survival after left ventricular assist device implantation. *Annals of Thoracic Surgery, 77*(4), 1321–1327. doi:10.1016/j.athoracsur.2003.09.089

Grady, K. L., & Shinn, J. A. (2008). Care of patients with circulatory assist devices. In D. K. Moser & B. Riegel (Eds.), *Cardiac nursing: A companion to Braunwald's heart disease* (pp. 977–997). St. Louis, MO: Saunders.

Hollenberg, S. M., & Parrillo, J. E. (2014). Cardiogenic shock. In J. E. Parrillo & R. P. Dellinger (Eds.), *Critical care medicine: Principles of diagnosis and management in the adult* (4th ed., pp. 325–337). Philadelphia, PA: Elsevier.

Hunt, S. A., Baker, D. W., Chin, M. H., Cinquegrani, M. P., Feldman, A. M., & Francis, G. S., . . . Smith, S. C. (2001a). ACC/AHA guidelines for the evaluation and management of chronic heart failure in the adult: Executive summary. A report of the American College of Cardiology/American Heart Association Task Force on Practice Guidelines (Committee to Revise the 1995 Guidelines for the Evaluation and Management of Heart Failure): Developed in collaboration with the International Society for Heart and Lung Transplantation; endorsed by the Heart Failure Society of America. *Circulation, 104*(24), 2996–3007.

Hunt, S. A., Baker, D. W., Chin, M. H., Cinquegrani, M. P., Feldman, A. M., Francis, G. S., . . . American College of Cardiology/American Heart Association. (2001b). ACC/AHA guidelines for the evaluation and management of chronic heart failure in the adult: Executive summary. A report of the American College of Cardiology/American Heart Association Task Force on Practice Guidelines (Committee to Revise the 1995 Guidelines for the Evaluation and Management of Heart Failure). *Journal of the American College of Cardiology, 38*(7), 2101–2113.

Interagency Registry for Mechanically Assisted Circulatory Support. (2017). Public statistical reports. Retrieved from https://www.uab.edu/medicine/intermacs/reports/public-statistical-reports

Lala, A., & Mehra, M. R. (2013). Durable mechanical circulatory support in advanced heart failure: A critical care cardiology perspective. *Cardiology Clinics, 31*(4), 581–593; viii–ix. doi:10.1016/j.ccl.2013.07.003

Maciver, J., & Ross, H. J. (2012). Quality of life and left ventricular assist device support. *Circulation, 126*(7), 866–874. doi:10.1161/CIRCULATIONAHA.111.040279

O'Shea, G. (2012). Ventricular assist devices: What intensive care unit nurses need to know about postoperative management. *AACN Advanced Critical Care, 23*(1), 69–83; quiz 84-65. doi:10.1097/NCI.0b013e318240aaa9

Rose, E. A., Gelijns, A. C., Moskowitz, A. J., Heitjan, D. F., Stevenson, L. W., Dembitsky, W.; Randomized Evaluation of Mechanical Assistance for the Treatment of Congestive Heart Failure Study Group. (2001). Long-term use of a left ventricular assist device for end-stage heart failure. *New England Journal of Medicine, 345*(20), 1435–1443. doi:10.1056/NEJMoa012175

Writing Group Members, Mozaffarian, D., Benjamin, E. J., Go, A. S., Arnett, D. K., Blaha, M. J., . . . Stroke Statistics Subcommittee. (2016). Heart disease and stroke statistics—2016 update: A report from the American Heart Association. *Circulation, 133*(4), e38–360. doi:10.1161/CIR.0000000000000350

■ THE VIOLENT PATIENT

Janet E. Reilly
Michael Wichowski

Overview

Direct patient-care providers, like nurses, are often the victims of violence, especially in the emergency department (ED) and critical care settings. The occurrence of workplace violence in health care settings is four times higher than the reported rates across nonhealth care sectors of the industry (Occupational Safety and Health Administration [OSHA], 2015b), and is often under reported by nurses. Workplace violence, classified as type II: customer/client violence, occurs when patients act violently toward health care workers, and is the most common type of workplace violence in health care settings (Centers for Disease Control and Prevention [CDC], n.d.). Workplace violence comes in many forms (e.g., physical assaults, threatening behavior, verbal abuse, and sexual harassment) and occurs on a spectrum from verbal statements that result in minor physical or psychological harm to physical assaults resulting in life-threatening injuries. Nurses need to be aware of precipitating factors of workplace violence, type II, as well as be able to accurately assess, prevent, and implement effective, evidence-based strategies that maximize safety for themselves, patients, and others.

Background

Violence within health care settings like the ED is escalating, with the number of violent acts against nurses and nursing assistants doubling between 2012 and 2014 (Gomaa et al., 2015). Violent behavior is often associated with patients who experience mental health crises, like substance abuse or extreme stress, both of which are increasing to almost epidemic levels. In 2014, over 20 million adults in the United States had substance abuse issues; half of these people also have underlying psychological disorders (U.S. Department of Health and Human Services, 2015). More psychological disorders continue to be identified, resulting in greater than one in six Americans being prescribed a psychiatric medication to optimize mental health (Moore & Mattison, 2016). Changes in the economy since 2008 have led to increased stress and negative health outcomes in individuals, as well as less funding for inpatient and outpatient mental health treatment nationwide (Mucci, Giorgi, Roncaioli, Perez, & Arcangeli, 2016; Nesper, Morris, Scher, & Holmes, 2016). These factors, plus the inherent stress from crowded environments and highly charged emotional and life-threatening situations that occur in intensive care units and EDs, can easily trigger a patient to become violent.

There are obvious legal consequences for violent patients, 37 out of 50 states have legislation (e.g., felony charges) for perpetrators of type II violence in health care settings (Jacobson, 2014). Type II violence compromises nurse safety, increases risk of injury, and decreases job satisfaction, which can lead to higher nurse turnover, nursing shortages, and a subsequent lower quality of nursing care. Financially speaking, health care systems can spend between $27,000 and $103,000 to replace a nurse (OSHA, 2015a). Recognizing and preventing violence in health care is key and nurses play a critical role in prevention. Furthermore, workplace violence in health care settings has significant impact on the nursing workforce, the financial status of health care systems, and state legislation and judicial processes have been instituted in most states to mitigate the negative consequences of workplace violence.

Clinical Aspects

ASSESSMENT

Nursing assessment, an essential step in the nursing process, should include situational awareness of the patient and environment for potential violence as well as physical and psychosocial evaluations of patients. Using situational awareness, nurses focus on everything happening around them; assess the situation; and identify abnormal data and unsafe conditions (Solon & Kratz, 2016). Nurses need to assess the clinical environment for unsafe practices or weapons, or objects that could be used to harm others in order to prevent type II violence. For example, some exam and patient rooms are arranged with the patient situated between where the nurse works and the door, which blocks a safe exit route for the health care worker, if violence erupts.

Nurses should also carefully assess the patients for risk factors and behaviors that could potentially lead to violence. Research indicates patients who act violently often have one or more of these common traits: male gender, aged 26 to 35 years; a history of violence; high-level stress or loss of control in the current situation; agitation or aggression; homelessness or unemployment; and low socioeconomic status (Arnetz et al., 2015; Tishler, Reiss, & Dundas, 2013; Villaire, 1995). Assessment of individual patients and their physical and psychological status is also critical. Many disorders can precipitate patient violence, particularly diseases of the brain causing cognitive impairment (e.g., dementia, intellectual disability); endocrine disorders (e.g., hyperthyroidism or hyperglycemia); diseases leading to oxygen deprivation to the brain, or hypoxia (e.g., seizures, chronic obstructive pulmonary disease [COPD], or carbon monoxide poisoning); head trauma; and infections (e.g., sepsis, HIV/AIDs, encephalitis, meningitis, etc.). Patients with a history of or current mental health/psychiatric disorders are also at risk for committing type II violence. Substance abuse, whether from alcohol, prescribed, or illegal substances, also puts patients at risk of acting violently. Violence can also be a result of adverse effects or polypharmacy from certain prescribed medications, such as antipsychotics, antidepressants, amphetamines, benzodiazepines, tobacco-cessation aides (i.e., varenicline), antimalarials (i.e., mefloquine), anticonvulsants, and sedatives (i.e., zolpidem), which have shown to enhance aggression or violent acts among individuals prescribed these medications in various combinations (Arnetz et al., 2015; Tishler, Reiss, & Dundas, 2013; Villaire, 1995).

In addition, nurses should be alert to and assess for patient behaviors that may indicate escalation in aggression or violence, such as pacing or restlessness; increasingly loud or rapid speech; insistence or demanding behavior; threats; use of profanity; intimidating or overly sexual language; clenched fists, throwing, or punching objects; or accusing health care workers of conspiracy (OSHA, n.d.; Tishler et al., 2013). Situations that often incite type II violence include patients who demand discharge against medical advice, patients undergoing painful procedures or transfers, patient transitions in care and use of patient restraints (Arnetz, et al., 2015).

NURSING INTERVENTIONS, MANAGEMENT AND IMPLICATIONS

Appropriate interventions and evaluation of their effectiveness are the next steps in the nursing process with the violent patient. Therapeutic communication can help patients feel understood, and, when coupled with patience while teaching/ explaining, can empower patients with better understanding. Simple interventions that address basic patient needs (i.e., offering food to a hungry or homeless patient) are other ways nurses can intervene to prevent patient violence. Utilizing proper nursing technique in procedures and creative interventions, like numbing cream or ice applied to the site before needle injections, can help decrease and manage pain associated with patient care and diffuse violence. When physical or chemical restraints (antipsychotics, benzodiazepines, etc.) are ordered, clear documentation of the indication for use and assessment at regular intervals of vital signs, neurological and extremity checks, Glasgow Coma Scale, and/ or sedation scale scores should be frequently assessed as indicators of agitation and therapeutic response. Nurses must never use patient restraints as punishment, and restraints must be discontinued as soon as the threat of violence has ended. Nurses need to be constantly aware of potential violence. If a situation does become violent and a nurse feels unsafe, every effort should be made by the nurse to leave the situation. In the event that an unsafe or violent situation has occurred, nurses should be offered debriefing and counseling to deal with the recent event and prepare better for future experiences (Tishler et al., 2013; Villaire, 1995).

OUTCOMES

Prevention and reduction of violence in heath care is the desired outcome. This can be achieved in many ways by nurses, but health system support and resources, like the appropriate use of security guards and video monitoring, are also needed. Other methods used to prevent and reduce violence include (a) active safety and health committees that can create nurses' awareness and sensitivity to violence and (b) the establishment of open and trusting health care work cultures that support and encourage the report of type II violence. Violence prevention programs are an upcoming trend in health care that also promote quality of care and safety for patients and nurses. Regular rehearsal and adoption of violence-prevention programs, like the OSHA (2015a) *Guidelines* for Prevention Workplace Violence for Healthcare and Social Service Workers, should be mandated for hospitals, as well as violence-reporting policies put in place to enact a cultural shift that type II violence in health care settings is unacceptable.

Summary

Violent acts committed by patients have been escalating in health care, particularly in the ED and critical care due to multiple intrapersonal and social factors. Prevention of violence is key and depends on effective use of accurate assessment and effective nursing interventions with patients who are at risk for violence. In addition to prevention, nurses need to be constantly aware of potential threats. Accurate assessment can identify patients with potential for violence and possibly prevent such acts. A systematic approach to antiviolence by nurses and health care organizations for violence prevention, management, and evaluation is needed. Although all violent acts cannot be prevented, with proper training, assessment, and system resources, they can be decreased.

Arnetz J., Hamblin L., Essenmacher L., Upfal M., Ager J., & Luborsky, M. (2015). Understanding patient-to-worker violence in hospitals: A qualitative analysis of documented incident reports. *Journal of Advanced Nursing, 71*(2), 338–348.

Centers for Disease Control and Prevention. (n.d.). Workplace safety and health: Workplace violence course. Retrieved from https://wwwn.cdc.gov/wpvhc/Course.aspx/Slide/Unit1_5

Gomaa, A. E., Tapp, L. C., Luckhaupt, S. E., Vanoli, K., Sarmiento, R. F., Raudabaugh, W. M., . . . Sprigg, S. M. (2015, April 24). Occupational traumatic injuries among workers in health care facilities—United States 2012–2014. *Morbidity and Mortality Weekly Report*. Retrieved from https://www.cdc.gov/mmwr/preview/mmwrhtml/mm6415a2.htm

Jacobson, R. (2014, December 31). Hospital administrations and the judicial system do little to prevent assaults against nurses and other caregivers by patients. *Scientific American*. Retrieved from https://www.scientific american.com/article/epidemic-of-violence-against-health-care-workers-plagues-hospitals

Moore, T., & Mattison, D. (2016). Adult utilizations of psychiatric drugs and differences by sex, age, and race. *JAMA Internal Medicine.* doi:10.1001/jamainternmed.2016.7507

Mucci, N., Girogi, G., Roncaioli, M., Perez, F., & Arcangeli, G. (2016). The correlation between stress and economic crisis: A systematic review. *Neuropsychiatric Disease and Treatment, 12*, 983–993. doi:10.2147/NDT.S98525

Nesper, A. C., Morris, B. A., Scher, L. M., & Holmes, J. F. (2016). Effect of decreasing county mental health services on the emergency department. *Health Policy/Brief Report, 67*(4), 525–530.

Occupational Safety and Health Administration. (n.d.). ICU: Workplace violence. Retrieved from https://www.osha.gov/SLTC/etools/hospital/icu/icu.html#WorkplaceViolence

Occupational Safety and Health Administration. (2015a). *Guidelines for prevention of workplace violence for healthcare and social service workers* (OSHA Report No. 3148-04R 2015). Washington, DC: U.S. Department of Labor.

Occupational Safety and Health Administration. (2015b). Workplace violence in healthcare: Understanding the challenge. Retrieved from: https://www.osha.gov/Publications/OSHA3826.pdf

Solon, R., & Kratz, R. (2016). How mindfulness and situational awareness training help workers. *Benefits Magazine, 53*(3), 30.

Tishler, C., Reiss, N., & Dundas, J. (2013). The assessment and management of the violent patient in critical hospital settings. *General Hospital Psychiatry, 35*, 181–185.

U.S. Department of Health and Human Services. (2015). Substance Abuse and Mental Health Services Administration: Results from the 2014 National Survey on Drug Use and Health: Mental Health Findings, NSDUH Series H-50 (HHS Publication No. [SMA] 15-4927). Retrieved from http://www.samhsa.gov/data/sites/default/files/NSDUH-FRR1-2014/NSDUH-FRR1-2014.pdf

Villaire, M. (1995). Peter De Blieux, MD: Violence: Living with the growing shadow. *Critical Care Nurses, 15*(5), 80–87.

Index